TINNITUS TOOLBOX HYPERACUSIS HANDBOOK

SECOND EDITION

JAN L. MAYES

Library & Archives Canada
eBook ISBN: 978-1-77252705-0-8
Paperback ISBN: 978-1-7752705-4-6

Flesch Reading Ease = 66

DEDICATION

To my husband for his unwavering love and support.
My daughters for my joy and inspiration.
My colleagues for their wisdom and dedication.
People with tinnitus and hyperacusis for their courage, humour, and
perseverance.

I would also like to thank everyone who has given me encouragement,
support, and helpful feedback while writing this book including
Charlotte Douglas, Andre Lafargue, Brad Mayes, Clarissa Mayes,
Gerry Slater, Glynnis Tidball, Anna Van Maanen, and Dennis
Wilkinson.

Special thanks to Samantha Mayes, without whom this book would
never have been possible.

CONTENTS

1

FORWARD

If I should pass the tomb of Jonah, I would stop and sit for a while. For I was buried one time deep in the dark and came out alive after all.

- Anonymous -

I hope this book helps at least one person find at least one coping tool that helps you have a better quality of life.

I hope it helps at least one person become a more informed consumer who can find your way more easily through the maze of tinnitus and hyperacusis healthcare. Helps you find practical solutions to help you cope better.

Don't forget that approaches to tinnitus and decreased sound tolerance like hyperacusis are always changing. New tools, new tech, new treatments, new products, new services. I come from the Dark Ages of the

1980s when nothing could be done. Now something can be done. You are not alone. It will only get better.

Quiet cheers, Jan

2

DREAM MACHINES

I dream of a machine
wired
brain to brain
they hear
exactly
what I hear

I dream of a machine
potato head inspired
ears snap off
new snap on
rewired brain
silence

INTRODUCTION

I have often lamented we cannot close our ears with as much ease as which we close our eyes.

-Richard Steele 1600s -

Noise is unwanted sound. Unwanted because the person doesn't like the sound, doesn't like the loudness, or doesn't like how it's there all the time. That's tinnitus and hyperacusis in a nutshell. Unwanted sound.

Treatments for tinnitus were first written on ancient Mesopotamian clay tablets. That's over 5,000 years ago. They used exorcisms for ear ghosts, spells or prayers whispered into ears, and herbal treatments. Tinnitus treatments continued through the ancient Greeks to the Victorian 1800s. And then tinnitus fell off the radar.

I found a 1974 dictionary; tinnitus wasn't in it. It's in dictionaries now, but most people don't know what it is. It's the name for noises in the ears that people hear when there is no outside sound source. In other words, you're hearing something nobody else can hear.

It's very common. Tinnitus is pronounced [tin-it-us] or [tin-night-us]. The correct Latin pronunciation is [tee-nee-toos] although most people don't say it that way. It comes from hyperactivity in the brain's hearing system.

Why don't people talk about it? Tinnitus is invisible. People with tinnitus often feel uncomfortable telling other people, "I hear noises, but nobody else can hear them." Tinnitus is hidden.

When people do talk about it, they describe tinnitus as different sound types—or combinations of sounds—including ring, roar, hiss, screech, whistle, buzz, click, hum. Tinnitus is Latin for jingling ear. Usually only the person with the tinnitus hears it. It can be in one ear, both ears, or in the head. It can be constant, occasional, or only once in a while.

Loudness can be any volume from low to high. Tinnitus often changes loudness or tone on its own for no reason you can figure out. It can do its own thing when you move your body (e.g. open mouth, yawn, chewing, change position of head, neck, shoulders). It can change depending on loudness of sounds around you. This is natural.

It's similar to living with chronic pain. Changing from day-to-day. Hour to hour. Morning to evening. Minute to minute. People feel they have no control over tinnitus, thinking nothing can be done. This makes people distressed, including frustrated, worried, upset, angry, sad, or hopeless.

Hyperacusis is decreased sound tolerance along with misophonia and phonophobia. Decreased sound tolerance is when people have negative reactions to sounds that don't bother the average person. Hyperacusis is a pain reaction to louder sounds. It comes from hyperactivity in the brain's hearing system so the person hears sound extra loud.

Sound hurts. Like jabbing needles through your eardrums. Sometimes all sounds hurt. Sometimes only certain sounds hurt, like a fork scraping on a plate, dishes clattering, a balloon popping, or ambulance siren. People of any age can have hyperacusis.

Misophonia is a strong dislike of specific sounds, like chewing, teeth sucking, whistling, clicking, crackling, or tapping on the keyboard of a phone. The term was first introduced around 2001. For people who only have misophonia, their hearing system works normally. Misophoia is not about the sound; it's about the person's reaction to the sound because of hyperactivity in the brain's emotion system.

Phonophobia is a type of misophonia where the person fears specific sounds, like an air horn, balloon pop, or unexpected bang. It's about the person's emotional reaction to the sounds more than the sound itself.

Fear and anxiety gets worse when the person thinks the trigger sound will happen. Symptoms include feelings of panic, terror or dread, rapid heartbeat, nausea, dry mouth, and trembling.

Hyperacusis, first defined in 1993, is a real thing. Why don't people talk about it? Hyper what? How do you pronounce that? How do you spell that? Like tinnitus, hyperacusis is invisible. Hidden. Sound is uncomfortable. The world's volume is stuck on high. It's not surprising headaches are common in people with hyperacusis.

Hyperacusis is the forgotten fraternal twin of tinnitus. They are two sides of the same coin, like chronic pain and chronic fatigue. Hyper ears. Hyper means hyperactive or too energetic. That's what's happening for people with tinnitus or hyperacusis. Similar hyperactive hearing systems. Similar coping tools and therapy options. Changes to the tinnitus toolbox help hyperacusis. Some tools work for misophonia.

Millions of people around the world have tinnitus. Men and women. Of every age and generation. About half the people with tinnitus have normal hearing and half have hearing loss. Members of the military and veterans have a much higher risk of tinnitus, especially with combat military experience.

Some people are born with tinnitus. As children, they report hearing tinnitus for as long as they can remember. This is normal. The children think it's strange everyone doesn't hear tinnitus. They don't understand why people get upset over it. It's just part of them. Like black hair or brown eyes. Like some people have dimples when they smile, and some people don't.

About 16% of children under 10 have tinnitus distress. Aged 10 and into adulthood, the percentage with tinnitus distress drops to around 10%. The difference is probably because childhood ear infections that cause tinnitus often stop by age 10.

About 9% of adults have hyperacusis. Nobody knows how many children have hyperacusis. About 30 to 40% of adults with tinnitus distress as their main concern also have hyperacusis. About 86% of people with hyperacusis as their main concern also have tinnitus distress. Lots of hyper ears.

About 60% of people with hyperacusis distress have misophonia. There's a wide range in stats for adults and children with only misophonia. Nobody knows how widespread it is.

Sometimes people hear a high pitch tinnitus in one or both ears that only lasts a few seconds. It's called Transient Spontaneous Tinnitus. It often gets louder before fading away. Sometimes the ears feel full or plugged before the sound starts.

Anyone with hyper ears might hear a spontaneous sound now and then. People with regular daily tinnitus can have spontaneous sounds too.

These sounds are louder and at a different pitch. People with decreased sound tolerance also hear these sounds.

Occasional spontaneous tinnitus is normal in humans. It's not hyper ears and doesn't mean hyper ears are getting worse.

Regular tinnitus has different causes. It's common with noise or acoustic trauma to the ears. Extreme noise trauma includes sudden loud blasts of noise. Causes of occasional or regular noise damage over time include environmental noise, work noise, or loud activities like shooting with no hearing protection.

Medical conditions linked with tinnitus include whiplash, concussion, closed head injury, skull fracture, high blood pressure, heart disease, stroke, thyroid disease, diabetes, anemia, and dental or jaw problems. Tinnitus can start after surgery or electrocution. It's a side effect of many drugs or medications. It could be from stress or genetics. People with chronic pain or migraines have more tinnitus than average. Tinnitus is linked with food allergies and mercury (amalgam) teeth fillings. Because so many things are related to tinnitus, audiologist Dr. van Maanen asks, "What doesn't cause tinnitus?"

Some people are born with decreased sound tolerance. It can be from the same causes as tinnitus, but acoustic trauma and closed head injuries are common. Causes include depression, post-traumatic stress disorder, and pain syndromes, e.g. fibromyalgia.

Sometimes people have only had tinnitus or decreased sound tolerance for a short time (acute). Other people have tinnitus or decreased sound tolerance that they've had for a long time, e.g. 6-12 months or longer (chronic). Often there's no medical cause for hyper ears: cause unknown or idiopathic. Whether or not there's a medical reason, non-medical coping tools and treatment options are similar for acute and chronic tinnitus or decreased sound tolerance.

After acoustic trauma or head injuries, it's common to take over a year for tinnitus or decreased sound tolerance improvement, so don't quit. No matter how long you've had hyper ears, keep using coping tools. After tinnitus or hyperacusis start, the sooner a person uses coping tools, the better.

Hyperacusis can be reversed. For chronic tinnitus, the goal is not to get rid of it. That's a cure. And there isn't one. Yet. The goal is less distress.

The same care applies for children as it does for older people. See the doctor as needed, e.g. newly started hyper ears. Is the child bothered by their tinnitus? If not, great. If yes, there are coping tools. Same for a child with decreased sound tolerance. Anybody can customize a toolbox for hyper ears, no matter their age or hearing ability.

This book covers current science and coping options so people with hyper ears can make informed decisions and use tools correctly. Know what to avoid. Know how to protect themselves from companies and people in it for the money.

With the right info, I believe anyone with hyper ears can put together his or her own toolbox. Including everyday tools or tools as needed for flare-ups. Including the latest tool combination trend.

People get the most benefit from a toolbox customized for their own needs: self-help, professional therapy or somewhere in between. Try tools as needed or recommended. Some won't work; some will. Keep using what helps you.

Since 2012, I've found new tools that help me. Always exciting after 30 years of coping with tinnitus and decreased sound tolerance. I've done bad tool experiments on myself. More things to avoid.

Hyper ears distress is complicated. Coping better takes time. It takes time to add changes into your daily life. It takes time to see results. The longer you've had hyper ears, the longer it takes to notice changes. But by trying different coping tools and customizing your own toolbox, you can have a better quality of life.

The goal is workable helpful solutions for tinnitus and decreased sound tolerance. Knowledge is power.

Jan's View

I've had misophonia since I was born. As a child, I didn't know what misophonia was; there was no name for it. Disliking trigger sounds that nobody else hated was my secret. I told no one, because I worried I was crazy. I didn't find out what it was until the late 1990s.

I've had hyperacusis since childhood. It happens when I get migraines, starting days before the headache, and lasting days after.

I joined tinnitus world in 1986 at age 21. I wanted to be an author. Or a journalist. But one spring day, I was driving in my 1967 VW Bug and there was the loudest noise I've ever heard. The speeding driver of a big truck was late for work. He got distracted and didn't see my car.

The focus was on my neck injury. And concussion. Nobody asked about my ears. I now heard a loud squealing. I worried, so I saw my family doctor. He referred me to an ear specialist. There were sounds I feared, like air horns. I worried they'd make my tinnitus worse.

The ear specialist told me, "It's tinnitus. Ear noise. Just learn to live with it."

I wasn't happy to hear that. "It's from the accident, right?"

"Total coincidence," he told me.

"But before the accident I didn't have it, and after the accident I did."

He shrugged.

Now I was mad. "What am I supposed to do now?"

"Nothing can be done."

I refused to accept that. I planned to spy from the inside, so I studied audiology.

"But what about tinnitus?" I'd ask. Over and over.

Shrugs.

I couldn't believe nothing could be done. Unless you had hearing loss; then you could get an analog hearing aid. Sound quality not good. Lots of static. There was nothing for anyone with normal hearing. That was when I got depressed.

Technology was different. Rotary phone connected to land line. A mobile phone was when you had a super long cord connecting your phone to the wall. Boxy black and white or colour TVs with rabbit ears and 3 channels. Knobs to change the channel or volume. No remote controls: the horror.

Games were played on boards. Or with decks of cards you could snazzy shuffle to impress and amaze on-lookers, even if you weren't a magician. Books were paper. Snail mail. Boxy personal computers arrived. No internet. No social media. No digital tech.

I had nothing to help me cope. My tinnitus got worse. Louder than other noises and voices around me. All day. All night. Sometimes it shrieked for a minute or two. I would panic. If it stayed like that, I wouldn't be able to stand it.

I listened and thought about it constantly. Everything

sounded too loud. I decided quiet was the answer. I fought with my partner over the radio and TV loudness. I stayed away from groups of people or "noisy" places like malls or restaurants.

I ended up off work because of chronic pain and fatigue. Despite months in the quiet of my home, my tinnitus didn't get better. I read about triggers and kept a detailed diary, searching for changes I could make in food or activities that might cure me. A year later I figured out that was a pointless waste of time. Tinnitus does what it wants. When it wants. It's the nature of the beast.

I tried anything to get better. Experimenting on myself. Nothing worked.   I had suicidal thoughts. Then I took an 8 week pain management self-help class. I tried my chronic pain, anxiety, and depression coping tools for my tinnitus. Especially the mental strategies. Mind therapy helped me cope better. And every bit helps. My first tinnitus coping tools.

There was science on new therapy approaches for people with hyper ears. I was too embarrassed to see an audiologist for an evaluation or therapy; I felt like a loser audiologist distressed by my own tinnitus. Sound therapy arrived at clinics. I learned choosing silence and always checking on my tinnitus was wrong. But I didn't want to listen to more sound.

Clients came in for follow-up appointments, telling me how much better they were doing after they used the sound therapy I recommended but didn't use myself. I felt like a hypocrite. So I used sound therapy too. It made my tinnitus softer. Less noticeable. More tools for my toolbox. I wished I hadn't been too stubborn to use sound therapy.

I kept trying new tools over the years. Some didn't help me, but they helped other people. Some helped me cope better, but didn't help other people. I put together a personal toolbox for coping better, one tool at a time, That I could add to whenever I wanted. Over time, I didn't notice my tinnitus unless I stopped to think about it.

I kept waiting for people with hyper ears to know there were coping options. Know something could be done. But it didn't happen. It was so strange. The days of nothing can be done ended in the 1990s. But most people with hyper ears didn't realize.

This book is an update to my 2010 book, Tinnitus Treatment Toolbox. It covers hyper ears coping options so people can learn enough to make informed decisions. I figured if anyone could learn something from what I went through and from what I knew as an audiologist, then it was worth it. Even if the book only helped one person.

4

COPING TOOLBOX

Through knowledge, creating health.

- University of British Columbia -

A tool is anything that helps you cope better and/or helps reduce brain hyperactivity. It's that simple and that hard. The focus of coping tools is to improve quality of life, whether used alone or with medical treatment.

Difficulty coping causes stress. Some speakers on stress management use the example of holding up a small glass full of water and asking people to guess how much it weighs. But the weight doesn't matter. What matters is how long you try to hold up the glass.

If you hold the glass for a minute that's not a problem. If you hold it for an hour, you'll have an ache in your arm. If you hold it for a day, you'll have to call an ambulance. In each case it's the same weight, but the longer you hold it, the heavier the burden.

It's the same for hyper ears. If we carry distress all the time without learning how to cope, it's too much to handle alone.

There's no tinnitus or decreased sound tolerance tool or therapy specific to a certain type of tinnitus or decreased sound tolerance . So the cause—if you know it—doesn't matter. This is like chronic pain where no matter what the cause is, options might include massage, physiotherapy, chiropractic treatments, acupuncture, pain creams, medications, counselling therapy.

Which hyper ears tools will work best for you? You don't know until you try.

MEDICAL ATTENTION

If you haven't already, see your family doctor if you have:

- Tinnitus in one ear only
- Pulse-like tinnitus
- Drainage, pain, or discomfort in one or both ears
- Better hearing in one ear than the other
- Dizziness (vertigo) or imbalance
- Chronic worry or sadness (anxiety; depression)

Get to emergency services as soon as possible if you have:

- Sudden onset tinnitus
- Sudden onset hyperacusis
- Tinnitus that sounds like voices
- Rapidly worsening tinnitus
- Rapidly worsening hearing loss in one or both ears
- Sudden onset hearing loss
- Thoughts of hurting yourself or suicide

Before using any tinnitus or decreased sound tolerance (hyperacusis, misophonia, phonophobia) coping tools, aids, devices, treatment, or therapy options, you need to get clearance first from your family doctor and/or ear specialist to make sure you have no medical conditions that need treating first.

THE CURE

Different manufacturers sell products claiming to cure tinnitus. There is no cure. Yet. Don't waste your money. These cure ale are false advertising.

Thirty years ago when my tinnitus started, there was no cure on the horizon. Now the cure is on the horizon and coming closer every year. Fantastic research is happening. Scientists are studying cures for hearing loss that could be available in the next 5 years. What will these cures do for tinnitus and hyperacusis? It will be exciting to find out when they start human trials. Cures for tinnitus and hyperacusis from specific causes are also being studied and tested in clinical trials.

6 TOOL CATEGORIES

It's hard to make toolbox decisions if you don't know what options are available. Hyper Ears World can be like a maze with people struggling to find answers. This book describes coping tools, with categories of tools organized into specific sections. Coping tools fall into one of these 6 categories. Combine tools when possible:

1. Sound Therapy Tools
2. Hearing Aids Tools
3. Mind Therapy Tools
4. Body Therapy Tools
5. Sleep Tools

6. Hearing Protection Tools

Don't feel like you have to read everything. This book has a lot of information and some content doesn't apply to each person. Some depends on how well you hear; for example, a coping tool useful for a Deaf person might be different than a coping tool for somebody who is hard of hearing.

Don't feel you have to read this book in order. If you want to try Sound Therapy, start with that section. If your tinnitus or hyperacusis is from sudden loud sound or acoustic trauma, start with the chapter on Noise Damage or Resting Hearing. If you're distressed by bad sleep, flip to the section on Sleep Tools. If you're struggling with stress, anxiety, or depression, flip to Mind Therapy Tools. You can always go back to read earlier chapters or sections after you've found starter coping tool options.

Tool Combos

You will need more than one tool in your toolbox. Using more than one tool at the same time helps people cope better. Using more than one tool in the same 24-hour period is also helpful; for example, a person might use one tool while having their morning tea and a different tool before falling asleep at night. When and how tools get combined depends on the individual person, their lifestyle, and how distressed they are.

The 6th Sense

Besides tool combos, tools that combine more than one sense help distract the brain and help people cope better. The 5 main senses include sight, smell, taste, touch, and hearing. What is the 6th sense? Thinking. If you're distressed, you'll need hyper ears tools that help switch your thoughts away from your hyper ears. A tool that gets you thinking about something different is a 6th sense tool that lowers brain hyperactivity and draws attention away from tinnitus and decreased sound tolerance.

TOOLBOX DECISIONS

Why can't I tell you specific tools to use? I can't endorse or recommend anything. Plus, I don't know you. You know yourself best. Your toolbox will be personal to you. Not the same as someone else. My goal is to share educational info. Not myths or wrong information. Facts. Science.

You might already use tools that help you cope better. I know there are tools that are products or devices you already own or activities you already do. I know there are many free and low cost tools available. Learn about professional therapy approaches. Learn about techniques, products, or services before deciding what's right for you. It's all about making informed decisions.

Personalize your toolbox with tools from different categories. Don't feel you have to try everything at once. Or rush into things. Go at your own pace. Coping tools should make you feel better. Not stress you out.

Cost-Benefit Analysis
When considering tools to try, it's good to do a cost-benefit analysis. What is the cost? Not just how much products, aids, devices, or therapy services cost in money. What does your time and effort cost?

Is it something you already have, use, or do? Is it available where you live? Does it involve travel or multiple appointments? Does the provider offer telephone or Skype appointments or answer email questions? If there's a trial or return period, how long is it? How much does it cost to return a product, aid, or device if you don't find it helpful?

Then weigh the cost against the benefit. How helpful is the tool based on science? How well does it fit with your own likes, interests, and lifestyle? Is it something you would use, for at least 3 months, to see what your results will be?

You can't just try something once or twice and then quit because you notice no difference. Re-adjusting hyperactivity takes time. You need to decide if the amount a tool could help is worth the cost.

After my tinnitus started started and everyone said no cure and nothing could be done, I refused to believe it. I became a guinea pig in my own experiments. Try this and see what it does. Try that. I found a coping tool that helped. Then another. Then combinations. Building up a tool-box. With tools I like. It was pretty hit and miss. Until science on different aids and therapies helped me pick better tool experiments to try.

Now science shows what helps up to 80% of people for various proven options. But nobody knows what specific tool or therapy helps who. People say, "I tried this, and it didn't work. I give up."

Care providers should tell you results aren't 100% guaranteed. There is no cure. About 20% of people notice no benefit from treatments that help up to 80% of other people. If one tool or approach doesn't help at all, that's normal. There are always other options.

Tool Experiments

For choosing coping tools, when do you think about your tinnitus or decreased sound tolerance? When do they bother you the most? If the answer is all the time, pick a situation and start there; for example, reading, concentrating, trying to fall asleep.

There are tools for any situation. It takes experimenting to find what works best. Guidance from professional care providers is helpful during this time.

When building a coping toolbox, you're the subject of your experiment. To be scientific, you'd have to try one tool at a time to see the result. Try another to see the result. Changing one tool at a time. You could spend ages experimenting to find out what helps the most. This doesn't help distress.

New combination products and therapies are being studied and available at clinics. No cure. No single bullet. Shotgun blast and see what sticks. Use tool combinations when you can. Once you're coping better, you can always remove tools from the mix and see what happens.

Coping Goals and To-Do Lists
It's important not to overload yourself with goals or to-do lists when you're putting together your coping toolbox. Start with coping tools you can use right away. Tools where you already have everything you need to use them. Then set practical goals you know you can do daily if you take the time and make the effort, e.g. use a relaxation technique at bedtime.

Don't set too many daily goals at once; people who do often give up because they feel overwhelmed. Most people with hyper ears say 1-3 goals is more than enough for new daily routines. It's better to start with one new coping tool or a combo of tools that go together, like a new bedtime routine, and use that tool or combo daily.

If you want to list things you need to do so you can use a new tool, like download a free app, you could make a Toolbox reminder list. Only set due dates if something must be done by a set date. Take things one step at a time.

I've always made to-do lists. They used to be analog. On a piece of paper with lists of things I would scratch off after doing them. When things didn't get done, and the list grew, I freaked out.

I switched to must-do and want-to-do lists. That helped. I must pay the bills. I must go to an appointment. I must refill my prescriptions. Not as many must-do. Want-to-do got done when possible. Turning into must-do if it got close to a deadline. This helped me cope better. Then I got a smartphone.

So I added lists of all my things to-do, and set due date reminders for every- thing. It was fine at first. One or two reminders. Sometimes I would get things done. Sometimes I didn't. The reminders would carry over to the next day. Blaring at me every time I checked my phone.

After a few days, I had about 15 to 20 reminders. I was freaking out. I couldn't keep up. Then I stopped myself and did deep breathing. I forgot must-do versus need or want-to-do. I went through the reminders. Turning due dates off when possible.

The things I want or need to do are still in reminder lists like my writing list, shopping list, projects list. So I can keep track of things I need to remember even if they're not happening for a while. I'm less anxious about trying to remember everything. I don't feel overloaded.

Another option is to write each goal or to-do item on an index card. Put them in order with the top priority at the top of the pile. Recycle the card when you've finished the to-do. Organize cards as needed so your next must-do item is at the top. You can only do one thing at a time.

Energy Management
Chronic stress from hyper ears drains physical and mental energy, e.g. memory, concentration, attention. Even if sleep seems fine, people with hyper ears are often more tired than other people. This is like people with chronic pain that need rest and refuel breaks.

If fatigue is a problem, look at how you spend energy in a day. Experts suggest breaking activities down into smaller chunks of time, separated by rest breaks, to keep your energy up.

For example, your energy is full in the morning. You vacuum for 1 hour. Your energy drops to 25%, and it takes 3 hours to rest and recover your energy. The lower the energy the longer it takes to refuel.

Or, you could vacuum for 20 minutes dropping your energy to 75%, rest for 10 minutes and bring energy back up; vacuum 20 minutes, rest 10 minutes, vacuum 20 minutes, rest 10 minutes. You'll have vacuumed for 1 hour. The 30 minutes of rest is enough because you didn't drain your energy from doing too much at once.

This was a big problem for me. I'd spend too long doing chores or activities without a break and exhaust myself. I couldn't do anything for at least a day or two because I didn't have the energy. I figured out 10 to 20 minute chunks of time work better for me. Whether it's vacuuming, laundry, gardening, or writing, I limit the time. I take rest and refuel breaks.

If you have chronic headaches, migraines, or pain disorders like fibromyalgia, you'll have less energy to start with than other people, including people with just hyper ears. Energy takes longer to recover. Planning and pacing activities with enough rest, before and after, is important to lower fatigue.

Less energy makes coping harder. Louder tinnitus and more tinnitus or hyperacusis distress go with fatigue. It's hard always weighing pros and cons of activities or social situations versus how much they'll flare up hyper ears. Harder to plan outings, accept invitations, or invite people over.

Will you have enough energy on the day? How long is the activity or visit? Is there time to rest and refuel before and after? Do visitors know not to stay longer than planned? So they don't leave you with no energy and complaining hyper ears?

Energy management is a challenge for people with hyper ears. Effective coping tools mean less stress, less hyper ears distress, and better energy from day-to-day. This means better quality of life.

Better Coping Trend

Hyper ears distress goes in waves, up and down, cycling from coping to   not coping and coping again. Doing nothing only makes distress last longer, leading to little or no long-term change for the better. Using coping tools is the best way to tackle distress. The goal is to find workable tools and solutions. To cope better. Spend more—if not all—of your time coping. Not bothered by hyper ears.

Even if something only helps a bit, every bit adds up towards better coping and quality of life. One step at a time. One tool at a time. One day at a time.

5

TOOLBOX EVOLUTION

It is only a noise...It is simply and utterly a noise.

- William Shatner -

People go through different stages with their coping toolbox from intensive care to flare-up care. Over time, tools used evolve or change for different reasons. But before using tools, the first step is getting through the stages of grief to reach acceptance.

This step means accepting hyper ears is a chronic condition and accepting that grief is a natural reaction. People with hyper ears often don't realize many of their emotional reactions are related to grief at diagnosis.

People are told they have a condition that isn't expected to go away. Natural reactions include sadness, anger, fear, worry, anxiety, and depression. These emotional reactions are the same for grief.

This isn't surprising. Grief happens with any loss people go through in life. Hyper ears can certainly cause a sense of loss, especially loss of silence and loss of comfortable hearing.

In his book Care of The Soul, Thomas Moore describes the role of depression through the ages. Humans have a range of emotions from sad to happy. In the past, depression or sadness was linked with the Roman god Saturn. But Saturn was also linked with wisdom, experience, and reflection. In ancient times depression wasn't good or bad. It was more a state of being and not a problem that needed to be fixed.

Moore describes how even up to Renaissance times, some gardens had areas dedicated to Saturn. These were usually shady isolated places where people could go to feel sadness or depression without being disturbed.

Our modern society expects people to be social. But our natural range of emotions means people still need places where they can be alone to have sad feelings. Especially when people are dealing with conditions needing visits to doctors, specialists, hospitals, or clinics. We might not be caring for ourselves properly if we don't accept this.

When learning to accept chronic hyper ears, people often move through stages of grieving: disbelief, distress, and caring. The disbelief stage starts with the diagnosis as something with no cure, not usually expected to go away although both tinnitus and hyperacusis can get better over time.

At this stage, people often think, "This can't be true" or "Why me?" This disbelief is a common reaction to unwanted news. It can last 1 or 2 months.

In the distress stage, negative emotions and feelings last longer, are more intense, and can seem overwhelming. During this painful distressing stage, people often get very focused on their hyper ears. This is where negative emotional reactions can grow.

The distress stage usually lasts about 4 months. But it can last longer if people don't get education, reassurance, and basic coping counselling. It can last longer until people learn how to manage their hyper ears.

In the caring stage, there will still be disbelief and moments of pain, sadness, worry, or anger. But people have more interest in what's going on around them, and can start planning ahead. This is the stage where people start using coping strategies and treatment recommendations so hyper ears moves away from being a central focus in their life.

Don't forget that sometimes no matter what you do, your hyper ears are going to go up and down on their own. That's what hyper ears do, like chronic pain or other chronic conditions. Learning to live with good days and bad days are a big part of coping.

BEFORE COPING TOOLS

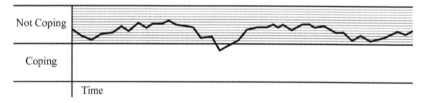

INTENSIVE CARE

Science proves people's quality of life gets better when they learn coping strategies for their hyper ears. Strategy is sometimes defined as a plan for reaching a goal. Strategy is also defined as military methods used to meet enemies under conditions beneficial to your own forces.

Intensive care gives you an individual plan to reach your end goal of better coping. With intensive care, you also create conditions beneficial to yourself to help overcome any hyper ears distress.

Starting off, tool combos are most common. Sound therapy, with wearable aids if needed. Mind therapy techniques. Body therapy. New sleep routine. Social hearing protection. Regular treatment or counselling sessions. Possibly prescription drugs.

Hyper ears distress doesn't get better instantly with intensive care. Some people start coping better quickly. Others might feel their hyper ears are mildly worse. This is similar to treatment for other injuries.

For example, imagine you're in severe pain from an injury. After physiotherapy appointments you also feel pain from treatments or exercises. But the pain is different. People describe it as a "good pain" as healing starts to take place.

If you notice some unexpected mild changes in sound pitch or loudness after starting intensive care, it can be a positive sign that your hearing system is responding by reacting differently. Let your care provider know. If your hyper ears or distress are much worse after starting treatment, talk to your care provider as soon as you can.

It can be exhausting to go through intensive care. Medical and audiology evaluations, treatment and therapy appointments, changing your routine with new aids, devices, or techniques to try.

Trial and error is also exhausting and challenging: figuring out what helps you and your individual hyper ears. Maybe something helps you like it helps other people. Maybe something helps you, but doesn't help other people. Maybe something helps other people, but doesn't help you. There's no way to know without trying. It's a big letdown when something doesn't work.

Even when something helps, it's normal for outcome measures to go up and down over months of treatment. That's OK. For example:

Appointment 1 = very severe distress.
Appointment 2 = severe distress; improved.
Appointment 3 = very severe distress again.

Don't worry if this happens. These measures are snapshots of distress at single moments in time along the up and down cycle of hyper ears. If outcome measures show significantly less distress at an appointment and then distress goes back up again at the next appointment, it doesn't mean you've wasted your time or treatment is useless.

Keep the big picture in mind. Over the long-term, if you stick with coping tools or keep following recommended treatment, you'll spend more time coping and less time distressed.

INTENSIVE CARE

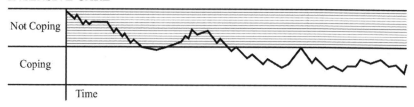

ONGOING CARE

Over time intensive care leads into ongoing care. You won't need your intensive care coping tools or won't need to use them as often. People won't need regular treatment or counselling appointments. They might use aids or devices less. They might forget or not need to use their sound therapy continuously 24/7. They might not think about mind therapy tools specifically for hyper ears during their daily routine. Wean off prescription drugs if possible.

This change is similar to coping with chronic pain. For example, a person with severe chronic pain may begin to cope with strong prescription painkillers, regular physiotherapy, braces, canes, specific exercises. Once they're coping better, they might use different or weaker prescription painkillers, over-the-counter painkillers, physio-therapy as needed, braces only for difficult activities, less intensive maintenance exercises.

The less distressed people are, the more likely they won't need to keep using any coping tools daily for ongoing care. The more distressed people are, the more likely they'll have coping tools they use regularly as part of their daily routine.

Coping will still be better on some days than others. It's the nature of the beast. But over time, the downs are not as bad and won't last as long. Coping and general well-being will get better overall with ongoing care.

WITH COPING TOOLS

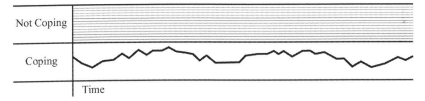

FLARE-UPS

Sometimes you'll do things that you know ahead of time will make your hyper ears worse. That's OK. You control what you want to do. Not your hyper ears. Don't stop doing something or avoid activities you'd like to do just because your hyper ears don't like it.

Planned Flare-Up

If I drive on the highway, it makes my tinnitus worse. Too bad. If I do yoga, my tinnitus goes crazy. Quit your whining. Put on your big tinnitus pants. If I play piano, my tinnitus gets loud. FU T. I'm not quitting piano because of hyper ears.

If I go to a concert, it makes my tinnitus worse even with musician's type hearing protection. If I like a band that's coming to town, I'm going. My tinnitus doesn't stop me. I tell my tinnitus ahead of time. "Guess what? I'm going to a concert, and you're going to flare-up, and I don't care. Talk to the hand, 'cause the face ain't listening."

Hopefully, I'm not the only person who talks to their hyper ears. After over 30 years, my tinnitus is like a horrible relative that's long over-stayed their welcome; but I still talk to them now and then.

If there are sudden very loud sounds when I'm out and about, it makes my hyperacusis worse. It's not stopping me from going out. I have coping tools like social hearing protection to use.

I might need coping tools to get through my daily routine. But at least I control my routine. Not my ears.

Then there's the social cost-benefit analysis. What if you know an activity will make your hyper ears worse, and it's not worth it to you?

For social events, if I know I'm going to enjoy myself, it's worth a hyper ears flare-up to me. For example, on big holidays, I know my hyper ears are going to get worse from running around more, being in more noisy places outside my home, going to social events, talking and straining to hear. If it's an activity I'm looking forward to, I tell my hyper ears, "Suck it up buttercups. I'm going to flare you up, and I don't care."

If I know I'm going to be around toxic negative people who make me upset and leave me feeling more down after the social event than before, it's not worth it. Toxic plus hyper ears equals higher distress. People might judge. But it's an individual decision whether to do the activity or not. Make decisions based on what's best for you to keep you coping as well as possible.

Unplanned Flare-Up

Even with intensive and ongoing care, there will be times a person's hyper ears flare-up and they have trouble coping again. The intensive coping tools that you dropped from regular use when you were coping better with hyper ears become your flare-up tools.

Flare-ups are common for people with hyper ears. If you have a flare-up, you're not alone. It happens to everyone at some point. Flare-ups can be from natural distress cycle ups and downs or be from different triggers.

Triggers include change in hearing, change in health (minor cold to major disease), loud music or noise exposure, bad news, death in family, change in work situation, financial worries. Personal triggers can increase stress and make it harder to cope.

People feel relief and satisfaction when they're coping better. Flare-ups can take people back to the sadness or other negative emotions they went through when they were diagnosed. When you're coping well, it's frustrating and depressing to go back to intensive care coping tools like more appointments, more aids or devices, more strategies and techniques. But this is part of coping. Learning how to handle flare-ups will only improve your coping ability over time.

Jan's View

Even after years of using coping tools, I still get flare-ups sometimes. Once, I had a severe increase in tinnitus distress and pain.

My usual support network all said, "Oh, you're just stressed out."

Knowing that stress is a trigger doesn't make the distress any less or make the flare-up go away any faster. It only made me feel all alone that most people don't understand.

After a month of using my usual intensive tools with no effect, I went to see my family doctor. A short term prescription drug was recommended for sleep. I tried some tools I hadn't tried before. These included a mind therapy technique, a different distraction tool I hadn't tried before, and a different relaxation tool at bedtime.

Gradually over time, this tool combination helped settle down the flare-up. I added the most useful tools to my toolbox so I can use them as needed for future flare-ups.

If you have a flare-up, and you're as distressed as you were before intensive care, don't panic. You already have coping tools in your toolbox that have helped you before. They'll help you again.

If necessary, make an appointment with your audiologist or tinnitus-decreased sound tolerance care provider. Care providers can help you work through flare-ups. Some providers call these "booster visits" since they can help boost you over a rough patch. Some people also have supportive family or friends they can reach out to during a flare-up.

I've noticed getting flare-ups to settle down with coping tools usually happens a lot faster than the time it takes to go from intensive care to coping.

For example, a woman panicked when she had a severe hyper ears flare-up. We talked about what was happening in her life. Her partner had just been diagnosed with cancer. Her job was in jeopardy. Stress was obviously a big factor.

"What tools have helped you before?" I asked. "Do you have any sound therapy you can add? Do you have any mind therapy techniques you could start doing again? Body therapy or sleep tools?"

She started listing off tools she hadn't been using regularly.

"Can you start using them again to help settle the flare-up down?"

She could.

"Do you need some in-depth telehealth counselling?"

She didn't think so. If she changed her mind, she'd get in touch

Knowing she had tools that worked before and could be used again, helped her feel less stressed out. After several weeks, the flare-up settled down. She was back to coping as usual.

Sometimes flare-ups are from trial and error experiments that make things worse instead of helping. A person with severe hearing loss, severe speech-in-noise loss, and very severe tinnitus distress had been through sound and mind therapy in the past, and was using combination hearing aids for day, and sleep sound therapy. They were mostly coping well. Their concern was they drove long hours between cities, and couldn't hear their front seat passenger. They couldn't chat. It was frustrating and upsetting.

I asked if they wanted to try a special microphone system that was compatible with their hearing aids. The passenger could talk into the microphone and their speech would go straight to the driver's hearing aids, cutting background noise. It seemed like a good idea. They agreed.

A local hearing aid professional fit the system. There were problems so the manufacturer's regional sales rep visited the clinic to help with the fitting. It was a disaster. It made the person's tinnitus so bad it was right back to the severity it was before their treatments.

When I talked to them, I apologized. I was so sorry the system made their T worse. Nobody had heard of that before, so it was a surprise. There was no way to know something like that would happen. This trial was an error.

We talked about coping. We talked about how the tinnitus severity had gone up and down before. They had stopped using ambient sound therapy while awake, so we talked about what they could use again for continuous daily sound therapy.

We talked about mental techniques that helped in the past, but weren't used daily any more. Deep breathing. Relaxation techniques.

They started coming up with more helpful tools they could use again. Flare-up toolbox tools. In less than a month, their tinnitus and tinnitus distress got better. They were back to how they were coping before the microphone system trial. This helped remind me that every coping tool trial is not a success. We're all individual.

Jan's View

When I started using coping tools, for months I tried not to pay attention or listen to my tinnitus. My distress went down significantly, and I was managing better. Then one day when I checked on it, I noticed a change in the volume and pitch. Suddenly my T was no longer screeching at me.

I went from not coping towards coping. But instead of feeling happy, I was surprised to feel an unexpected sense of loss. I don't know if this is common because I've never seen any mention of this by anybody else with tinnitus.

I started listening to see if my tinnitus had completely disappeared. It was still there, and within days had gone right back up to its original screeching. Once again I wasn't coping. I felt frustrated, disappointed, and angry that after months of coping tools, there didn't seem to be any lasting benefit.

Then I took a deep breath and kept on using my coping tools. Within a month, my tinnitus distress went back down again. My tinnitus is always there when I check on it. I can't help it. I still do. But now after months and years of using my toolbox, I'm rarely distressed by my tinnitus anymore.

FLARE-UPS

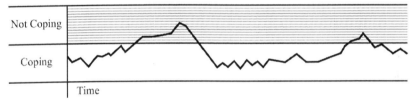

NEW COPING TOOLS

Many tools today are not the same even as recently as ten years ago. When my tinnitus was the most distressing in the 1980s, there was no internet and tech was analog with horrible sound quality and limited features. No eHealth, telehealth, or online courses and programs.

Aids and devices have been transformed by digital tech into good sound quality products with many helpful features. Combination hearing aids are much better than past wearable tech, and will only improve as manufacturers add and update features over time.

Mobile apps and wireless connectivity are some of the biggest changes, and in my opinion, some of the most helpful. They make it easy to find and use your favourite sound type, or help you with cognitive, relaxation, distraction or guided imagery exercises while on a waitlist, or to keep up routines during and after therapy.

In my opinion, the best apps for tinnitus-decreased sound tolerance will have different sound options, and mind therapy options will be text based and/or open captioned as well as having trained speakers with deep distinct voices for the audio. Options could include:

- Tinnitus-decreased sound tolerance learning.
- Cognitive techniques.
- Deep breathing exercise with visual indicator for inhale/exhale timing.
- Relaxation techniques, e.g. progressive muscle relaxation.
- Meditation and mindful meditation techniques.
- Guided imagery.
- Relax and sleep sounds, e.g. white, pink, brown noise, nature sounds.
- Relax music, e.g. no percussion.
- Sound mixing and sound libraries.
- Peer support online .

Over time, reading materials have evolved to include ebooks. Cards and games are now on apps, gaming systems, and online games. Black and white TVs have evolved to Smart TVs. Rotary phones to smartphones. Tape cassettes and Sony Walkmans to LPs, CDs, and digital music.

Entertainment now includes podcasts and YouTube videos. People around the world can socialize with each other using email, texts, Facebook, Twitter, and other social media that also continues to evolve over time.

Tools in your toolbox will reflect these changes and technology upgrades. We don't know exactly what future tech will look like yet. But it will definitely change the tools in your toolbox.

This book can't describe every tool in the world. There are always new products, technologies, and techniques targeted to people with hyper ears. Different countries have different tools available.

When you see or hear about a new tool, is there any science to it? What specific features does it offer? Was it developed by somebody with skills and experience in hyper ears management?

What coping tool category or categories does it fall into? Sound, mind, or body therapy? Something to help you sleep better? A different way to protect your hearing?

Does your family doctor or ear specialist think it's medically safe for you to try? What does your audiologist think? What is your cost-benefit analysis?

TOOLBOX EVOLUTION SUMMARY

Toolbox evolution is a normal part of coping with hyper ears. Something can be done. The exact something changes with new science and knowledge about hyper ears. In the end the goal isn't to be a happier person. The goal is to cope better.

The Happiness Experiment by YouTuber Boyinaband shows how routine can be helpful. He's very open about his struggle with depression. At the height of success, he quit YouTube. A year later in 2017,

the first video he did when he returned was The Happiness
Experiment.

He set up a daily routine. Charting out a daily calendar of activities for
work time and personal time. Doing the activities as planned with
encouragement from his sister. In the end, this routine didn't make him
feel happier. But he got more done. The routine made him more
productive. Which helped him feel less depressed.

Your toolbox is not going to stay the same forever. Society and technology are always advancing and improving. Some of your tools may
fall by the wayside. Some tools will develop into better versions. New
tools may become available in your country or community, or be something you happen to find that you didn't know about before.

Think outside Hyper Ears World for your coping toolbox. Sometimes
tools weren't meant for tinnitus or decreased sound tolerance; but if it
helps you cope safely, it's something to consider, including new
approaches for sleep, chronic pain, anxiety or depression, and wellness.

Sometimes a tool will stick in your toolbox for ages. A certain sound
type. A certain mental technique. But using the same tool over and
over again can get boring. Especially if you've been using it for years.
If you get bored with a tool, it's fine to switch things up and try something different. As long as it ends up having the same helpful effect as
the original tool.

A great idea, shared in a 2018 article in the Evening Edinburgh News,
comes from 11 year old Amy McLaughlin. She made a chart of things
she likes doing. When her tinnitus is bad, she randomly picks something from the chart, and does whatever it is "whether that's playing on
the Xbox or going on her trampoline." I really like this idea, because
it's an easy way to pick a coping tool, and also stops boredom from
using the same coping tool over and over again.

It's a hopeful time for people with hyper ears. There has never been so much science on underlying mechanisms and treatments. There is hope that scientists will find a treatment or approach that will cure tinnitus and make decreased sound tolerance go away completely.

Harriet Beecher Stowe once said, "When you get into a tight place and everything goes against you, till it seems as though you could not hang on a minute longer, never give up then, for that is just the place and time that the tide will turn."

Treatment has come a long way from trying to get rid of ear ghosts. While we wait for cures, use the coping tools available now to lower distress and turn the tide. There are workable helpful solutions for tinnitus and decreased sound tolerance. By trying different coping tools and customizing your own toolbox, you can have a better quality of life.

6

CARE PROVIDERS

The future depends on what we do in the present.

- Mahatma Ghandi -

Care provider options depend on each person's hearing and tinnitus or decreased sound tolerance distress. They could include family doctor, ear specialist or ENT, audiologist, hearing healthcare professional, and/or psychologist.

FAMILY DOCTORS

The family doctor, or general practitioner, is the first care provider people see for tinnitus or decreased sound tolerance. Family doctor appointments are about 15 minutes long. The family doctor tests, diagnoses, and treats medical ear conditions. If the person says they can't hear because of tinnitus, that's a sign of hearing loss. The family doctor can refer for a hearing evaluation. Otherwise, people with tinnitus or decreased sound tolerance need basic counselling:

Education & Reassurance

- Tinnitus = hyperactive hearing system.
- Tinnitus = common benign symptom.
- Used to it? Great, carry on as usual.
- Hyperacusis or decreased sound tolerance = hyperactive hearing system.

Basic Coping

- Avoid silence. A lit candle is much more noticeable in a dark room than in a bright room. Tinnitus is more noticeable in quiet than when other sound is going on, e.g. music, podcast, YouTube video, TV, radio. Sound enrichment lowers hearing system hyperactivity.
- Shun. If you ignore your hyper ears, it will reduce hyperactivity. Don't listen to it or think about it. Don't restrict your life because of it.
- There are tinnitus and decreased sound tolerance management options for coping better.
- Tinnitus Distress: can refer for tinnitus evaluation.
- Decreased Sound Tolerance Distress = can refer for decreased sound tolerance evaluation.

A 2017 survey found 92% of people with tinnitus distress were unhappy after seeing their family doctor. Problems included limited tinnitus and decreased sound tolerance awareness. Family doctors showed no concern, sympathy, or sensitivity to tinnitus impact on people's quality of life. The British Tinnitus Association website shares

Tinnitus Guidance for GPs (General Practitioners). Family doctors who use available guidelines give consistent care and counselling.

If you're distressed, a family doctor can make recommendations or referrals. They could refer you to an ear specialist for medical investigation. They could refer you to an audiologist for hearing-tinnitus-decreased sound tolerance evaluation.

But it takes a few months for those appointments to happen. Time for people to worry and get more distressed if they're not given basic counselling by their family doctor. The 2017 survey found 85% of people weren't given any education, reassurance, coping information, or any other support from their family doctor while they waited to see an ear specialist or audiologist.

If they don't have time, family doctors could give people an informational tinnitus or decreased sound tolerance handout so people needing coping options or resources don't walk out with nothing more than they walked in with.

A survey of UK tinnitus services published in 2018 found most people see their family doctor and get referred for ear specialist evaluation or audiology hearing evaluation. About 33% of these people were referred for tinnitus evaluation and therapy.

Of the rest, 40% saw their family doctor again within 1 year. Over 33% of these people were referred again to ear specialist or audiology services for hearing evaluation. The survey researchers called this an *"unsatisfactory and expensive revolving-door pattern of healthcare."* Tinnitus and decreased sound tolerance services are available, but it's difficult for people to access them.

EAR SPECIALISTS

Ear specialists—sometimes called otologists, otolaryngologists, or ENTs—are medical doctors who specialize in ear, hearing, and balance disorders. Ear specialist appointments are short. If they say "nothing can be done", they mean nothing medically. People need ear specialist medical clearance before starting tinnitus or decreased sound tolerance non-medical treatment.

There are ear specialist guidelines available for tinnitus or decreased sound tolerance patients. Consistent approaches help specialists provide better diagnosis and treatment. The Tinnitus Research Initiative shares a science-based Tinnitus Flowchart for Patient Management. The interactive flowchart is updated as needed. It's available for worldwide use at tinnitusresearch.net.

Like family doctors, ear specialists should give basic hyper ears counselling: education, reassurance, and basic coping information. Some ear specialists take advanced courses in tinnitus and decreased sound tolerance management and offer therapy services. If they don't have time, ear specialist offices could develop and share an informational handout on coping options and local resources.

MRI Testing

Sometimes ear specialists recommend an MRI to help diagnose different conditions, including causes of hearing problems. MRI machines use magnetism, radio waves, and a computer to create images of hearing and/or balance structures. People with pacemakers, metal chips, or metal implants in their body can't have MRIs, because metal interferes with the magnetism.

In 2018, scientists found noise levels of modern MRI machines are high enough to cause noise-induced hearing loss. MRI machines have average noise like a jackhammer or chainsaw loudness and pulses of noise as loud as gunfire. Many people report new or worse tinnitus and hyperacusis after MRI testing. This is a serious concern, especially for people who need more than one MRI over time.

Sometimes staff give people MRI safe—no metal—earplugs or earmuffs to wear during the MRI. Sometimes people bring their own MRI safe hearing protection. But earplugs or earmuffs are not enough for high MRI noise. This is a rare situation where the public should protect their hearing with double hearing protection: earmuffs plus high noise reduction foam or formable earplugs.

MRI departments should always provide double hearing protection and have a variety of MRI safe earplugs and earmuffs to fit different shapes and sizes of ears including children and adults. For some people with hyperacusis, noise during MRI testing will still be painful even with double hearing protection.

New more powerful MRI machines have higher noise levels than older machines: louder than military jets taking off from aircraft carriers. There is high risk of hearing loss, tinnitus, and hyperacusis even when people use double hearing protection. Medical experts are asking MRI manufacturers to make quieter machines with much lower noise to prevent hearing system damage when people get MRIs.

HEARING AID PROFESSIONALS

Hearing aid professionals are licensed to do hearing testing, fit hearing aids, and custom fit hearing protection. They can offer basic counselling on hearing loss, tinnitus and decreased sound tolerance, hearing aids, and coping strategies. They can refer to an audiologist for more in-depth evaluation, counselling, or therapy.

AUDIOLOGISTS

Audiologists are the primary non-medical hearing healthcare provider for people with hyper ears. Many audiologists are licensed hearing aid professionals. Audiologists often work at hospitals, hearing aid, or tinnitus-decreased sound tolerance clinics. They specialize in hearing healthcare like optometrists specialize in vision healthcare.

Audiologists evaluate, prescribe, and provide treatment for hearing loss and/or tinnitus-decreased sound tolerance. This might include counselling on communication and coping strategies. They fit prescription hearing aids and custom fit hearing protection. Services might include auditory retraining programs, communication management classes, and/or tinnitus-decreased sound tolerance management counselling. The counselling, aids, devices, or therapy recommended depend on the hyper ears distress severity.

Audiologists can also do paperwork needed to get income tax disability credits or to help get funding from third party providers like Medicare or worker's compensation systems.

The most trusted professionals are knowledgeable and use a Shared Treatment Decision Making approach to decide on options together and make sure the treatment plan meets what their patient or client wants. This helps people cope better and gives them hope for the future. As Tom Kalinske of Sega once said, "The only thing they [consumers] valued more than making the right decision was making their own decision."

Tinnitus is typically a long-term condition, and hyperacusis or decreased sound tolerance takes time to treat. Tinnitus-hyperacusis management to help people cope better usually takes at least 3 months, and ongoing check-ups or "booster" appointments are often needed.

Choose a care provider you can be comfortable with over the long-term, just like you do with a family doctor.

Choose an audiologist who gives you time to talk about concerns whether you're starting out with a treatment plan or working through a flare-up. Some providers are uncomfortable talking about feelings or distress, and might give pep talks, e.g. it's not that bad, it could be worse, etc. Look for audiologists who really listen and have empathy. Empathy is when a person can relate to your feelings or situation.

Jan's View

Sometimes I was too empathetic with clients. I remember a man with tinnitus who felt nobody really understood what he was going through. I decided to share that I had tinnitus too.

I told him, "I have tinnitus and cope with tinnitus distress. I get it. Often other people don't get that it's there all the time, 24/7. Every day and every night. Non-stop. Up and down. There's no silence, you can't concentrate, you can't sleep..."

He smiled with relief. "Oh. Mine isn't that bad at all. I feel so much better now."

We talked about coping tools, but he wasn't bothered enough to make any changes to his daily routines. On his way out, he was feeling so much better than when he arrived, he was whistling a cheery tune, almost skipping.

I was unprofessional to talk about my emotions. But it did help that client.

There's nothing worse than going to a provider and walking out of an appointment feeling as if the person didn't listen or the person didn't seem interested in working on your concerns.

Sometimes questions aren't answered because the standard appointment isn't long enough. If needed, the provider can schedule another appointment by telehealth or in clinic.

If your appointment is for an annual hearing test or hearing aid adjustments but you also want to discuss your hyper ears coping, it's good to let the clinic know so staff can schedule extra time.

TINNITUS CLINICS

More and more specialty tinnitus and hyperacusis or decreased sound tolerance clinics are starting up. Some specialize in certain therapy approaches or products. Some offer a combination of services, including sound, mind, and/or body therapy.

More and more audiologists around the world are getting certified as tinnitus (and decreased sound tolerance) management care providers. Certificates require course work, exams, and continuing education about every 5 years. That's about how long it takes for there to be enough new tinnitus-decreased sound tolerance science to make it worth another course.

For example, in 2017, the American Board of Audiology introduced a continuing education Certificate Program in Tinnitus Management. Audiologists who complete it include CH-TM (Certificate Holder– Tinnitus Management) in their professional designations. The program includes decreased sound tolerance management.

The European Tinnitus Course is one of the longest running tinnitus courses in the world. It was developed by Dr. R. Coles in the late 1970s. In 2018, it ran for the 29th time. It covers the latest tinnitus-decreased sound tolerance science, evidence-based evaluation, and clinical treatment approaches for audiologists, psychologists, ear specialists, and scientific researchers.

HEARING AID CLINICS

The most common way for people to get tinnitus-hyperacusis management help is from a local hearing aid clinic. The hearing healthcare provider could be hearing aid professionals and/or audiologists. The word "tinnitus" might not be in the name of their clinic. But that doesn't mean they don't offer tinnitus or decreased sound tolerance services, or aren't up to date with at least sound enrichment.

If you have hyperacusis, misophonia, or phonophobia, it's usually best to see an audiologist. Some people with tinnitus don't have a local audiologist, so they see a local hearing aid professional.

Sometimes people with tinnitus already have a local hearing aid professional and want to stick with them. That's fine, as long as the care provider is knowledgeable about tinnitus and sound enrichment.

Find another hearing healthcare provider if the person's counselling is negative, e.g. nothing can be done, or it's catastrophic. They should at least be able to give counselling with basic education, reassurance, and coping info.

Find another hearing healthcare provider if they waste follow-up appointment time doing yet another full hearing test if your last test was less than a year ago, and you haven't noticed any hearing problems or changes. The professional can always do a quick hearing screening if needed. Then use the extra appointment time talking about how you're managing, any current issues, possible new coping tool options, referrals if needed.

Sometimes people need to weigh a good relationship over experience with a specific approach, especially with so many new options available that are also newer to care providers. When deciding on a provider, you can find a lot of this info on clinic websites or ask your local hearing healthcare provider:

- What tinnitus-decreased sound tolerance management approaches does their clinic offer?
- What brands of hearing aids or combination hearing aids do they sell?
- Are they an audiologist and/or hearing aid professional?
- Do they know about current treatment options, including cost and availability?
- What treatment or approach do they recommend and why?
- What treatment outcome measures do they use?
- What is the provider's success rate with recommended approach?
- Do they work with, or refer to, other local professionals as needed, e.g. psychologists, physiotherapists?
- Will they share decision making, problem solving, and work together with you on an individual management plan?

They should also explain results and findings clearly. You should feel comfortable sharing concerns. And they should make you feel hopeful about coping better over time.

AUDIOLOGY & EAR SPECIALISTS

Audiologists and ear specialists often work together at hospitals or specialized clinics. They see children or more difficult tinnitus-decreased sound tolerance cases. Some governments are shutting these departments down so people have to go to private clinics.

Can your hearing clinic afford specialized equipment—or trained staff to use it—like an MRI machine? Would they have specialized audio-vestibular testing for people with dizziness or imbalance? Can they run

a cochlear implant program? Do they have someone on staff with
surgical privileges for cases where that is an option?

Is there an audiologist and ear specialist to consult on diagnosis and
treatment for complicated cases? How much would you end up paying
for testing or treatment from a private clinic? Keep an eye on your
local hospital audiology and ear specialist departments. Fight cuts that
hurt hearing and hyper ears healthcare.

PSYCHOLOGISTS

Psychologists study people's thoughts, emotions, and behaviours.
Depending on their specialty, psychologists do different therapies to
help people cope better with tinnitus-decreased sound tolerance. Sometimes audiologists and psychologists team up to offer more options for
tinnitus-decreased sound tolerance management services.

Some psychologists take advanced courses in tinnitus-decreased sound
tolerance management. Most don't specialize in hyper ears. Look for
psychologists who specialize in helping people cope with chronic pain
or chronic conditions.

PEER SUPPORT

There are some negative places on line where people talk about tinnitus
and decreased sound tolerance. There are other supportive places to
find other people dealing with the same feelings, sharing information,
and helping problem solve. Popular websites include Tinnitus Talk
Support Forum (includes hyperacusis support) and The Hyperacusis
Network.

PEOPLE WITH HYPER EARS

People often choose a self-help approach after their hyper ears evaluation, counselling, and medical clearance. Some people choose guided self-help. Guidance is usually from an audiologist or psychologist. Self-help programs or courses are available. The more distressed a person is, the more likely they'll need professional tinnitus-decreased sound tolerance management services.

You are the decider. The consumer target market. Professionals can describe options available, make recommendations, or give guidance. But you have to decide what tools to try. Based on your individual needs, cost, availability, preferences, and lifestyle. What coping tools do you want in your toolbox?

7

HEARING SOUND SYSTEM

Myth: If you have tinnitus, you will lose your hearing.

To better understand hyper ears, it's helpful to know some basics on how humans hear sound. This is also important for self-help or treatments to better understand certain approaches. Treatments or cures will depend on where tinnitus or hyperacusis is starting or happening in the hearing system.

Human hearing systems are most tuned for speech and music sound waves. This makes sense because speech and music are part of every culture dating as far back as recorded history.

Acoustics is the science of sound, and how the environment changes how sound waves travel. If you drop a pebble in a pool of water, it will make ripples that travel out from where the pebble fell in. Sound also travels in waves. Rippling out from whatever made the sound. Sound waves are biggest at the start. Getting smaller fast as they travel farther away from the sound source.

If something is in the way, if possible, sound waves break around it and keep travelling. Like if a person was standing up to their neck in the ocean, waves of water would break around and over their head and keep going.

If there is a wall, tree or something blocking the way, sound waves will echo by reflecting off the surface and travelling in a new direction. The amount of sound wave that reflects and keeps going depends on what it hits. The harder the surface, the higher the echo. Sound waves hit and reflect without losing much of the volume they had before they hit the hard surface.

With softer surfaces, some sound wave energy is absorbed each time it hits, leaving less of the sound wave to reflect and echo. Sound waves get smaller and quieter every time they reflect off a soft surface.

Sound waves can also travel through liquids, but not as easily as through air. When moving from air to liquid, the size of the sound wave drops making it softer. That's why if you're swimming, sound is more muffled when your head is underwater.

Sound waves can also change from travelling through air to vibrating through skull bones to reach the hearing system. This happens for very loud sound.

PITCH (Hz)

Sound frequency is measured in Hertz (Hz): how fast sound waves travel in a period of time. Pitch is our subjective sensation of the sound. For example, when sound waves move slowly, we hear a low deep tone. When sound waves move fast, we hear a high squeaky tone. The full frequency range of human hearing is 20 to 20,000 Hz.

Low pitches are much louder and travel longer distances than high

pitches. When the person on the other side of a wall is blasting music
or a car stereo goes blaring by, that's why you hear the boom, boom,
boom of the bass. That's why if you're hiding and need to get somebody's attention, you whisper a high pitched psst. Or use sign
language.

Humans can't hear infrasonic sound waves <20 Hz. Humans can't hear
ultrasonic sounds waves >20,000 Hz. Buying a stereo system that does
something above 20,000 Hz is nice for your dog (hearing up to 45,000
Hz), or your cat (hearing up to 64,000 Hz). But it doesn't improve
sound quality for human ears.

Pure tones are a single frequency tone or note mainly heard in music or
hearing testing. Most sounds are combinations of different pure tones.
Hz can be shortened to kHz for higher frequencies. For example, 500
Hz = 0.5 kHz, 4000 Hz = 4 kHz, 20,000 Hz = 20 kHz, and so on.

<20 Hz—infrasonic
20 Hz—thunder
264 Hz—music, middle C
27 Hz-4,186 Hz—music, 88 key piano range
250 Hz-8 kHz—music, speech communication
8 kHz-20 kHz—fine-tuning music, speech; birds
>20 kHz—ultrasonic

VOLUME (dB)

Amplification or gain turns sound wave volume into a bigger louder
sound. Intensity or volume is measured in decibels (dB). The bigger
the sound wave, the louder the sound. The smaller the sound wave, the
softer the sound. The dB scale is logarithmic like the Richter scale for
earthquakes. Small differences in numbers mean big differences in
sound wave size and power. You can't do math using dB numbers
unless you're using a logarithmic equation.

3 dB Doubling Rule = Plus 3 dB = Twice as Loud

80 dB is twice as loud as 77 dB, 77 dB is twice as loud as 74 dB, 74 dB is twice as loud as 71 dB, and so on. If one vacuum cleaner is 80 dB, two vacuum cleaners together would be 83 dB. The general volume or dynamic range of human ears is 0 dB to 140 dB: softest to painfully loud signals heard across 20 Hz to 20 kHz. Usually only younger ears or highly sensitive adults have very good hearing.

-10 dB—very good hearing
0 dB—softest young adult can hear (historical)
10 dB—breathing
20 dB—whisper
30 dB—rustling leaves, babbling brook
40 dB—birds singing, refrigerator humming
50 dB—quiet office
60 dB—conversational speech, laughing
70 dB—shower, dishwasher

Entering Hearing Hazard Zone

75 dB—loud restaurant/store, vacuum cleaner
80 dB—blender, garbage disposal
90 dB—lawnmower
100 dB—motorcycle, public hand dryers
110 dB—jackhammer, rock concert, MRI
120 dB—thunderclap, chainsaw
130 dB—professional DJ system, .22 caliber rifle
140 dB—military jet departing aircraft carrier

The louder the volume, the shorter the safe listening time.

PAIRED EARS

Hearing in only one ear or hearing much worse in one ear than the other makes it much harder to hear. People with single-sided or unilateral HL can't tell what direction sound is coming from. It's much harder to understand speech-in-noise or difficult listening situations. Music doesn't sound as good.

Humans are born with a pair of ears or bilateral hearing. A pair of ears gives natural hearing. There are reasons humans have two ears. We need a pair of ears with working stereo sound for safety, communication, and music sound quality.

With paired ears, the brain can use sound signal differences between the left and right ears. This gives directionality or location. People with paired ears know where sound is coming from. With one ear there's no way to know; that's a problem whether you're moving through a forest or walking down the street.

A single ear is like having only one eye. No visual depth perception. In 1881, Clément Ader at the Paris Opera demonstrated the first stereo sound, described as auditive perception. Auditory depth perception is as important as visual depth perception for humans.

Directionality from paired ears also helps speech understanding. People with paired ears can face who they want to listen to and pick words out from background noise better.

Sound only heard in one ear has strange effects. If a person with hearing only in their left ear had somebody talking at their right side, it sounds as if the person is standing on their left side. With a single ear, speech and noise blur together into one distorted sound signal. Communication is a lot harder. You should use communication strategies in difficult listening situations to help anyone with single-sided hearing; for example, only one ear with useable hearing, one hearing aid, one cochlear implant.

For music, the history of mono systems changing to stereophonic proves people prefer to hear in stereo. In 1925, the BBC did an experimental first radio stereo broadcast of a concert in Manchester, England. British engineer Alan Blumlein invented modern stereo technology in the 1930s.

Stereo sound was first used in the US by the Philadelphia Orchestra in 1933, and then at Carnegie Hall in the 1940's. Walt Disney Studio's Fantasia was the first movie to use stereo sound. Television had the first stereo broadcast from the New York Metropolitan Opera House.

Ask a musician if they would give up hearing in one ear. No more paired hearing. You'd have trouble getting any musician to say yes. Same for music lovers and audiophiles. Nobody chooses to listen to music in one ear, with nothing useable coming from the other side. Paired hearing gives much better sound quality for music, communication, and daily life.

OUTER EARS - SOUND CONDUCTION

Sound waves arrive at the visible outer part of the ears also called the auricle or pinna. Outer ears are as unique as fingerprints. Earprints aren't easy to do, so police still use fingerprints to identify criminals. People use outer ears for earrings, piercings, ear gauges, or to hang glasses or hearing aids on.

For sound aimed directly at one outer ear, the volume difference or head shadow effect between outer ears is around 3 dB: half as loud from one ear to the other. Adult heads are only about 8 inches or 20 centimetres wide; that's a short distance between ears. A small volume

drop when sound waves travel between 1 ear and the ear on the other
side of the same head.

If you can hear, imagine you're surrounded by a circle of hearing
ability with you in the exact middle. Sound waves from behind you
will reflect off the back of your outer ears and head. Making the
volume behind you softer.

Sound from front and sides is louder than the back. This pinna effect
helps people tell what direction a sound is coming from. It helps with
communication in noisy places. But if someone is missing an outer ear,
it won't hurt communication as much as missing more important parts
of the hearing sound system.

The outer ears work to collect sound waves and funnel them into the
ear canals. Cupping a hand behind the ear to hear better by making the
funnel bigger, makes the sound about 3 dB or twice as loud as an
uncupped ear.

This was the idea behind ear horns or ear trumpets. These were funnel
shaped devices people could listen through to help them hear better.
Ear trumpets were first sold to the public in London in 1800. They
worked better than some early analog hearing aids.

Sound travels down the short tube-like ear canals to the middle ears.
Each ear canal is about 1 inch or 2.5 cm long and 0.3 inch or 0.7 cm
diameter. Ear canals come in different shapes and sizes. Narrow or
wide. Straighter or curvy. The ear canals are where hair and earwax
happen. Tinnitus often happens when earwax, even a flake, is touching
the eardrum.

The hair and wax help protect the eardrum from dirt and bugs. Objects
found in ear canals include small toys, crayons, and unwanted
creatures.

Warning: Do not use ear candling or ear coning!

Alternative healers say ear candling or coning removes earwax. Ear candling uses a special cone shaped candle in the ear canal while a person is lying on their side. The burning wick and smoke are said to remove earwax and impurities from the ear. Some people say impurities are drawn out of the head and sinus cavities while candling but this is physically (anatomically) impossible.

Science proves all "residue" comes from the candle itself. Risks include outer ear burns, wax blockages in the ear canal, and burn holes in the eardrum.

Earwax comes out of ear canals on its own. If needed, qualified trained professionals can remove excess earwax safely.

For cleaning by irrigation, care providers aim a body temp stream of water against the side of the ear canal. Water runs past the wax and brings wax with it when it washes back out. If the care provider shoots the water at the eardrum, the wax can get caught against the eardrum.

This method can be too loud for some people with hyper ears. If necessary, there are other methods to remove earwax. Discuss any earwax concerns with your family doctor or audiologist. In some cases, you might need to see an ear specialist.

Anyone can have outer ear problems no matter what their hearing is like. Often outer ear problems can be treated medically.

There's a rumour that Vincent Van Gogh cut off his ear in an attempt to get rid of his tinnitus. Or was it a gift for his lady love? The debate continues. Either way, it would not have cured his tinnitus.

MIDDLE EARS - SOUND CONDUCTION AMPLIFIERS

Conductive hearing loss is from outer or middle ear problems that change how sound is conducted down the ear canal and through the middle ear system. At the end of the ear canal, the sound wave hits the very tiny eardrum (tympanic membrane). It's a thin, flexible, round sheet of tissue. Each eardrum moves back and forth independently. Vibrating at the pitch and volume of incoming sound waves. There are tiny sound wave differences between the eardrums because of the head shadow effect.

In 2017, American scientists at Duke University found our eardrums move with our eyes. Eyeballs and eardrums move in the same directions. This gives directionality so we know where sounds are coming from. Kind of like how with animals, their eyes turn and ears swivel towards the direction of a sound e.g. cat hearing can of food being opened.

The brain uses this vision-hearing link to compare sound wave differences between ears. Sound will be faster and louder in one ear; reach the 2nd ear later at a softer volume because it had to travel a little farther. These tiny differences between sound waves reaching each eardrum plus outer ear differences give directional information to the brain. You know where sounds are coming from because of paired ears.

The eardrum is so sensitive it picks up sound wave movements as small as the diameter of a hydrogen atom.

Experts usually say when sound is loud enough, people with middle ear problems can hear and understand speech fine. But based on the Duke University study, directional information is lost when middle ears don't work as a pair. This makes it harder to tell where sounds are coming from and makes it harder to understand speech in background noise. People with conductive hearing loss could have more difficulty understanding speech than previously expected.

Behind the eardrum, there is a chain of 3 connected middle ear bones or ossicles. Middle ear bones sit in an air-filled space between the eardrums and the inner ears. The eardrum's inside surface attaches to the hammer (malleus). The hammer connects to the anvil (incus) and it connects to the stirrup (stapes).

The stirrup is the smallest bone in the body, about the size of a grain of rice. Sometimes this comes up on Jeopardy in case you're ever a contestant. Other middle ear bones are not much bigger. These are the only bones to reach adult size before birth.

Acoustic Reflex

Loud sound triggers a tiny muscle reflex that pulls on the stirrup middle ear bone, tightens the eardrum, and makes hearing worse briefly. This is the acoustic or tympanic reflex. It's like the patellar reflex that doctors check when they hit below the kneecap to see if they can make your leg kick out.

The acoustic reflex is a quick action that needs another tap of loud sound to happen again. Constant sound will trigger the reflex at the start, but the effect goes away just like the knee drops back down after kicking out from the patellar reflex.

The big difference between knees and ears is the acoustic reflex is paired. Loud sound hitting one middle ear system makes the acoustic reflex happen in both ears. Paired ears work together for incoming sound signals.

Eustachian Tubes

The middle ear space behind the eardrum gets outside air flow through the Eustachian tube. The Eustachian tube leads from the middle ear space to the back of the throat. This tube lies more flat at birth, but slopes downward towards the throat as children grow. It keeps the air pressure equal between the middle ear space and outside air.

The Eustachian tube stays closed. It only opens briefly during yawning or swallowing. Temporary tinnitus changes can happen when yawning, e.g. louder.

Some people notice pops or crackles when their Eustachian tube(s) open and close. The Eustachian tube can get stuck closed because of infections, allergies, or sudden changes in air pressure, e.g. airplane landing. This causes ear fullness and severe pain.

The most common middle ear problem is ear infections or ear fluid in the middle ear space behind the eardrum. This can be caused by Eustachian tube problems. When it doesn't open properly, fluid can fill up the space behind the eardrum. This fluid can get infected, causing an inflamed, bulging red eardrum. When the fluid gets thick, it's called glue ear. Glue ear doesn't hurt but it causes hearing loss because it stops the eardrum from moving.

> 30% of kids age birth to 3 have ear infections.
> 8% of kids age 3 to pre-teen have ear infections.

If there's too much pressure behind the eardrum, and it can't leave out the Eustachian tube, there is only one other option. The eardrum bursts which is painful like stabbing a knife through the eardrum. Ear infections can happen to anyone in the normal hearing, hearing loss, or Deaf communities.

Eardrum holes should heal on their own. If not, ear specialists like ENTs can patch the hole or insert tiny pressure equalization (PE) tubes. PE tubes keep air pressure in the middle ear space the same as outside air pressure to stop ear infections until the Eustachian tube works again. Infections often stop once the child has grown enough that their

Eustachian tubes are more downward sloped, around age 7 and up. Some people have chronic ear infections into adulthood.

Sound from Middle Ears to Inner Ears

The middle ear system changes sound wave energy from air conduction (outer and middle ears) to fluids in the inner ears. The middle ears have to power amplify so the sound wave pitch and volume stays the same when the signal moves from air to fluid.

First the middle ear turns sound waves travelling down the ear canal into a mechanical vibration. The eardrum vibrates to incoming sound waves. Vibration flows through the middle ear bones. The stapes moves like a piston, sending sound to inner ear fluids. Middle ear systems are strong. They don't break even when chronic sound is loud enough to cause noise damage to the hearing system's sensory-neural sections.

INNER EARS - BALANCE

The inner ears include a hearing system and a balance or vestibular system. This is basic information on the balance system. People in the normal hearing, hearing loss, and Deaf communities can have problems with imbalance or dizziness (vertigo). People with hearing problems are more likely to have balance problems than people with normal hearing.

The balance part of each inner ear has 3 semi-circular canals and other structures sensitive to head movement. Two separate fluids fill the balance system: endolymph and perilymph. Endolymph is only in the inner ears. Perilymph is like CSF (cerebrospinal fluid). The motion of these fluids give people their sense of balance.

The balance system works in pairs so the brain compares and analyzes small differences between the left and right sides. Each side gives the brain information on direction and amount of head movements. The inner ears detect forward-back, up-down and left-right movements. Rollercoasters and speedy amusement park rides use twists, turns, and loop-de-loops to throw off the balance system and make people feel dizzy.

The paired balance system is linked to our paired vision system. If you spin in a circle and then stop, it takes a few seconds for your balance system fluids to stop spinning. Your eyes tell your brain you're not spinning. Your balance system briefly tells your brain you're still spinning. Who's your brain going to believe? In this situation, your balance system. So after you stop spinning, the world still spins past your eyes.

If you have imbalance or dizziness, it's often because your balance system is telling your brain something different from your vision. Or the balance system in one ear is telling the brain something different from the other ear. In-depth balance testing includes ENG (electro-video-nystagmogrophy). Other tests include rotation tests, CDP (computerized dynamic posturography) and balance system scans, e.g. MRI, CT scan.

Vestibular Hyperacusis
Vestibular hyperacusis is when sounds make a person fall or lose their balance. Sound can be painful, like regular hyperacusis, but also causes severe dizziness. Sometimes there's nausea, headache, fatigue, severe confusion, and in more severe cases, people pass out.

Ear specialists and neurologists diagnose and treat vestibular hyperacusis. Treatment includes low-salt diet, anti-nausea drugs, and anti-inflammatory drugs sent into the vestibular system.

Vestibular hyperacusis audiology evaluation procedures are still being developed. In one test, audiologists present a low frequency 500 Hz tone and slowly raise the volume. Once loud enough, the tone can cause vestibular hyperacusis for care providers to see.

Vibronoise or Low Frequency Noise

Vibronoise is high vibration Low Frequency Noise (LFN) below 500 Hz. Vibronoise is less heard and more felt. People who can hear it say it sounds like hissing or electrical sparks. Some jobs and environmental noise pollution from transit or transportation can cause vibronoise. Effects include ear pain, imbalance or vertigo, tinnitus, hyperacusis, and worse noise-induced hearing loss than from noise alone.

Scientists debate if LFN and infrasound from wind turbines or wind farms causes vibronoise pathology or vibroacoustic disease. Vibronoise effects include physical changes in body cells, heart disease, and mental health problems. The effects of vibronoise and infrasound on the hearing and balance systems are not completely understood yet. Recent science found low frequency noise caused significant damage to vestibular system function.

Persistent Postural Perceptual Dizziness

Persistent Postural Perceptual Dizziness (PPPD) was called Phobic Postural Vertigo and Chronic Subjective Dizziness. Scientists believed people with PPPD were anxious, depressed, and Obsessive Compulsive. Now scientists think PPPD is a neurological condition.

People with PPPD get dizzy or lose their balance from their own movement. PPPD can happen in busy places where other people are moving. It can happen with high visual focus like reading or computer work. PPPD is worst when walking or standing, moderate when sitting, and mild or not noticeable when lying down. The World Health Organization is including PPPD for the first time in their 2018 edition of International Classification of Diseases.

Jan's View

Around 2011, I had sudden onset balance loss. Doctors thought it was neurological, but had no diagnosis. Now I know I have

PPPD. I get dizzy when sitting in a car at a stoplight and I see
other cars or pedestrians move. I fall on stairs or uneven ground
if I move the wrong way or too many people are moving around
me. Using a cane or walking sticks helps.

INNER EARS - SENSORY

Inner ears or cochleas look like small bony snail shells the size of peas.
They're protected by thick skull bones. What happens to inner ears
after birth depends on different things like genetics, ear health, and
preventable damage.

Hearing loss: 56% males — 44% females.

The mystery of why males have worse hearing than females is still
unknown. In the past, people thought it was because males had more
work noise-related noise-induced hearing loss. But that doesn't seem to
be the case anymore.

Special fluids called endolymph and perilymph fill the cochleas.
Multiple membranes keep these electrically charged fluids separate.
There is total hearing loss if fluids mix or leak out, e.g. head trauma
fractures bony part of cochlea. It's difficult to impossible for experts to
get at the cochleas without destroying hearing.

Inside the fluids, each cochlea has structural supports and over 20,000
sensory cells or hair cells. There's a large blood flow to the cochleas.
Circulating blood brings high oxygen levels needed for the cochleas to
stay healthy.

Imagine each cochlea is a keyboard 1.18 inches or 30 mm long. Turn it
into a snail shell by starting at the low pitch keys and rolling them up
toward the high pitch end of the keyboard. The 20 kHz high pitch keys

end up at the opening or base of the snail shell. The rest of the keyboard is a space-saving snail shell spiral ending at the low pitch keys of 20 Hz.

The cochlea is like a 20–20,000 Hz
digital keyboard.

Sound travels one way through the middle ears to the cochleas. The middle ear stirrup bone attaches to the cochlea entrance or base at a spot called the oval window.

Sound ripples up the cochlea keyboard like the flick of a whip. There are 15,000 hair cells in each cochlea tuned to the pitch and volume of incoming sound waves.

After hair cells convert sound waves, the electrical signals travel up the hearing nerves to the brain for processing. Cochleas (sensory) work together with hearing nerves (neural). Hearing loss is often called sensorineural whether the damage is sensory, neural, or both.

Inner ear strength might be related to skin colour and cochlea pigmentation. The US National Center for Health Statistics analyzed hearing loss data for over 200 million people. Ethnicity made a difference; Black and Hispanic adults had better hearing with only 4.2% having hearing loss. White adults had worse hearing with 9.4% having hearing loss.

Somebody looking down the ear canal can't see the cochlea. It's hidden behind the middle ear space. Inner ear damage is invisible and painless.

Hearing loss can happen from birth. Sometimes hearing loss will get worse in the first 5 years for children born with inner ear hearing loss, so regular hearing testing is important. But even with no recent family history, inner ear hearing loss can start at any age including in toddlers, children, teens, young adults, and adults. Around age 55 is when mild age-related inner ear hearing loss starts.

If you have tinnitus, it doesn't mean you're losing your hearing. Sensorineural hearing loss can happen independently from tinnitus. Hearing changes are usually from whatever is causing the hearing loss.

Stats show many babies are born Deaf or with severe hearing loss. Good hearing healthcare includes universal infant hearing screening. Every newborn needs their hearing screened before they leave the hospital or as soon as possible for home births.

Treatment for premature babies often includes hearing toxic antibiotics to help protect them from germs and infections. The antibiotics can cause profound hearing loss after even one dose depending on genetic risk. Scientists in the United Kingdom at the University of Manchester are developing a quick, genetic clinical screening test to see which babies are at risk, so doctors can use different antibiotics instead.

Some babies are born with normal hearing that turns into progressive hearing loss when they get older. Good hearing healthcare includes yearly hearing tests. The earlier hearing loss is identified, the earlier treatment can happen.

- 3 newborns in 1000 are born Deaf or with severe hearing loss.
- 90% of Deaf children are born to hearing parents.
- 0.23% of people are Deaf—can't hear or understand any speech.
- Sudden deafness is 5 to 20 cases per 100,000 people annually.
- 5.4% of people develop hearing loss before age 3.
- 14.2% of people develop hearing loss between ages 3-19.
- Depending on the country, 10% of people 15 and older have hearing loss.

High Pitch Inner Ear Doormats

The high pitches are the doormats of the inner ears. The middle ear connects to the high pitch end of the cochlea, so all sound has to cross the high pitch sensory cells. High pitch sound waves ripple across the high pitch sensory cells then turn into electrical impulses sent up the hearing nerve.

Mid pitch sounds ripple across the high and mid pitch sensory cells then turn into electrical impulses sent up the hearing nerve. Low pitch sounds ripple across the high, mid and low pitch sensory cells then turn into electrical impulses sent up the hearing nerve. That's a lot of action at the front end of the cochlea. Every incoming sound or noise—no matter what pitch or volume—crosses the high pitch doormat.

It's believed this could be why many people have a high frequency pattern of hearing loss. It's why people are often diagnosed with idiopathic hearing loss or cause unknown because the pattern doesn't' automatically tell you the cause.

Age-related and noise-induced hearing loss start with a high frequency pattern of loss but there are definite differences. Genetic hearing loss and other causes can mimic the typical age and noise patterns. Although patterns can look similar on a hearing test, age-related and noise-induced hearing loss are not at all the same inside the hearing sound system.

Age-Related Mild Hearing Changes

Human hearing stays fairly good into older age if no other hearing loss causes happen. With age, sensory cells in the inner ears gradually stop working. In mammals like humans, sensory cells do not regrow after damage like they do in fish, reptiles, and amphibians.

Age norms collected since the 1970s show age-related hearing loss starts at 20 kHz: the top of the pitch range for human hearing sensitivity. Over time, this hearing loss spreads in a domino effect from 20 kHz down to each lower adjacent pitch. Like starting at the right high pitched end of a keyboard and making keys softer before taking out keys in order, one after another.

Over time, age-related hearing loss spreads from the higher frequencies to the mid and low frequencies ; the loss is usually mild. People usually find out they have age-related hearing loss when they have significant speech frequency hearing loss that makes it hard to communicate.

Some people say people's hearing was much better in the past. How age-related hearing loss is really hearing loss from our modern noisy industrialized communities. Their proof is an old urban legend. How because they were quietly safe in South Africa's Kalahari Desert, the Kalahari Bushmen had "supernatural" hearing so good, they could hear single-engine airplanes flying 70 miles away.

In 1969, scientists figured out why Kalahari Bushmen had the super-natural hearing reputation. As children, Bushmen teach their children to always say yes. Do you hear it? Yes. It could partly explain why people thought the Bushmen could hear so well.

Professional hearing testing of Kalahari Bushmen in 1969 found they had mild high frequency hearing loss starting when they were older. It's believed metabolic and structural changes inside the inner ears causes age-related loss. These types of changes would affect Bushmen of the Kalahari in 1969 the same way they happen to modern humans.

Even though age-related hearing loss is a separate cause from noise-induced hearing loss, age alone can't account for much worse hearing loss seen in younger and younger people living in our modern noisy society. A lot of hearing loss, especially for people younger than 60, is from noise damage. Not natural aging.

Dead Zones and Musical Paracusis
Sometimes there are dead zones in the cochlea. Areas with no sensory

cells or no connection to the auditory nerve; no sound can travel up the hearing nerves to the brain. Dead zones are like missing keys from a keyboard. Adjacent keys are out of tune or off pitch. This is called musical paracusis.

Diplacusis is when musical paracusis is worse in one ear than the other; so people hear tones as different pitches in each ear. Paracusis and diplacusis make it very hard to enjoy music especially for musicians or very musical types.

Dead zones cause high hearing system distortion. Genetics can cause dead zones. Noise or high volume sound also causes dead zones and musical paracusis or diplacusis. People with inner ear dead zones have a harder time understanding speech in background noise or difficult listening situations. Sound quality is bad even if listening to crisp clear audio or music.

INNER EARS - NEURAL

The hearing nerves are like electrical cables between the cochlea and the brain. There are 30,000 nerve fibers or wires in each hearing nerve.

The hearing nerves carry paired electrical impulses from the inner ears up to the brain for processing. The brain compares and analyzes incoming data from each ear. This gives humans auditory depth perception and the ability to communicate and enjoy music.

The biggest cause of hearing system neural damage is unhealthy noise exposure during everyday life including personal listening, consumer products, work, play, school, and entertainment.

Hidden Hearing Loss
Scientists used to think noise damage started in the inner ears or cochleas. But science since 2009 proves occasional or regular noise

causes broken synapses or connections between the inner ears and hearing nerves. The scientific name for it is cochlear synaptopathy. It triggers rips and tears in the hearing nerves. The hearing nerve degeneration is progressive, getting worse for months after noise ends.

Scientists identify cochlear synaptopathy by doing hearing system autopsies using cadavers or animal models. It's called hidden hearing loss because there are no symptoms and hearing thresholds still test within the normal range.

The only test now that's sensitive to hidden hearing loss is speech-in-noise testing. If a person's hearing seems normal, but they've lost their understanding of speech in noisy environments, it can be a sign of hidden hearing loss.

Noise-induced hidden hearing loss could be the underlying cause for some cases of tinnitus or hyperacusis when hearing thresholds seem normal. Temporary or permanent tinnitus or hyperacusis can happen before the person notices any problems with speech understanding in difficult listening situations.

Temporary Threshold Shift
The first sign of later stage noise-induced hearing loss is temporary sensorineural hearing changes after occasional or regular noise damage. Hearing ability returns to pre-exposure levels, typically within 16 to 24 hours after the hazardous exposure ends. Temporary threshold shifts can happen along with temporary or permanent tinnitus and hyperacusis.

For example, after a concert with no hearing protection, a person might notice muffled hearing. It goes away in about a day. Leaving permanent progressive hidden hearing loss behind.

Temporary threshold shifts are linked to early sensorineural hearing loss before age 40—even if hearing recovered to normal after the temporary threshold shift. Every episode of temporary threshold shift increases the risk of early hearing loss with problems enjoying music or understanding conversations in noisy places.

Long ago, scientists used the Temporary Threshold Shift Method for noise research. This method uses noise damage on unprotected humans to cause temporary threshold shift; it gave scientists a way to study noise-induced hearing loss. But later science since 2009 has proven temporary threshold shift is not harmless.

Ethical scientists don't use vision damage on humans to study vision loss, or damage humans to study other health conditions. Ethical scientists don't use noise damage on human subjects to study even temporary noise-induced hearing loss.

Warning:
Never join clinical trials using noise damage on unprotected humans!

Permanent Threshold Shift
With occasional or regular noise exposure, permanent inner ear damage happens. Sensory cells in the cochlea die and the structures start to break. This is on top of the permanent progressive cochlear synaptopathy, hearing nerve degeneration, and hidden hearing loss. Noise trauma causes a mostly invisible to hidden neural hearing loss with sensory hearing loss not showing up until later.

Other hearing loss causes like aging are mainly a sensory loss without the high amount of neural damage seen after noise exposure. The preventable noise-induced result is high distortion for sound, music, and speech communication.

Early noise-induced hearing loss can first appear as a high frequency notched pattern. People can have normal hearing with a notch that isn't noticeable in day-to-day life. Early noise damage is often identified in hearing screening programs for people who work in hazardous noise.

Better hearing screening programs are also needed for the general public.

By the time a person notices communication problems from noise-induced hearing loss, there is no notch left. Other causes, including genetics and age, can mimic a notched pattern of loss. A notch alone is not evidence of noise trauma. The person must also have a history of hazardous noise exposure. Nowadays, that's pretty much everybody.

Noise damage does not cause profound hearing loss or Deafness. Noise-induced hearing loss stops getting worse when unprotected exposure to hazardous noise stops. If a person is using well fit hearing protection and their hearing loss keeps getting worse, it's likely not noise-induced hearing loss. In these cases, often the hearing loss is from genetic causes. If there is noise trauma plus vibration or high echo, noise-induced hearing loss is worse than from noise alone.

Acoustic Trauma
After high volume noise or acoustic trauma, it can take up to 18 months for hearing thresholds to partly or completely recover. If you have tinnitus or hyperacusis too, use coping tools as soon as you can and don't give up using them too soon. Even if tinnitus or hyperacusis don't change after 18 months, keep using the coping tools that help you. For more info, see the chapters on noise damage and resting hearing after acoustic trauma.

HEARING SOUND SYSTEM SUMMARY

Outer Ear(s):

- Conductive hearing loss: one or both ears.
- Tinnitus possible, hyperacusis more uncommon.
- Without an outer ear, the maximum hearing loss is minimal to

mild, but it will be harder to locate sounds or understand speech-in-noise.

- Causes include outer ear infections, trauma, too much earwax, objects stuck in ear canals, bony growths from swimming in cold water, genetic malformations.
- Medical treatment possible: medicine or surgery.

Middle Ear(s):

- Conductive hearing loss: one or both ears, amount of hearing loss depends on which part of the middle ear isn't working (eardrum and/or middle ear bones). It also depends if the problem is temporary, repeated, or progressive.
- Tinnitus often, hyperacusis more uncommon.
- Without a working middle ear, the maximum amount of hearing loss is moderate. Conductive hearing loss is a loss of volume, directionality, and ability to understand speech in background noise.
- Causes include middle ear infections, scarring, holes or perforations in eardrum(s), allergies, damage or dislocation of middle ear bones, genetic malformations, cholesteatoma, otosclerosis (hereditary bony growth stopping movement of middle ear bones). Sometimes otosclerosis spreads to the inner ear causing sensory hearing loss.
- Medical treatment (medicine or surgery) is possible to partially or completely fix middle ear problems. Sometimes people need communication strategies and hearing aids. Some people with more severe conductive or mixed hearing loss use bone conduction hearing aids.

Inner Ear(s) Balance:

- Tinnitus or hyperacusis are common.
- Causes of imbalance or vertigo include Benign Paroxysmal Positional Vertigo, head injury, concussion, neck injury,

cervicogenic (neck) syndrome, Persistent Postural Perceptual
Dizziness, Meniere's disease, labyrinthitis (inner ear
infection), vestibular hyperacusis, vibronoise, Mal de
Debarquement (feeling movement or sickness after getting off
transportation including boats, ships, airplanes, trains, cars),
migraine associated vertigo, vestibular schwannoma, age-
related imbalance, perilymph fistula, cholesteatoma,
otosclerosis, medications, ototoxic drugs, anesthesia, heart
disease.
- Treatment includes Exercise-based therapy, Balance
Retraining, surgery, medication.

Inner Ear(s) Sensory:

- Tinnitus or hyperacusis are common.
- Most commonly sensorineural (e.g. age) or neurosensory (e.g.
noise) related hearing loss usually in both ears.
- Without a working inner ear, the maximum hearing loss is
total or profound.
- Other causes of inner ear hearing loss in one or both ears
include genetics, heart disease, diabetes, inner ear infections
or viruses, head trauma, acoustic neuroma, cochlear
otosclerosis, Meniere's disease, ototoxic drugs, vape juice
with propylene glycol, meningitis, infectious diseases, ear
surgery, idiopathic or unknown.
- Treatment includes hearing aids, assistive listening devices,
cochlear implants, communication strategies, sign language.
- Because inner ear hearing loss is a loss of sensory cells, it
makes audible sound distorted and unclear. Noise damage
caused much higher distortion for sound, music, and speech
than many other causes.

Inner Ear(s) Neural:

- Tinnitus or hyperacusis are common.

- Neurosensory or sensorineural hearing loss, one or both ears, the more hearing nerve damage, the higher the distortion.
- Causes include noise damage, age-related, genetic, head trauma, acoustic neuroma.
- Treatment is the same as sensorineural loss except communication is much harder because of higher distortion, and music will sound worse than for sensory loss alone.

8

TINNITUS HYPERACUSIS SOUND SYSTEM

What shall possess them with the heaviest sound that ever yet they heard?

- Macbeth (Shakespeare) -

Cutting the hearing nerve does not stop tinnitus. Because we hear with our brain. It's the central processing hub of our hearing system. It's why 33% of Deaf people hear tinnitus.

After travelling through the ears, the brain starts processing sounds. Each hearing nerve's 30,000 nerve fibers lead into 10 million fibers in the brain's hearing system networks. This is basically a computer processing system for hearing.

There are fibers tuned for left ear information and fibers tuned for the right ear. Fibers tuned for loudness and timing differences between ears. Fibers tuned for overall pitch and volume. Tuned to every feature of sound including location and sound type like speech or music.

The hearing system in the brain is always ready. Nerve fibers are never completely quiet. Like a car in neutral, there's background activity. When system activity increases like an accelerating engine, more processing happens to check if the activity is important or not.

The brain interprets these patterns of increased nerve fiber activity as our sound environment. Sounds have their own unique pattern inside the hearing system, e.g. dog barking, voice, raindrops, birdsong. When nerve fiber activity matching known patterns comes through the hearing system, it's heard as that sound.

Different patterns of nerve fiber activity happen for silence. Our hearing system is designed to let us hear sound and no sound. Many nerve fibers are more active for softer sound input.

Day and night, our hearing systems process a constant stream of sound environment information. First it happens subconsciously. The hearing system screens incoming activity and delivers only the most important signals to the brain.

Imagine the hearing system works like an elevator stopping at each floor in a tall building. The basement may be full of potential sound environment information. But as information flows up the elevator, nerve fibers at each floor are working to check for patterns.

If patterns are identified as unimportant, the information is filtered out; for example, the hum of a refrigerator. This information does not make it to the next floor. If patterns are recognized as potentially important, this information does make it to higher levels as the nerve fibers continue trying to check out the pattern.

1. Outside Sound > Ears
2. Brain Activity > Processing
3. Sound Heard

Once past the subconscious networks, the higher levels of the hearing system in the brain analyze the nerve fiber pattern. More areas of the brain like those needed for language can become active. At this point, a person finally becomes aware of their sound environment. Processing at this level includes identifying that a sound is heard and recognizing the sound, e.g. car horn, music, speech. The sound is interpreted if necessary, e.g. understanding what was said.

Synesthesia

There is an interesting condition called synesthesia that shows how interconnected the nerve systems are in the brain. Synesthesia is when one sense is perceived as more than one sense. If a person has hearing synesthesia, sounds are heard and sensed as a colour or smell. For example, a person might taste banana every time they hear *Hallelujah* sung by Leonard Cohen. Another person might see the sung words and music as blue. Scientists think synesthesia is from cross-wiring between brain pathways for different senses.

Some people with synesthesia say they hear their tinnitus and see it as a colour. Experts suggest some tinnitus might be from synesthesia. For example, every time a person sees the colour brown, they hear tinnitus, or every time a person eats black licorice, they hear tinnitus. This can't explain every tinnitus case, but it's possible some cases of tinnitus are from synesthesia, especially cases where the usual tools and therapies don't help.

HEARING SYSTEM HYPERACTIVITY

There's an old philosophy question that asks: If a tree falls in a forest, does it make a sound? The most common answer is that it can't make a sound if nobody is there to hear it. Hearing system nerve fiber networks in the brain make sound waves heard. If there's no working hearing system near the tree, then there was no sound.

There is a rare hearing loss where sound waves travel through the ears, but the brain can't process it. If sound travels through the ears but the hearing system in the brain doesn't work, people can't hear sound.

The opposite is also true. If no tree falls in a forest, does it make a sound? Yes.

Sometimes the brain gets too busy or hyperactive. Processing information coming from itself. If the hearing system in the brain gets active enough, people hear sound even when there was no outside sound coming in through the ears. Tinnitus is sound from brain activity. That's why some Deaf people can hear tinnitus. The hearing problem is from their inner ears. The tinnitus is from the brain's hearing system.

Science shows in a quiet enough place most people can hear tinnitus. But it's hidden under background sounds so most people don't notice it. In 1953, Heller and Bergman did an experiment called *Tinnitus In Normally Hearing Persons*. Everyone had normal hearing and no tinnitus.

Each person was in a sound proof booth for 5 minutes. They thought they were getting a hearing test, but there was only 5 minutes of silence. After 5 minutes, most of the people reported hearing sounds in the head or in their ears identical to sounds reported by people with tinnitus. This experiment showed when it's quiet enough, most people can hear the brain's hearing pathways background activity. This is the sound called tinnitus.

It's not surprising tinnitus sounds different for different people, e.g. ring, buzz, hiss, beep, whistle. Each of these sounds will have its own pattern in the nerve fiber networks. The brain tries to check for activity patterns that match patterns it knows.

Tinnitus isn't generated from the same nerve fiber patterns in everyone or it would sound the same for everybody. With tinnitus, different nerve fibers patterns and combos of patterns are likely active for different people. Because the nerve fiber activity is happening within the hearing system, people hear tinnitus as sound. The specific tinnitus sound will change from person to person.

Tinnitus is normal for humans. Nobody said our brains work perfect all the time. Sometimes our hearing systems send an extra "sound message" through our brain. In quiet enough places, anybody can hear it.

Before I test a client's hearing, I ask questions to get their case history. One question I ask every person is: Do you ever hear any sounds or noises in your ears? Many people say no.

During the hearing test in a sound proof booth, my clients listen and signal me if they hear even the softest beeps or tones. This is a repeat of Heller and Bergman's 1953 study except with real sounds.

Everyone getting a hearing test signals at least once they heard a sound when there was no sound. Even people who reported no tinnitus. Tinnitus is human. Almost everybody hears an extra noise in their ears every now and then.

Quiet places or too much silence, like having hearing loss, increase the chances a person will hear tinnitus. Brain nerve fibers are active for sound and no sound. When there's no sound, nerve fiber activity for no sound increases.

No sound is important, because silence or soft sounds in the environment can signal danger for humans. Did the birds stop singing? If everything in the forest goes quiet, is there a bear or wolf nearby? Are you prey? Do you need to fight or flee by running away?

Extra Sound–Tinnitus

People in the Heller and Bergman experiment left with no lasting tinnitus. Why not?

Most people's brains tune out extra sounds coming from background activity. These sound messages don't make it past the subconscious networks. But sometimes the extra activity doesn't get tuned out. The brain gets hyper or overactive, and keeps processing this nerve fiber activity as lasting tinnitus.

Because tinnitus is from the brain's central hub for both ears, it's common to hear it in both ears or in the head. When people have single-sided tinnitus, brain activity in the central hub still pairs the ears. Over time, single-sided tinnitus can change so people hear it in both ears. They get scared and worried that the problem in one ear has spread to the other side. But it's normal. It's the way tinnitus hyperactivity works.

Scientists compare tinnitus to phantom limb pain. Tinnitus is sound when there's no sound signal. Phantom limb pain is pain when there's no body signal from missing or amputated limbs. Tinnitus and phantom limb pain happen with no ear or limb input. Both are from brain hyperactivity.

1. No Outside Sound > Ears
2. Brain Hyperactivity > Processing
3. Extra Sound Heard > Tinnitus

Extra Loud Sound–Hyperacusis
With hyperacusis, the hearing system is hyperactive for regular everyday sounds. Sounds like utensils scraping on plates, doors closing, running water, cooking noises, or normal conversation are too loud for comfort. Hyperacusis hurts. It's like banging your elbows if sound is the bang and ears are the elbows.

With tinnitus, brain hyperactivity turns up the volume of no sound.

With hyperacusis, brain hyperactivity turns up the volume of sound—louder than the outside sound waves were. A lot louder than other people hear the same sound. When people have hyperacusis, the inner ear also sends the brain a pain signal.

1. Outside Sound > Ears
2. Brain Hyperactivity> Processing
3. Extra Loud Sound Heard> Hyperacusis

Highly Sensitive Person
Dr. Elaine Aron has been researching and writing about highly sensitive people since the 1990s. The technical name is Sensory-Processing Sensitivity. It happens in an estimated 15 to 20% of people, and certain insects, birds, fish, dogs, or horses. People are born with it. Being highly sensitive means you can be overstimulated more easily than other people.

Have you been told, "Don't be so sensitive." Were you considered shy or sensitive as a child? Are you overwhelmed by sensing too much: too much light, too much smell, too much texture against your skin, too much sound? Do you get upset if you have too much to do in too short a time? When things get busy, do you need to take breaks for private rest time? If yes, you could be a highly sensitive person.

Are highly sensitive people more likely to have hyper ears? It seems possible. I wonder sometimes if some highly sensitive people are misdiagnosed with hyperacusis. Maybe some people need to learn how to cope better with overall sensitivity and not just hyper sensitive hearing.

Dr. Aron's website hsperson.com has self-tests for highly sensitive people. Her books include The Highly Sensitive Person and The Highly Sensitive Child.

Jan's View

I'm a highly sensitive person. I've never liked loud sounds, bright or flashy lights, or busy, crowded places. If I get overwhelmed, I have meltdowns. You could say I'm shy. At the end of kindergarden, the teacher asked my mother if I was mute, since she had never heard me say a word to anyone. I think the teacher could have asked before the last day of kindergarten, but what do I know.

Psychosomatic

Some doctors and scientists call tinnitus or decreased sound tolerance psychosomatic. It's not an insult. It doesn't mean they think people are faking. Psychosomatic definition is a physical illness or other condition caused or made worse by a mental factor such as stress. Tinnitus and decreased sound tolerance like hyperacusis are physical conditions. They get worse from stress and distress. Ears (physical) + distress (mental) = psychosomatic.

EMOTION SYSTEM HYPERACTIVITY

While tinnitus and hyperacusis start with hearing system hyperactivity, distress from hyper ears is from a hyperactive emotion system. The problem isn't if the person has hyper ears. Millions of people do. The problem happens when the person becomes distressed.

Tinnitus Distress

About 85% of adults who hear tinnitus aren't distressed. They notice their tinnitus if they pay attention to it, but it doesn't bother them. The other 10 to 15% have mild to very severe distress.

Science on how many children have tinnitus distress is inconsistent because scientists are inconsistent. They study different age ranges. They use different definitions of tinnitus. For example, can you hear a sound in your head now, inside a sound proof booth?

In 2016, Huffington Post reported on science showing 50% of children aged 11 to 17 have tinnitus. But the 50% was for children who had heard tinnitus at least once in the past year. That's not the definition of chronic tinnitus. Don't believe all the Hyper Ears World stats you read in the media.

A UK study analyzed 2002 to 2011 healthcare data on 4.7 million people. The tinnitus definition was if the hospital discharged people with main diagnosis of tinnitus or their primary care provider saw them for tinnitus with medical follow-up within 28 days. This is what they found:

Estimated Tinnitus Distress by Gender

Males = 50.9%
Females = 49.1%

Estimated Tinnitus Distress by Age (in years)

<10 = 0.3%
10-19 = 1.9%
20-29 = 4.9%
30-39 = 10.3%
40-49 = 18%
50-59 = 26%
60-60 = 23%
70-79 = 13%
80-84 = 3%

Tinnitus distress depends on the person's reaction to the tinnitus sound. Reactions are tied to sound meaning.

Some sounds are positive or pleasant like the sound of a loved one's voice or a favourite song. Some are negative or unpleasant like screeching nails on a blackboard or noise from aircraft.

There are lots of neutral sounds with no negative or positive meaning. They're not liked or disliked; they're just ignored in the background, e.g. sound of refrigerator running. If a sound, including tinnitus, has no negative meaning, it's easy to tune out or ignore. Even when people notice it, they aren't distressed.

But sound meaning is different for different people. Pleasant or neutral for one person can be unpleasant for somebody else.

I love the sound of wind chimes; a good friend of mine hates the sound of wind chimes. The sound of wind chimes from her neighbour's yard makes her unhappy. She has no control over that sound, and it has a negative meaning.

When sounds have a negative meaning, scientists think they trigger a fight-or-flight emotion system reaction. There are 3 things humans can do:

- Fight. But can't touch tinnitus. You can punch a pillow. But no direct hits to tinnitus.
- Flight. Can't run away from tinnitus; it goes where you go.
- Do nothing. When humans don't fight and don't flee, the emotion system gets hyperactive.

My partner and I were thrilled when we moved into our first home. The first night at 2:00 a.m. we woke up to the sound of train whistles. We didn't know the house was close to a railway line with a whistle crossing. The trains ran nightly.

We didn't mind the sound of train whistles. It wasn't unpleasant or negative. It wasn't important. Within a few weeks, we were sleeping through the night.

Our hearing systems were still processing the sound when we slept. But it was tuned out so it never reached our conscious awareness.

A negative emotional reaction to the sound of train whistles would activate the hearing system to process this sound whenever it happened. The hearing system would signal the brain about this important sound, causing sleepless nights and distress.

Distress increases a sound's importance. Instead of being a meaningless extra sound message, tinnitus becomes an important sound message for the hearing and emotion systems. While the hearing system makes us hear tinnitus, the emotion system determines if we become distressed.

It's interesting to see how animals handle distress, pain, fear, or anxiety. Animals often release their emotions physically. For example, a deer distressed by an attacking wolf often pronks after escaping. Pronking is when the deer makes high leaps that help discharge fight-or-flight chemicals and calm the deer's system.

Maybe people might cope better with tinnitus distress if they released their emotions physically. Cry. Punch a pillow. Run and jump around. Comedian Phyllis Diller once said, "*My recipe for dealing with anger and frustration: set the kitchen timer for twenty minutes, cry, rant, and rave, and at the sound of the bell, simmer down and go about business as usual.*" Releasing emotions could lower emotion system hyperactivity and help people cope better.

It's not surprising that tinnitus can have a negative sound meaning. It can be as annoying as any other endless or repeating noise. If tinnitus is sudden onset, it's more likely for people to have a negative reaction. For chronic tinnitus, people often wait years before trying to get help.

Many people think they're going Deaf, crazy, or have a serious medical problem. Then when people try to get help, they're told there's no cure. Too often, that's all the info they get.

Once a person realizes there's no quick fix, grief or distress can set in if they aren't told about coping tools and resources. Grief is linked with feelings of sadness, anger, fear, worry, anxiety, and depression. These are the same feelings tinnitus can trigger in the brain's emotion system.

These feelings are a normal reaction. But they can keep tinnitus happening and make tinnitus worse if distress lasts.

Tinnitus Distress Cycle

1. Negative emotional reaction.
2. Hearing system stays hyperactive: tinnitus sound lasts or gets worse.
3. Emotion system stays hyperactive: distress lasts or gets worse.
4. Repeat from step 1 or use coping tools to stop the cycle.

There is no difference in tinnitus between people who have tinnitus and people with tinnitus distress. Some have loud tinnitus with no distress. Others have soft tinnitus with severe distress. People with identical tinnitus loudness and pitch, and identical hearing, may or may not be distressed.

It's not the tinnitus sound itself that causes distress. It's the person's reaction to their tinnitus that causes distress. Distress can be for certain activities, e.g. feeling annoyed by tinnitus when trying to read in a quiet room. Difficulties with sleep, concentration, and relaxation are common. In severe cases, Tinnitus distress can affect a person's whole life including personal, work, and social situations.

For most people, emotions are reflected in their thoughts. We all have a running stream of thoughts in our heads. This background flow is made up of random thoughts that pop in our heads as we go through our day. When people have a negative reaction to their tinnitus, typical thoughts include:

What if I have a serious illness?
What if the tinnitus gets worse?
What if I lose my hearing?
What if I can never enjoy peace and quiet?
What if I go out and there's a loud sound?
What if I can't work?
What if I can't live with it?

Hyperacusis Pain

Hyperacusis distress depends on how people react to sound and—more importantly—how much they're avoiding sound. Hyperacusis can trigger the emotion system fight-or-flight reaction the same as tinnitus.

- Fight. Can't touch hyperacusis. You can hit a punching bag. But no direct hits to hyperacusis.
- Flight. Can't run away from hyperacusis; it goes where you go.
- Do nothing. Emotion system hyperactivity.

In mild cases, a person might avoid certain sounds, jump at loud or unexpected sounds, or worry about sounds that might happen. There are situations where the person with hyperacusis is uncomfortable from the loudness but other people aren't, e.g. walking along a busy street, at a restaurant, or shopping mall. Other painful sounds include cars honking, shouts, loud children, etc. In severe cases, hyperacusis distress can affect a person's personal, work, and social life.

Not much is known about hyperacusis and a high startle reflex. This is a big body twitch or spasm after sudden loud sound. Causes of the startle reflex include anxiety or depression, traumatic events, and brain activity when under stress. A startle response body jerk makes heart rate and anxiety go up, and can cause trembling. Coping strategies for hyperacusis can help.

Jan's View

I have hyperacusis during lifelong headaches and migraines; the worse my headache, the worse my hyperacusis. I also have a big startle reflex. Sudden loud sound. I jump. Things fly from my hands. Sometimes I squeak when my body jerks. My heart pounds. People think it's funny, because the sound doesn't startle them. I can't say it's funny for me.

Science still doesn't know how many people have hyperacusis because there's no single definition of hyperacusis or universal method of measuring hyperacusis severity for adults or children. Scientists use different age ranges in studies. This makes it very hard to pool data or compare findings. Based on available science:

Estimated Hyperacusis by Gender

Males = 12.5%
Females = 17.6%

Estimated Hyperacusis by Age (in years)

5-12 = 3.2%
13-17 = ?
18-25 = 6%
26-79 = 8.6%

If a person reacts negatively to sounds they hear, or possible unwanted future sounds, it causes distress, e.g. worry, fear, anger, and depression.

When a person has a negative reaction to hyperacusis, typical thoughts might include:

> What if the hyperacusis gets worse?
> What if I go out and there's a loud sound?
> What if I can never be around sound?
> What if I can't work?
> What if I can't live with it?

Hyperacusis Distress Cycle

1. Negative emotional reaction.
2. Overprotecting hearing.
3. Hearing system stays hyperactive: hyperacusis lasts or gets worse.
4. Emotion system stays hyperactive: distress lasts or gets worse.
5. Repeat from step 1 or use coping tools to stop the cycle.

People with hyperacusis need accurate information on how to reverse it. How to lower hyperactivity. How to become comfortable with sound again. How to avoid overprotecting their ears. Learn which coping tools help reduce the fight-or-flight reaction. The same tools that help tinnitus help hyperacusis with a few differences.

Misophonia Dislike

Remember misophonia is not about the pitch or loudness of a sound. It's about the emotional reaction. With misophonia, it's fight-or-flight. The person strongly dislikes certain sounds that don't bother the average person.

Not loud sounds. Soft repeated sounds, often quiet mouth, eating, or chewing sounds made by polite eaters. Other disliked sounds include humming, pen clicking, tapping on a keyboard, breathing noises, etc. Being trapped near the sound and not being able to leave makes the misophonia reaction worse. Some tinnitus and hyperacusis coping tools can help people cope better with misophonia.

People say misophonia is hate for certain sounds. But that's not the right definition. Dr. P.J. Jastreboff introduced the term misophonia as part of his neurophysiological model of tinnitus and decreased sound tolerance. In a 2015 interview with the American Tinnitus Association, Dr. Jastreboff said he decided on the name from the Latin translation for disliking sound and because he loves miso soup.

Words have power. If I hate a sound, my shoulders tense, heart beats faster, breathing gets tight. If I dislike a sound, I don't have as strong an emotional or physical reaction. In this book, I use Dr. Jastreboff's definition and describe misophonia as dislike. This small change in thinking helps retrain the emotion system to be less hyperactive.

Misophonia Distress Cycle

1. Negative emotional reaction.
2. Brain's emotion system stays hyperactive: misophonia distress lasts or gets worse.
3. Repeat from step 1 or use coping tools to stop the cycle.

A person with misophonia might dislike whatever makes the sound. For example, if a person with misophonia sees somebody getting ready to eat gum, they might still get upset or angry. These are visual triggers.

One coping strategy if you can't get away is to avoid the visual trigger. Don't look at it. Look away, look down—anywhere but the trigger. The emotional reaction will still happen, but sometimes it's not as severe as hearing plus watching the sound being made.

Misophonia is not getting annoyed or hating sounds like fingers on a blackboard, car alarms, blowers, or babies screaming. Many people hate these sounds. It's a natural reaction to an unpleasant pitch or loudness.

Misophonia has become a thing online. Loads of people say they have misophonia because they're disgusted and "hate it" when somebody eats gross, mouth open, chomping and slurping. But that's not miso-phonia. With eyes closed, do they dislike the sounds enough to get upset? Do they have strong urges to murder the chewer if misophonia is severe? No. Disgusted people just never want to see that person eating again.

Nobody knows how many children or adults have misophonia. It's not something people talk about. It's not ok to scream at people to shut up for chewing or breathing.

No child at school will say they're having problems because other kids are being too noisy chewing gum or tapping on cell phones in class. This can cause serious problems with learning, concentration, and taking tests. Gum chewing and mobile devices should be banned in classrooms.

Jan's View

It drives me crazy when it's quiet indoors and people sitting near me tap ticka tap tap on a mobile phone to text, email, or play games. After several minutes pass by, I hope they'll finish soon to stop the rage from building as if I'm the Incredible Hulk. Sometimes I can leave so I don't have to hear the sound anymore. But there are situations where the person with misophonia can't walk away.

I've always hated the sound of people eating, even when it's soft and polite. Pudding can be too loud, never mind potato chips or corn nuts. Growing up I thought I was crazy. I'd listen to my family eating meals, hating the sounds, and plotting how to kill them so I never had to listen to that sound again.

I realized I couldn't kill everybody who made chewing sounds, so I never put my plans into action. The distraction helped me cope better when I imagined the pros and cons of poison versus cutting the brake line in the car, or other murder methods.

I homicidally hate—I mean really dislike—the sound of teeth sucking. I think only somebody else with misophonia could understand. Once on a flight from Paris to London, I almost killed my teeth sucking seatmate. He was lucky it was only a 30 minute flight, never knowing how close he came to being strangled. I'm not joking. My fingers were twitching. Five more minutes and I'd have been guilty until proven innocent.

Phonophobia Fear

The phonophobia type of misophonia is a hyperactive emotional reaction that is more fright-or-flight than fight-or-flight. With phonophobia, the person fears the sound and whatever makes it. Treatment and coping tool options are very similar for phonophobia and hyperacusis. In this book, phonophobia won't be specifically mentioned unless info is different from coping with hyperacusis.

Balloons fill me with fright. There's been many an event where it would be rude to leave as soon as I arrived and saw balloons. I've had to stick around and stress over whether a balloon will pop. I feel sick when I see people carrying balloon bouquets to hospitals or parties.

Many children, teens, and older people are afraid of balloon gifts or decorations in case they pop. People who don't like being around balloons get called whiners or crybabies.

Sudden impulse or impact noise BANG, can damage the inner ears and the connections between the inner ears and hearing nerves. Canadian audiologists found popping balloons with a pin or blowing up a balloon until it explodes are louder than a shotgun and almost as loud as a 357 magnum handgun.

So nobody is being a whiner or crybaby. Balloons can cause hearing health damage. So can other sound sources that trigger phonophobia. Which is often why even seeing the sound source can trigger phonophobia like the sight of air horns or other noise sources that panic the person with decreased sound tolerance.

Distressed Personality (Type D)

People are divided into four general personality types. Type A people are active. Competitive. High achievers. Sometimes doing as much as they can as fast as they can. Type B people are relaxed. They don't get stressed out. They procrastinate when there are things to do. Type C people put others before themselves even if it's not good for them. They get bogged down by details when trying to get things done. They struggle with stress and depression.

Some experts say people with severe hyper ears distress are more likely to have Type D or Distressed personality. More likely to experience worry, depression, and other negative emotions. More social isolation. The glass is half empty.

But isn't it possible for people with a Type A, B, or C personality to have hyper ears distress? Lots of different personalities get hyper ears. Making links between personality types and specific medical conditions is dodgy. For example, experts used to say Type A people had a higher risk for heart disease; large-scale studies found no link.

Jan's View

I've taken an online personality type test. And no surprise, I'm

Type D. I'm wound a little tight. I struggle with anxiety and depression.

When I was desperate for hyper ears answers, different care providers gave me unhelpful advice. If I wasn't so anxious I could cope. I needed to get on with my life and forget my hyper ears. The message was quit whining. Suck it up, buttercup. My frustration was that my hyper ears were making me anxious and upset.

As an audiologist I saw it in medical reports for people having their hyper ears evaluated. "This anxious man..." "This anxious woman..." Labelling the personality as the problem.

When you're searching for answers and feel blamed for your personality, it's not a good thing. I know people struggling with hyper ears who were told they must have a mental illness. Others who have been psycho-analyzed back to their childhood. Newsflash: they're distressed because they're struggling with hyper ears. It makes it worse when care providers treat hyper ear related anxiety or distress as a personality flaw instead of something people can learn to manage so they aren't anxious or distressed anymore.

Prior Mental Illness

My favourite quote by anonymous is, *"If I should pass the tomb of Jonah, I would stop and sit for a while. For I was buried one time deep in the dark and came out alive after all."* I've had anxiety, panic attacks, and bouts of depression since I was a child. I tried to murder myself when I was fifteen. I've been buried more than once and come out alive.

Scientists ask, "Are people with a prior history of mental illness more likely to become distressed when they get hyper ears?

I ask, "What difference does it make?"

If someone is distressed, they need tools to help them cope better. Whether they've had mental health problems before or not.

BRAIN PROCESSING SUMMARY

Hyperactive hearing system:

- Tinnitus.
- Hyperacusis.

Hyperactive emotion system:

- Tinnitus distres.s
- Hyperacusis distress.
- Misophonia and phonophobia distress.

Neuroplasticity or brain plasticity means our brain can change over our lifetime. Pathways can rewire and systems can get less hyperactive. The goal of tinnitus and decreased sound tolerance treatments is to lower hearing system and/or emotion system hyperactivity. That's why changes on brain imaging are so important as a treatment outcome measure.

Negative emotional reactions can be changed for any distress. For example, I live in Vancouver, British Columbia, Canada. It has many illegal cannabis growing operations. These drug homes are in residential neighbourhoods. Rival criminals often target grow ops for drive-by shootings and armed robbery invasions. Sometimes these criminals get the address wrong and hit the neighbour's house instead.

The most common sign of a grow op is a house where windows stay covered day and night, and there's no activity. We once lived next to a house where we never saw our neighbour. Window coverings were always closed. Sometimes someone would enter or exit the home, but very early in the morning or late at night.

We worried. Had we moved next to a drug house? What if there was a drive-by shooting? What if our family or house was targeted by mistake? We were hyper aware of any activity next door. We constantly watched and worried about a possible dangerous situation. The constant worry took over our lives.

One day we were talking with a different neighbour. We found out the owner of the house next door was extremely shy and didn't like being outdoors. She worked long hours. When she was home, she stayed inside and spent time with her cat. There was zero chance she was growing drugs. Our anxiety and fear disappeared.

Nothing changed about our next door neighbour or her house. But our reaction was no longer negative. No more distress.

It's much much harder to change negative reactions to tinnitus and decreased sound tolerance. But people can become less distressed and cope well.

Changing how you react to tinnitus or outside sound can be as hard as learning to write with your left hand if you're right handed. The good news is by using coping tools, the emotional meaning of the tinnitus or sound trigger can change. The sound might stay the same. But the distress connection between the hearing system and the emotion system in the brain can be reset.

Much better coping happens when people change their reaction. People have successfully used various approaches and coping tools. The longer the hyperactivity or distress has been there, the longer it will take to see positive changes, sometimes up to 3 to 6 months. Change can't happen overnight or after trying a coping tool only once or twice. But it can happen.

9

TINNITUS-DECREASED SOUND TOLERANCE EVALUATION

Myth: If your tinnitus is really loud, hearing test results are not accurate.

Hearing testing or audiometry became widely used after World War II when many military veterans had hearing loss from combat noise. Audiologists customize evaluations for each individual person's hearing and hyper ears. They could include an interview, hearing testing, tinnitus testing, hyperacusis testing (if needed), distress measures, and counselling.

Keep in mind that evaluation makes people focus on their tinnitus or hyperacusis. This starts before the appointment when people rehearse what they want to share with their care provider.

People strain to hear during testing. Is that my tinnitus? Is that a test tone? During the interview and counselling the focus is the person's hearing, tinnitus or hyperacusis, and any related concerns. What you focus on increases.

It's common for tinnitus or hyperacusis to get worse temporarily after the evaluation appointment. This is normal. Over time, within a day or two, tinnitus or hyperacusis settles back to usual.

There's no hearing test for misophonia or phonophobia. They're diagnosed based on a person's description of their symptoms.

Online Hearing Tests
Hearing tests online or on apps are a hearing screening like the eye chart used in a doctor's office for vision screening. Some websites say you can calibrate your headphones with your computer to do accurate hearing tests online. This is not true.

Hearing tests are only accurate when done by a trained professional inside a soundproof booth using calibrated equipment and standardized test procedures. For yearly work hearing tests, under occupational noise regulations, it's illegal to use online hearing tests.

If a hearing screening shows hearing loss, you need professional evaluation, especially if you have hyper ears distress.

INTERVIEW

In the interview, audiologists ask about your health history, including tinnitus description, medical conditions, family history of hearing loss, and history of exposure to personal listening, music, or noise. Some providers will use a quick screening survey to check for hearing, tinnitus, or decreased sound tolerance difficulties.

There's a proper way to ask about tinnitus distress. The care provider shouldn't ask negative questions like, "How much does your tinnitus bother you?" Which makes a person think their tinnitus should bother them.

Neutral question:
How do you feel about your tinnitus?

When I ask this question—and I wait for an answer before speaking
again—I get two types of answers. Either people say they're used to it,
or there is a long pause and then people talk about the difficulties
they're having. There can be no concerns, concerns in specific situations, or widespread concerns in daily activities.

The audiologist should check if average everyday sound loudness is
uncomfortable to see if hyperacusis testing is needed. They'll ask about
fear or dislike for certain sounds.

OTOSCOPIC EAR CANAL EXAM

Otoscopes have special magnification and lighting to check the ear
canals and eardrums. This visual check identifies physical problems,
e.g. foreign objects, inflammation, infection, scarring or holes in the
eardrum, bugs. It also checks the size and shape of the ear canal, since
this can affect fit of any recommended aids or devices.

Some care providers have video otoscopes so people can see what the
care provider is seeing on a computer screen. It's very interesting for
people to see what's down their own ear canals, especially if there's
something unexpected going on in there. Yes, I have video-otoscoped
my own ears. Given the opportunity, who wouldn't?

MIDDLE EAR FUNCTION TESTING

Tympanometry is middle ear system testing done on a machine that
automatically measures how the middle ear system is moving. It also
measures air pressure behind the eardrum. Tympanometry can detect
holes or other problems with the eardrum or middle ear bones, e.g.

moving too much, moving too little, bulging into the ear canal from too much positive pressure, or sucked in towards the middle ear space from too much negative pressure. Equipment can also test Eustachian tube function.

Warning:
Acoustic reflex testing is not recommended!

The tympanometry machine can do acoustic reflex testing at different frequencies in each ear. It's an automatic reflex that pulls on the stirrup or stapes when loud sound waves hit the middle ear system. The loudness that triggers the reflex helps show type, amount, and pattern of hearing loss.

The acoustic reflex is present or absent. If present, there is no more than mild hearing loss. An absent reflex is inconclusive. Maybe the plug in the ear isn't sealing off the ear canal enough to pick up this small reflex. Maybe there's a problem with the middle ear system. Maybe there's some hearing loss of any type or amount.

If the acoustic reflex is absent, testing can go up to 110 dB. This is painfully loud for people with hyperacusis. And loud enough to cause temporary tinnitus or make tinnitus temporarily worse. Then results are often inconclusive. Other softer hearing testing can detect problems in the middle ear system and measure conductive hearing loss.

Jan's View

Back in the 1980s, my audiology class divided into groups of 3 to practice acoustic reflex testing on each other. Back then, we used signals up to 120 dB to look for reflexes. Nobody had heard of H. Nobody cared about using this test on people with T. Not even me until the testing started.

BEEP. My classmates chatted. Was that a reflex? Try again.

BEEP. Try louder. BEEP. BEEP. Louder BEEP. Over and over again. In both ears. I thought, Hurry up. Ouch. I don't like this. Hurry up, already. Afterwards, my tinnitus kicked up a big fuss. I was not a fan of acoustic reflex testing.

In the clinic, I wouldn't do this test on anyone with hyperacusis. But audiologists used it for people with tinnitus. I couldn't blast people when I knew it might make their tinnitus worse. On their hearing test results form or audiogram, I wrote DNT. Did not test. Nobody ever complained. Nobody ever asked why.

Around 2002, scientists recommended no acoustic reflex testing for people with tinnitus or hyperacusis. I was so happy. Other audiologists disagreed. We would argue.

"But it's so useful diagnostically," they would insist.

"But it's too loud for people with hyper ears," I would insist.

Experts recommend acoustic reflex testing if care providers suspect middle ear problems. Care providers should wait until after Loudness Discomfort Level testing to make sure there's no tolerance problem for the high acoustic reflex test sound levels.

Audiologists should adapt tinnitus-decreased sound tolerance evaluations for people with hyper ears the same as they adapt evaluations for people with other hearing conditions. Testing should only use soft comfortable sound signals. Before tympanometry starts, you might need to ask your care provider not to do acoustic reflex testing because you have tinnitus or hyperacusis.

INNER EAR FUNCTION TESTING

With modern test equipment, we can now test hair cell health inside the cochleas. Soft automatic otoacoustic emissions testing sends different frequency tones down the ear canal, through the middle ear system, and to the inner ear. The machine measures any response or emission sent back from the inner ear.

Healthy inner ears have healthy otoacoustic emissions. This is the test used for newborn and infant hearing screening programs. It's also a screening test for noise-induced hearing loss.

The pattern of otoacoustic emission results matches the pattern of any hearing loss. Responses only appear with a normal middle ear system and healthy inner ear. Small or absent responses can mean there's inner ear damage or hearing loss.

Noise-induced inner ear damage can show as absent emissions before noise-induced hearing loss is detectable by hearing testing.

HEARING THRESHOLD TESTING

People of any age can have their hearing tested, from newborn to elderly. You don't need hearing testing repeated if you've been tested within the last 12 months. Keep copies of your hearing tests so providers can see your results and don't test hearing again if they don't need to. Sometimes a quick hearing threshold screening can confirm if you need another full test, or whether time is better spent on tinnitus-decreased sound tolerance counselling.

Standard Audiometry
Standard audiometry is used to test hearing for pure tone thresholds starting around age 4 to 5 years old, depending on the child. The pure tone frequencies tested are .25-8 kHz since this is an important range for speech communication. Many children and adults with tinnitus-decreased sound tolerance have normal hearing for standard audiometry frequencies.

Hearing should be similar in both ears. Threshold definition is the softest loudness or intensity a person can hear a pure tone at a specific frequency. Hearing threshold changes of ≤10 dB from test to test are not significant.

Testing uses air conduction and bone conduction signals. For air conduction, sound signals travel through air down the ear canal and through the middle ear system to get to the inner ear.

Bone conduction signals travel through the skull to get to the inner ear. Low frequency bone conduction sound is often more felt than heard. Comparing air and bone conduction thresholds shows if hearing loss is conductive, sensorineural, or mixed (conductive and sensorineural).

For pure tone testing, people signal when they hear very soft tones. Care providers something think people with tinnitus are difficult to test because they have trouble telling the difference between their tinnitus and the test tones.

Pulsed Tones
Typical test tones or warbled tones are continuous beeps lasting about 3 seconds (e.g. beeeeeep). These beeps can sound like tinnitus at certain pitches or frequencies. But care providers can change from continuous to pulsed tones.

Pulsed tones are a series of short repeated tones (e.g. bip bip bip). Thresholds are the same for pulsed and continuous tones. Pulsed tones make it easier for people to tell when they're hearing a test tone and not their tinnitus.

Jan's View

I hate having my hearing tested. I hear multiple beeps and rings inside my head. When I sit in a soundproof booth and listen hard for test tones, my tinnitus takes off. I've often had the audiologist walk into the booth—while no test signal is being sent—as I sat signalling responses to my own tinnitus. When I have my hearing tested, I ask for pulsed tones.

As an audiologist, I always use pulsed tones for hearing testing. The pulsed tones sound different enough from tinnitus, making testing easier. People with tinnitus can request pulsed tones for pure tone threshold testing if needed.

Tone Break
Audiologist training includes not letting the client know a tone happens. Moving only our fingertips on the audiometer. No eye, head, or body movement to help the person guess when there's a sound. Poker face.

If someone is constantly pressing the button for their own tinnitus, I break the rules. I stop sending any test tones for a few minutes. Next time the person signals they heard something, I shake my head. No. Every time they signal. No. They stop pressing the button for their tinnitus.

The next time I send a test tone, I make sure it's a volume they can hear easily. When they respond, I nod. Yes. It's a reminder of the tones they're listening for. I go back to poker face. People seem to find testing easier after tone breaks.

Hearing Loss Severity
The pure tone average is an average of hearing thresholds at important frequencies for understanding speech. There is no single pure tone average definition. It depends on the age of the person tested, and what the pure tone average is being used for. When you see hearing loss statistics reported, what definition of hearing loss was used?

For children and adults, hearing loss severity depends on expected communication problems during daily activities, including conversations in quiet or difficult listening situations.

Some people think definitions of hearing loss severity should be more sensitive for children. But even slight hearing loss can cause problems for children and adults for understanding speech in noise.

Severity can be based on individual hearing thresholds at specific test tones or a pure tone average. These are some current hearing loss severity definitions for children and adults:

Degree of Hearing Loss

Normal = 0 – 15 dB
Slight = 16 – 25 dB
Mild = 26 – 40 dB
Moderate = 41-55 dB
Severe = 56 – 70 dB
Profound >70 dB

A person with a 50 dB pure tone average has moderate hearing loss. Sometimes people turn the pure tone average into a percentage of hearing loss: 50 dB pure tone average = 50% hearing loss. That's wrong. Only severity descriptions are used.

Since hearing loss severity can be different at different frequencies, care providers describe hearing loss based on the pattern and type of hearing loss. For example, moderate flat conductive hearing loss in one ear, or normal low frequency hearing sloping to moderately-severe high frequency sensorineural hearing loss in both ears.

Tinnitus or hyperacusis-distress is not related to the type, severity, or frequency pattern of hearing loss. People with any hearing loss can have tinnitus or hyperacusis distress. But some people are told their hearing is "normal" when they have slight hearing loss that could causing hearing difficulties noticed in everyday life.

People with normal hearing often think tinnitus interferes with their hearing in difficult listening situations. The problem is divided attention.

Scientists found young adults with normal hearing and tinnitus have a harder time with a listening task than young adults with normal hearing but no tinnitus. Having tinnitus divides our attention. Our brain automatically attends to tinnitus plus whatever else we're listening to.

If you have hearing loss and tinnitus, you'll have more trouble with a listening task than someone with only hearing loss . Your communication ability will be mildly worse than what hearing healthcare or medical professionals expect if they only consider your hearing loss severity.

Extended High Frequency Audiometry

Extended high frequency audiometry tests if people can hear air conduction frequencies above the 8 kHz upper limit of standard audiometry. Frequencies tested include 10, 11, 12, 14, and 16 kHz. It's not significant if people can't hear 20 kHz; it's often from equipment issues.

Extended high frequency thresholds can be more like an electrical sensation than heard. This type of testing is used to monitor hearing in people treated with ototoxic drugs needed for life saving measures like cancer treatment or severe infections. It's a sensitive screening test to detect early hearing loss in people at risk, e.g. genetic, early noise damage.

It's best when there are baseline extended high frequency audiometry results from before ototoxic drug treatment or noise exposure. Extended high frequency audiometry thresholds can be very different from person to person, so individual threshold results compared to individual baseline are the best way to see if hearing is changing.

Online extended high frequency audiometry tests are not accurate. It's very hard even for audiometer manufacturers to make equipment that can produce consistent extended high frequency pure tone test signals. The higher the frequency, the harder it is to manufacture. Your computer can't play extended high frequency tones accurately enough even for a hearing screening.

Jan's View

I tried doing an online extended high frequency hearing test, out of curiosity. I turned the volume as low as possible on my computer first. The constant tone quickly went up from can't hear it to OUCH. It was like a horrible high pitched tinnitus that got louder fast before I fumbled with my laptop's volume control and turned it off. I don't recommend it.

Online extended high frequency testing could make hyper ears worse. In a professional evaluation, care providers start very soft and slowly increase loudness of extended high frequency tones to find thresholds. Threshold is identified long before the tone gets to an uncomfortable loudness.

For people with tinnitus or hyperacusis, including children, extended high frequency hearing loss can be an underlying reason for tinnitus or hyperacusis. Maybe hearing isn't as normal as assumed by standard testing.

Extended High Frequency Hearing Ability

4-17 years old: 10-11-12-14-16-kHz

18-49 years old: 10-11-12-14-kHz
50-59 years old: 10-11-12-kHz
60+ years old: 10-11-kHz

The older the person, the worse the expected extended high frequency hearing thresholds. Based on estimated hearing ability, a 35 year old who can only hear up to 11 kHz would have early onset extended high frequency hearing loss.

People with a history of chronic noise exposure have worse extended high frequency hearing thresholds than people of the same age with no noise exposure history. Noise-induced damage usually starts at 11-14 kHz.

With age, extended high frequency hearing for different frequencies are not out of order. For example, if a 45 year old person with tinnitus or hyperacusis could hear below 10 kHz, had hearing loss at 10 to 14 kHz but normal hearing at 16 kHz, something besides age is the cause, e.g. noise damage, genetics.

SPEECH COMMUNICATION TESTING

Hearing health is about more than hearing thresholds. Normal hearing includes understanding speech in different listening situations.

Speech communication testing identifies hearing system distortion that makes it harder for people to understand speech even when their hearing thresholds fall within the normal range.

Hearing healthcare providers should use digitally recorded test materials so words and speech are completely the same from test to test.

Most Comfortable Loudness

This is the loudness level where speech is most comfortable. Speech testing is done based on each person's most comfortable loudness.

Word Recognition (WR) in Quiet

This testing uses standard lists of one syllable words, e.g. chew, knees. The words are presented one word at a time with no background noise. The lists are designed to pick up common mistakes made by people with hearing loss. For example, a person might hear "knees" as "knee" or "me".

Scores are the percentage of words repeated correctly. The worse the WR in quiet, the worse the hearing system distortion. For example, if a person's WR score is 50%, they're only catching about 50% of words in quiet.

Score—Word Recognition

90 – 100% = Normal
76 – 88% = Good
60 – 74% = Fair
50 – 60% = Poor
50% or less = Very Poor

Speech-in-Noise Testing

This tests how well a person understands sentences in different volumes of background noise. For speech-in-noise, speech is the primary signal, and the noise is running speech mixed together, sometimes called speech babble. People are scored on how many of the sentence's key words they can pick out using only their hearing.

Testing is done at different volumes of noise to find each person's degree of speech-in-noise loss. This helps give information on a person's speech communication abilities in daily life when they're trying to understand conversations in difficult listening situations, e.g. restaurant, retail store.

Most people can't easily understand conversations when ambient noise is louder than who they're trying to listen to. People with normal hearing health can understand speech even when it's about the same loudness as background noise. People with speech-in-noise loss need speech at least 50% louder than background noise to understand conversations. Some people have more severe speech-in-noise loss than others.

Depending on the cause, some people have speech-in-noise loss even when their hearing thresholds fall within the normal range. This includes almost everybody with tinnitus and hyperacusis who have "normal" hearing.

People with normal hearing health and no speech-in-noise loss can even do fine when the background noise is louder than the speech. This is really common in retail stores or restaurants, especially when there are people talking plus background music playing. I've been in restaurants where the average background noise was much higher than speech conversations without raised voices or shouting. Everyone with speech-in-noise loss is going to struggle to communicate.

Most people have never heard of hearing system processing distortion or speech-in-noise loss. Maybe because not enough care providers are using best practice guidelines by doing speech-in-noise testing for all evaluations.

Speech-In-Noise Loss Severity
At 0 dB speech-in-noise ratio, speech is the same loudness as background noise. The dB increase is for the level of test sentences over the level of speech babble needed for a person to understand speech-in-noise.

Normal (0 to +3 dB): Understands when speech is 0 to 3 dB louder than background noise.

Mild (+4 to +7 dB): Understands when speech is 4 to 7 dB louder than background noise.

Moderate (+8 to +15 dB): Understands when speech is 8 to 15 dB louder than background noise.

Severe (>15 dB): Understands when speech is > 15 dB louder than background noise.

Speech-in-noise loss can be from different causes. It can't be predicted by hearing thresholds. Two people can have the same hearing thresholds, but very different speech-in-noise loss severity.

For example, one person might have severe hearing loss but only mild difficulties understanding speech-in-noise. Another might have severe hearing loss and severe problems understanding speech in the same amount of background noise.

Hearing impaired people with severe degree of hearing loss and severe degree of speech-in-noise loss have the most speech communication difficulties. Especially if they also have tinnitus or hyperacusis.

TINNITUS-HYPERACUSIS TESTING

These are some of the common tests used in tinnitus and hyperacusis evaluations. Some are for tinnitus, and some for hyperacusis. There are no specific tests for misophonia or phonophobia.

Pitch & Loudness Match

This is a test where people compare their tinnitus to a tone presented through the audiometer. Care providers adjust pitch and loudness as needed to find the best match.

Pitch matches are often high frequency. With hearing loss, pitch matches can be close to the frequency of greatest hearing loss but not always. It's common for pitch matches to change from test to test. This is interesting since certain sound therapy approaches use tinnitus pitch matches.

Loudness matches are measured at the tinnitus pitch match. They stay about the same over time. People with normal hearing pick louder matches than people with hearing loss. Loudness matches are often within 10 dB of a person's hearing threshold at the pitch match. For example, a person's hearing threshold might be 60 dB, and their tinnitus loudness match 65 dB.

Some people are surprised when their loudness match is close to their hearing threshold. It doesn't mean their tinnitus is soft or faint.

With the 3 dB doubling rule; small dB differences equal big volume differences. A person's tinnitus can sound loud regardless of the loudness match.

Minimum Masking Level
This is the softest level of white noise needed to mask or cover up tinnitus so it's not heard. White noise has equal sound energy at all frequencies.

Minimum masking levels show how helpful sound might be to make tinnitus less noticeable, and the amount of sound needed. If treatment makes tinnitus softer, minimum masking levels will also be softer. But tinnitus loudness will still go up and down over time.

Tinnitus pitch loudness matches and minimum masking levels measure tinnitus characteristics at the time of testing. They don't identify distress.

Jan's View

My tinnitus isn't one sound. There's constant squealing like a dump truck slamming on the brakes, a pulsing sh-sh-sh, and extra tones and noises that come and go as they please. Why is the smoke alarm going? Is the phone ringing? Oh, just my tinnitus.

Because my tinnitus isn't tonal or a single frequency, my tinnitus matches and minimum masking levels would only be roughly the same from appointment to appointment. If my minimum masking level was softer than before, it could be from using coping tools that are helping. Or it could be because my tinnitus gets louder and softer for its own reasons.

Residual Inhibition

This test measures if a person's tinnitus changes after listening to white noise or other sound for a set time. If there's residual inhibition, tinnitus gets softer or stops while the sound is on. Residual inhibition only lasts for a few seconds to a few minutes after the sound is turned off. This test helps show people sound can be helpful for tinnitus. Some tinnitus sound therapy treatments are based on residual inhibition.

Loudness Discomfort Levels

These are sometimes called Uncomfortable Loudness Levels. This test checks hearing at each frequency to find when sound loudness is uncomfortable. Volume is increased in very small steps. Loudness comfort averages 100 dB for people with normal hearing.

Discomfort levels <70 dB at a particular frequency are a sign of hyper-acusis. But loudness discomfort levels are not the same across frequencies tested.They can average 60 to 85 dB across frequencies for people with hyperacusis. For example, some people might find lower deeper frequencies more uncomfortable, and other people might have more loudness discomfort from higher frequencies. Some people are so sensitive to sound, loudness discomfort level testing can't be done.

Loudness discomfort can go up and down over time. Some experts don't recommend loudness discomfort level testing routinely, but it's difficult to identify hyperacusis or fit therapy devices without loudness discomfort level results.

Noise Floor

Noise floor is the volume of background noise in your environment. In a stereo system, a high noise floor means you hear noise coming from the system itself, just from turning it on. The hearing system can also have a high noise floor. This is called central gain. If the noise floor is too high at one or more frequencies, people can hear it as the sound of tinnitus.

Normal Hearing   Tinnitus

Noise Floor   **Noise Floor**

Dynamic Range

Dynamic range is the amount of audible comfortable hearing between a person's hearing thresholds (hearing system noise floor) and their loudness discomfort levels.

People with tinnitus (T) might have normal dynamic ranges. But people with hyperacusis have smaller dynamic ranges because there is less listening room between their hearing thresholds and softer-than-normal loudness discomfort levels (LDL).

Normal Hearing

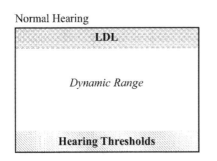

Hyperacusis

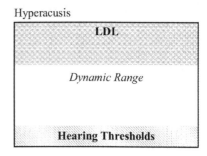

Tinnitus

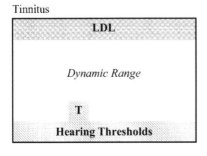

Tinnitus & Hyperacusis

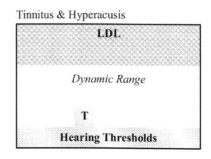

Recruitment is when loud sounds bother people with hearing loss the same as people with normal hearing, e.g. babies screaming, fire alarms, loud movies at cinemas. hearing loss is for softer sounds. The louder sounds get, the more similar loudness discomfort levels (LDL) are for people with hearing loss and people with normal hearing.

Normal Hearing

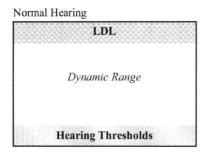

Hearing Loss Recruitment

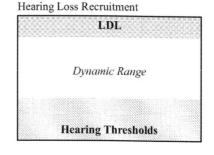

People with hearing loss recruitment have a smaller dynamic range because there's less listening room between their elevated hearing loss thresholds and loudness discomfort levels (LDL).

People with hearing loss and hyperacusis have the smallest dynamic range.

Hearing Loss

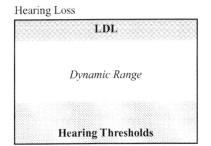

Hearing Loss & Hyperacusis

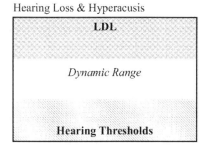

DISTRESS MEASURES

At the evaluation, audiologists use distress measure questionnaires to check tinnitus or hyperacusis severity. Distress measures are also used as treatment outcome measures. Severity should be significantly lower after treatment if the treatment helped.

Some people think treatment outcomes should only be measured with tests like tinnitus matches, minimum masking levels, or loudness discomfort levels. Minimum masking levels needed to mask or cover up tinnitus should be softer. Loudness comfort levels should be higher than before treatment.

But these tests don't measure distress. If a person's minimum masking levels are softer after treatment than before, does that mean they're not as distressed? Not necessarily. The loudness isn't the issue. The person's reaction to their tinnitus is the issue.

Distress measures are also important when people can't be tested. Some people have such severe hyperacusis, they can't do loudness discomfort level testing. Deaf people or people with very severe hearing loss can't hear tinnitus or hyperacusis test tones or sounds.

That's where distress or treatment outcome measures are key. The problem is too many different questionnaires are being used by scientists, product manufacturers, and care providers.

It's a problem because you can't compare treatment outcomes for different products or therapies if they don't measure distress the same way. What if science Team 1 and science Team 2 both find 20% improvement when people use their tinnitus-hyperacusis products? But Team 1 used Questionnaire A for their product and Team 2 used Questionnaire B for their product.

Which product lowers distress the most? Nobody knows because it's comparing apples to oranges unless they use the same distress questionnaire. Same problem for clinics offering therapy services. If you improve 50% at Clinic 1 with Measure C and 50% at Clinic 2 with Measure D, there's no way to know which therapy helped lower distress more.

Imagine if this was blood pressure testing. Dr. A uses a blood pressure test used by most doctors; Dr. B uses a different blood pressure test. Dr. B. treats you using a new approach and says your blood pressure has significantly improved. But there's no way to know when results can't be compared to treatment by other doctors. Everybody should use the same test.

Tinnitus Handicap Inventory
Experts are asking international scientists to use one universal adult treatment outcome questionnaire for their research. Not the over 70 questionnaires used now. If everyone uses the same questionnaire,

scientists can pool research data and compare data from different approaches. Apples to apples.

At a 2006 Tinnitus Research Initiative meeting in Regensberg, Germany, experts found the Tinnitus Handicap Inventory is most commonly used for adults, and could be used as an international standard.

As of 2020, scientists are working on a universal evidence-based distress or treatment outcome questionnaire for children.

The Tinnitus Handicap Inventory uses 25 questions to measure different factors causing distress, e.g. sleep, anxiety, concentration, depression. Tinnitus Handicap Inventory scores can be tracked before, during, and after therapy to identify any improvement. Changes ≥ 20% are significant.

Tinnitus Handicap Inventory Score

0 – 16%. Slight
18 – 36% Mild
38 – 56% Moderate
58 – 76% Severe
78 – 100% ~~Catastrophic~~ Very Severe

Catastrophic Very Severe Tinnitus Distress
There was no Tinnitus Handicap Inventory when my tinnitus started. But I know my tinnitus distress would score catastrophic. If anyone told me that at the time, I'd have killed myself. I was teetering on the edge as it was.

The Tinnitus Handicap Inventory is on multiple websites including tinnitus associations, hearing and tinnitus clinics, and tinnitus product manufacturers. What if somebody at home uses an online Tinnitus

Handicap Inventory to check their distress severity? And finds out their
tinnitus is catastrophic: causing great damage or suffering. With
nobody to reassure them they are not alone and something can be done.

Negative emotional reactions increase brain hyperactivity that makes
tinnitus worse. Outside of scientific research, can't Hyper Ears World
use a less negative word to describe level of tinnitus distress? If they
wanted to know, I told clients their tinnitus was very severe. Isn't that
bad enough? Changing a Tinnitus Handicap Inventory severity description adjective doesn't change the science.

The Tinnitus Handicap Inventory has been widely studied for decades
and is a valid and reliable treatment outcome measure for tinnitus
distress. It's free to use without copyright infringement. It's used
worldwide, translated into many languages, and still found valid and
reliable.

Tinnitus Handicap Inventory–Screening
The Tinnitus Handicap Inventory is very useful because it is one of the
very rare questionnaires that comes in a short 10 question version for
clinics and care providers to use. Research shows the Tinnitus Handicap Inventory-Screening version is as valid and reliable as the Tinnitus
Handicap Inventory, even when translated into other languages.

Jan's View

When science proved the 10 question Tinnitus Handicap
Inventory-Screening was science-based for clinics to use, I
switched right away. Why make a person do 25 questions when
10 are just as good? I used the time I saved for counselling and
treatment planning.

In my opinion, public websites should use the Tinnitus Handicap
Inventory-Screening, not the full Tinnitus Handicap Inventory
science or research version. I also think they should update their

description. To me, it seems negligent for websites to use a questionnaire that describes very severe tinnitus distress as catastrophic.

The Tinnitus Handicap Inventory-Screening is scored from 0 to 100% to determine distress levels, same as the Tinnitus Handicap Inventory. Answers of yes = 10; sometimes = 5; no = 0. Changes ≥ 20% are significant.

1. Because of your tinnitus, do you feel frustrated?
2. Does your tinnitus make you upset?
3. Because of your tinnitus, do you feel depressed?
4. Does your tinnitus make you feel anxious?
5. Because of your tinnitus, is it difficult for you to concentrate?
6. Does your tinnitus make it difficult for you to enjoy life?
7. Do you find it difficult to focus your attention away from your tinnitus and on other things?
8. Because of your tinnitus, do you often feel tired?
9. Do you feel as though you cannot escape your tinnitus?
10. Do you feel that you can no longer cope with your tinnitus?

Tinnitus Handicap Inventory-Screening Score

0 – 25% Mild
26 – 50% Moderate
51 – 75% Severe
76 – 100% ~~Catastrophic~~ Very Severe

Decreased Sound Tolerance Questionnaire
There are no questions used consistently across clinics to determine if a person's decreased sound tolerance is mild, moderate, or severe. Many questionnaires are used including the Hyperacusis Handicap Inventory. Greenberg and a newly developed 25 question Inventory of Hypera-

cusis Symptoms for scientific and clinical use. People with decreased sound tolerance need one universal decreased sound tolerance distress or treatment outcome questionnaire for children and adults.

Scientists are working on a decreased sound tolerance questionnaire for children. For adults, scientists and providers internationally need to use one valid and reliable short questionnaire so results can be pooled and compared across research studies and clinics. Examples of adult questions include:

- Are you bothered by sounds others are not?
- Are you afraid of sounds others are not?
- Do sounds ever cause you worry, stress, irritation, or annoyance?
- Are you emotionally drained by daily sounds?
- Do you ever not go out because you would be exposed to bothersome sound?
- Do you ever isolate yourself in quiet environments so you won't be exposed to bothersome sound?
- Do you ever use earplugs or earmuffs to reduce loudness of sound around you (when it is not hazardously loud)?

DST Questionnaire – Screening
There isn't anything universally used by scientists or clinics for children or adults.

Visual Analog Scale
There are no consistent visual analog scales used among tinnitus or decreased sound tolerance scientists or care providers. One popular type, used for older children or adults, is to have the person rank their tinnitus distress or decreased sound tolerance severity on a scale of 1 to 10 with 10 being the worst possible. People might also be asked to rank each distress factor on a scale of 1 to 10, e.g. concentration, sleep, anxiety.

These types of ranking scales are mainly used because they're easy and fast for care providers to use. But, if you're going for professional therapy, these simple scales alone are not specific or detailed enough to highlight key concerns or really compare treatment progress over time.

Another problem is that a scale of 1 to 10 isn't wide enough to account for day-to-day fluctuations. It doesn't help lower distress if a person rates their tinnitus or decreased sound tolerance as 10 (worst possible) and every day it's at a 10. A scale of 1 to 100 is better. A visual analog ranking scale can be used no matter what your hearing is like.

Happy Face-Sad Face Scale
Another scale that could be useful is a happy face–sad face scale like the Wong-Baker scale used for pain. Care providers could use something similar for children or adults distressed by tinnitus or decreased sound tolerance (DST).

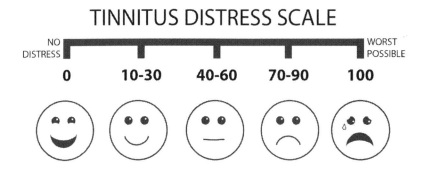

DST DISTRESS SCALE

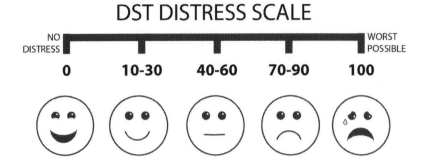

NO
DISTRESS

0   10-30   40-60   70-90   100

WORST
POSSIBLE

TINNITUS-DECREASED SOUND TOLERANCE EVALUATION SUMMARY

- Interview.
- Otoscopic examination.
- Tympanometry.
- No acoustic reflex testing.
- Otoacoustic emissions, if available.
- Pure Tone Thresholds (.25–8 kHz): air and bone conduction.
- Extended High Frequency Audiometry (10 – 16 kHz): air conduction.
- Tinnitus Testing: pitch and loudness matches, minimum masking levels, residual inhibition.
- Hyperacusis Testing: loudness discomfort levels.
- Tinnitus or decreased sound tolerance distress or treatment outcome measures: e.g. Tinnitus Handicap Inventory-Screening visual analog scales.

An important research goal is to divide people into subtypes of tinnitus or hyperacusis to identify which treatment approach works best for individual cases. This could include dividing people with tinnitus and/or hyperacusis into distinct hearing loss categories based on standard and extended high frequency hearing. Subtypes could be fine-tuned more if people have misophonia or phoonophobia.

Hopefully more science is being done on how to divide people with hyper ears into categories or subtypes based on hearing abilities and different causes. To find treatment differences between people in the different categories. Getting scientists closer to identifying which specific treatment approach is best for each individual person. And one day, find the cures we've been waiting for so long.

COUNSELLING

Audiologist counselling after tinnitus or decreased sound tolerance evaluation is in-depth. It covers results, education and reassurance, specific concerns, and individual recommendations. The 6 tool category options to consider include:

1. Sound therapy tools.
2. Hearing aid tools (normal hearing or hearing loss).
3. Mind therapy tools.
4. Body therapy tools.
5. Sleep tools.
6. Hearing protection tools.

Some people don't need more coping tools or professional treatment. Others might be using helpful coping tools. If needed, the care provider can recommend fine-tuning or changing tools for more benefit. Care providers can tell people with empty toolboxes that there are helpful coping tools and treatments available. More distressed means bigger toolbox.

Sometimes care providers refer people for more testing after their evaluation. Tests could include Auditory Brainstem Response (ABR) for detailed info on how sound travels up the hearing nerves. ABR is a very loud test, hearing protection can't be used, and an MRI might still be needed after ABR.

The final decision to go ahead with treatment or coping tools is up to you. People must be motivated to make changes in their daily life. For treatment to help, they need to follow instructions and use aids or devices as recommended. Coping tools won't give a quick fix or cure. But over time an individual coping toolbox can lower distress and improve your quality of life.

PART I

SOUND THERAPY TOOLS

1

SOUND THERAPY BASICS

Why is it that the buzzing in the ear ceases if one makes a sound?
Is it because the greater sound drives out the less?

- Hippocrates -

Sound therapy or sound enrichment is the specific use of soft sound to treat tinnitus or hyperacusis. Experts believe sound therapy helps exercise the hearing system and lower hyperactivity. This therapy keeps your hearing system busy with sound coming from outside your body.

This is the sound your hearing system should process. You can use sound therapy to take control and get relief. For many people, this means better coping.

One of the best ways not to listen to tinnitus is to listen to something else. People with tinnitus listen to sounds that are more comfortable and make tinnitus less noticeable or less a focus of attention. This makes the hearing system less hyperactive. By using sound therapy, people's tinnitus can get softer. Even a tiny drop in tinnitus loudness helps people cope better.

Sound therapy helps people with hyperacusis adjust to hearing sound more comfortably as their hearing system becomes less hyperactive. Using sound therapy regularly can have a positive long-term effect.

Extra sound can help people cope better with misophonia by making it harder to hear the disliked sound although sound therapy alone will not change the misophonia emotional reaction.

People use sound therapy for relaxation or distraction. Relaxation sound is common. Imagine you go to the spa for a massage. Soothing sounds will often play in the background to help improve relaxation. Imagine you go to the dentist for an appointment. Soothing music is often playing in the background to help people relax and feel less anxiety, fear, or stress. Comfortable pleasant relaxation sound works best when people can easily tune the sound out.

Distraction sound can draw attention away from tinnitus or misophonia. It's hard for people to pay close attention to more than one sound at a time. Multiple sounds divide the brain's attention and divides listening attention.

Imagine you're having a conversation or listening to a sound. It's harder to pay attention to tinnitus or misophonia when you're focussing on another sound or voice. Less awareness helps people cope better. Distraction sound works best when the sound is comfortably loud, interesting, and pleasant.

People with profound Deafness or severely impaired unaidable hearing can turn on cochlear implants for sound therapy. When their cochlear implant is turned on, most people notice their tinnitus less. In about

10% of implants, people who didn't have tinnitus hear it after the implant. Scientists are studying why this happens.

Some people with hyperacusis get sudden onset single-sided hearing loss and severe tinnitus. In these cases, a cochlear implant can lower hyperacusis and tinnitus severity. But cochlear implant surgery is a last resort when other treatments haven't helped.

People with structural problems in the cochlea or hearing nerve can't get a cochlear implant. Scientists are studying brain implants or auditory prostheses. So far cochlear implants help hearing more. Scientists don't know why yet. If you use a cochlear implant, try using sound therapy. Also use coping tool options that aren't hearing or sound-based.

SELF-HELP SOUND THERAPY

People with mild distress often just need basic education and reassurance counselling after their tinnitus or decreased sound tolerance evaluation. Some people start self-help sound therapy after their evaluation and medical clearance. The less distressed a person is, the easier it is to do.

GUIDED SELF-HELP SOUND THERAPY

With guided self-help, care providers guide people on how to use sound therapy. Sometimes audiologists offer telehealth, giving counselling and guidance with phone call appointments instead of office visits. Providers sometimes use Skype, email, or other communication methods.

Guided self-help can happen as needed or at scheduled appointments.

Self-help workbooks can be a useful way to learn sound therapy tools and how to use them. Audiologists can give added guidance as needed.

Jan's Case

I always found people liked telehealth guided self-help if it was right for their needs. After their tinnitus or decreased sound tolerance evaluation and counselling, some people liked having a scheduled appointment by telephone a week or two later so I could check how they were doing, answer questions, and give more counselling as needed.

These appointments could be as short as 15 minutes long. Audiologists doing this can pro-rate their tinnitus or decreased sound tolerance counselling rate, e.g. charge 25% of their hourly rate for a 15 minute appointment.

SOUND TYPES

Relaxation and distraction sound therapy uses different sound types. There is no single sound type that works best for everyone. If there was, we'd know by now. I thought it was a crazy idea when science on sound therapy first came out in the 1990s. But my personal and professional experience and decades of science prove sound therapy helps hyper ears.

Coloured Noise
This is a common sound type for therapy. It's described as the sound of wind or waterfalls. When care providers tell people with hyper ears that therapy uses noise, the first reaction is, "No thanks. I have enough noise to listen to."

For communication, noise is defined as unwanted sound. For sound therapy, sound is wanted to lower hearing system hyperactivity. Sound therapy noise definitions are acoustic definitions that define noise by colour. The colour of noise depends on the pitch or frequency range.

It would be nice if we could call coloured noise something different instead of noise. But that would make the acoustics folks very unhappy and confuse things even more in Hyper Ears World. Certain types of coloured noise are best.

White Noise

This was the first sound type used for sound therapy. White or broadband noise—shhhh—contains all tones or frequencies like white light contains all colours. With flat or equal power at all frequencies, white noise stimulates a good cross section of nerve fibers when processed through our hearing system. This always includes the frequency range of a person's tinnitus.

White noise is a neutral background sound people can easily ignore. It helps make people feel more relaxed. Often products advertising white noise actually play pink noise.

Pink Noise

This sound has more power at lower frequencies making it similar to the range of everyday sound. This means pink noise could help improve tolerance for regular daily sounds. With less high frequency power, pink noise—deeper pitched shhhh—is often more comfortable than white noise for people with hyperacusis. Pink noise can slow brain waves and help with better sleep.

Brown Noise

This is sometimes called red noise. It has more low frequency power than pink noise. It's sometimes called Brownian after Robert Brown, the discoverer of Brownian motion. Brown noise—deeper pitched shhhh than pink noise—is helpful for blocking out annoying sounds. It's comfortable for people with tinnitus and hyperacusis.

Desensitization Sound
This sound is sometimes used for misophonia. Therapy uses the disliked sound to make the person with misophonia less bothered or angered by the sound. Decreased sound tolerance experts say desensitization sound doesn't help. People with misophonia agree. Some clinics offer desensitization treatment for tinnitus or hyperacusis. It's usually a fancy name for sound therapy and/or mind therapy.

Low Frequency Sound
Most people with hyper ears like listening to low frequency sound more than high frequency emphasis sounds. It's easier to hear for people with hearing loss who have better hearing in the low frequencies.

Music
Most people enjoy music, and own machines or devices that play music. Music stimulates the hearing system and brain. Try listening to different genres of soft music to see what's helpful for your hyper ears.

Music is relaxation sound if it's pleasant and easily ignored. Instrumental music is useful as relaxing background sound. Any enjoyable music can give a comfortable, pleasant, relaxing sound environment.

It's easy to use music as distraction sound by listening more closely. Music with lyrics is helpful. People can memorize lyrics or sing along to a favourite song to distract their focus from tinnitus.

Jan's Case

Music was the first sound type I used for sound therapy in quiet places. I turned on music whenever I was in a quiet environment.

Fractal Music

This soothing music is created using a math algorithm or calculation. It has notes at a constant loudness repeating in melody patterns that sound similar but aren't exactly the same. It sounds like wind chimes or Zen music used for yoga or meditation.

Science shows fractal music helps with relaxation, lowering stress, and coping better, although some people have reported worse tinnitus after using it. Sometimes people with hyper ears who don't like coloured noise use fractal music for sound therapy.

No Percussion Music

This music style doesn't include instruments hit or scraped like drums, cymbals, triangles, or tambourines. It can be much more comfortable to listen to for people with hyper ears. Some singer-songwriters with hyperacusis only write and play no percussion music, e.g. Chris Singleton from Ireland.

No Percussion Relaxation Music

This no percussion music is specifically for relaxation. It is low or no percussion plus no vocals. It's very similar to fractal music. There are repetitive notes and melodies with small variations, and the music is an even consistent volume so there's nothing sudden or jarring. If you set a comfortable loudness for the music, it should stay comfortable for the whole song.

Nature Sounds

Soothing natural sounds include moving water, e.g. ocean waves, streams, rivers, waterfalls, or fountains. People use bird or animal sounds, e.g. birdsong, crickets. Weather sounds are helpful, e.g. wind, raindrops, thunderstorms.

Nature sounds are available by opening a window, spending time outside in natural areas, or enjoying the outdoors by going to a quiet park or secluded haven. Garden sounds like wind chimes, fountains, or water features can give a pleasant background soundscape.

Jan's Case

I love the sound of Pacific Northwest storming waves crashing against the shore. I love sitting in the garden and listening to birds singing and chirping. I like the sound of bees. In the spring I stick my head into my raspberry patch to listen to the drone of bumble and honey bees. I can't find this sound online or on apps.

I was once at a posh wedding in a fancy house with water features running through every room. The ceremony was in a large open space with a narrow stream. It wasn't long before all my attention was on the tinkling water sound and not the words. All my attention was on my uncomfortable need to pee.

A small child in front of me shifted and squirmed. They tugged on their parent's arm. "I have to go pee," they said in a loud voice.

Everyone chuckled. I wasn't the only one there feeling the pee effect from the sound. Tinkling stream sound type is not in my toolbox.

Pitch Match

This type of sound therapy increases sound energy in the frequency range of a person's tinnitus pitch match. This stimulates the hearing system in linked nerve fiber networks. Some scientists are developing hidden object games using audio signals that include a person's pitch match. The aim of the game is to ignore sounds matching the person's tinnitus.

Notched Sound

This therapy approach uses white noise or music with lower sound energy around the person's tinnitus pitch match. This gives less stimulation to linked nerve fiber networks. Experts say notched sound is best for people with tinnitus and sensorineural hearing loss, not conductive hearing loss.

Processed Sound
Different manufacturers digitally process therapy sounds in different ways. Processed music or nature sounds are mathematically processed or changed for tinnitus or hyperacusis sound therapy.

Specific Sounds
People have their own sound likes and dislikes. For example, some people find the humming bubbling sounds from a fish tank soothing. There was a case where the sound of a train whistle helped a man cope better with his tinnitus. A helpful sound for one person might not be comfortable, pleasant, or easily ignored by someone else. Consider your own hobbies, likes, and dislikes. Find the sounds that help create a comfortable sound environment for you.

Jan's Case

My house has a 150 gallon fish tank full of tropical fish. There's bubble and filter noise. Sometimes I think it's annoying when the filter isn't working properly, but it's a good background sound to raise the noise floor in my family room and combine with other sounds I have turned on.

One of my favourite sounds is sports events on TV: pro golf tournaments and pro tennis matches. There's something I like about the thunk of the ball, the low murmur of the announcers, the fans gently clapping. Sometimes I have the sound on soft in the background for relaxation while I do other things. Sometimes I use the sound as a distraction when I pay attention to what's happening. No expert or anybody else ever said, "Jan, you need to use pro sports for sound therapy. It will help you cope."

I had to figure it out for myself.

Speech Sound
Speech can be used for distraction or relaxation. Distraction options
include movies, comedy shows, podcasts, TED talks, radio, news,
sports announcers, audio books, YouTube. It's very important to avoid
subjects or topics that cause a negative emotional reaction. Interesting,
pleasant, or funny topics are most helpful.

Conversation is a good way of paying attention to other people instead
of hyper ears. Speech relaxation options include using speech as a
background sound, e.g. show, video, or podcast playing so a person can
hear it but isn't paying attention to what's being said.

Tapping
This is an unusual option for misophonia (not phonophobia). Never
look at the soft trigger sound source. When the trigger sound is
happening, make a tapping noise at the same time just loud enough to
help cover the trigger up. Are you holding a pen or pencil you can tap?
A small pebble or crystal you carry with you? Can you click your
tongue inside your mouth? Hum in your throat? Tap the toes of your
shoes or click your heels on the ground?

Are you near a hard surface? I use one hand for this. Rest your wrist on
something solid. Tap the surface with the fingernail of your index
finger. Lightly tap the pads of all your fingers onto the solid surface.
Play air piano or different finger patterns. Practice making tapping
softer or louder depending on how you hold your fingers. When there's
a trigger sound, tap to mask it.

Task-Related Sounds
Many jobs need some listening to different sounds, equipment, or
people, e.g. doctor, sales, teacher. Many hobbies include listening to
specific sounds. For example, if you play a musical instrument or

dance, then you need to listen while practicing or performing. If you take a class or course you need to focus on the instructor, e.g. golf, new language, yoga, meditation, pottery, photography.

A helpful sound for one person might not be comfortable, pleasant, or interesting for someone else. Consider your own hobbies, likes, and dislikes. It helps people relax when they do things they enjoy.

People sometimes stop playing their musical instruments because they have hyper ears. With coping tools and treatment, they play again. I enjoy playing the piano. My tinnitus gets louder after, but that's a cost I'm prepared to live with.

SOUND LOUDNESS

Never use loud sound. Only use soft to moderate volume sound. More moderate loudness can be helpful for distraction sound therapy, and softer sound is helpful for relaxation sound therapy.

The term "masking" was first used to describe covering up the sound of tinnitus with another sound. Partial masking is the lowest volume, increasing to complete masking.

Partial Masking Loudness

- Both outside sound and tinnitus (T) heard clearly.
- Outside sound does not mask or cover up tinnitus.

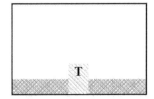

Mixing Loudness

- Outside sound and tinnitus (T) sound mix or blend together.
- Outside sound does not mask, change, or cover up tinnitus.
- Sometimes tinnitus sounds quieter or different in some way.

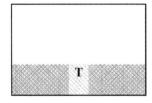

Complete Masking Loudness

- Outside sound completely covers up tinnitus (T).
- Tinnitus not heard.

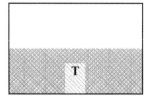

Most people can't turn the volume of outside sound up loud enough to mask their tinnitus without the sound going over their loudness discomfort level.

Partial to mixing loudness is the most common volume recommended for tinnitus and hyperacusis sound therapy.

For people with hyperacusis, some outside sound, no matter how faint, is better than no sound. They should gradually increase volume as comfortable over a period of days, weeks, or months once hyperactivity is less and the person with hyperacusis can tolerate sound better.

Using soft sound therapy for hyperacusis will also help phonophobia since people won't be as afraid of sounds when they're not as painful.

Sound therapy will not lower emotion system hyperactivity causing misophonia. I've used tinnitus and hyperacusis sound therapy for decades, but my misophonia dislike for certain sounds has never changed. Tools that target the emotional reaction, described in the section Mind Therapy Tools, are most helpful for misophonia.

People with misophonia can still use sound to cope better by using distraction sound as needed in difficult situations and using relaxation sound to help with general relaxation.

Mixing, partial, or complete masking loudness are options, depending on the sound and the person with misophonia (M) as long as it's not too loud.

Mixing

Masking

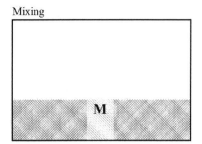

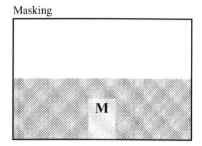

Jan's Case

One trick I've learned for chewing sounds from loud food is to eat the same thing at the same time, if possible. I hear my chewing sounds much louder than other people's trigger sounds.

For example, if somebody near me is eating crunchy tortilla chips, I eat them too. Timing my chewing with the noisy eater. Nobody has ever noticed when I chew in sync with them.

I also chew loud food when misophonia triggers are happening. If I'm munching raw carrot sticks, it makes it harder to hear trigger sounds. Humming or singing can also work for sound enrichment.

There's no soft or moderate loudness that works best for everyone. The actual volume used depends on the individual person, and can change over time as people cope better and get less sensitive to sound. Choose a comfortable non-annoying loudness. If you're in professional therapy, use the volume of sound therapy recommended by your care provider.

People with hyper ears often have strong likes and dislikes for how much sound they want to use. The goal is to find the loudness where you get the greatest sense of relief. The volume should be fine to listen to for long periods of time. If the loudness is annoying, it's better to turn down the volume than turn off the sound. It's worth repeating that some sound is better than no sound.

Because coloured noise is a steady constant sound, it's easier to set the volume. Other sound types like music can fluctuate in loudness, so it's more difficult to pick a volume. If this happens, choose a comfortable, pleasant listening level.

Don't keep adjusting or fiddling with the volume; it makes people focus attention on hyper ears and can make hyperactivity worse. Set a comfortable loudness, then don't think about it.

SOUND DURATION

Sound duration is how much time a person uses sound therapy daily. Regular, consistent listening to sound can lower the hearing system hyperactivity causing tinnitus or hyperacusis.

There's debate over what sound duration is best, ranging from as needed to up to 24 hours a day for certain professional therapy approaches. Info on how to use sleep sound is in the chapter Sleep Tools.

Listening Time Options

- As needed.
- Awake.
- Asleep.
- Awake and asleep.
- As recommended by care provider.

For tinnitus or hyperacusis, some experts recommend at least 6 hours a day of sound therapy at least to start. People break up their sound therapy into shorter chunks, e.g. 2 hours for 3 times a day. People might listen more at the start of treatment and less for ongoing hyper ears management.

I've seen sound therapy products targeted at people with hyper ears instructing the user to listen for 5 minutes a day. It reminds me of the movie There's Something About Mary when the psychotic hitch-hiker argues his 5 minute abs exercise video idea is a better product than 6 minute abs. Why do 6 minutes if 5 minutes works as well? Because when exercising the hearing system, longer is typically better.

Jan's Case

In the 1990s, my first sound therapy tool was simple. I still use it. If it's quiet around me, I turn on soft music. It can be any genre from indie metal to classical. Whatever fits my mood, as needed, while awake. I thought using sleep sound therapy was crazy. I didn't use sleep sound for many years. If I knew what a difference sleep sound would make to my hyper ears, I'd have used it a lot sooner.

After so many years of using sound enrichment, it sounds strange when I'm in a quiet room with no sound of any type playing. I avoid silence now. Science and my professional and personal experience prove sound therapy helps people cope better with distressing tinnitus or hyperacusis.

The length of time people listen to sound daily depends on their individual needs. The more severe the hyper ears, then the longer the sound duration in a 24-hour period, the better.

Make sure you use your sound therapy every day for best results. Don't skip days. Don't expect overnight results. Sound therapy takes time to have a helpful effect, often from three to six months, although some people notice an immediate improvement.

SOUND THERAPY DEVICES

Sound can be ambient from a device playing sound therapy in your environment. Some people use personal listening or personal audio systems for portable sound therapy. There are professional sound therapy approaches that use specific ambient, personal listening, or wearable devices. Others use personal amplifiers or hearing aids which often have built-in music or sound libraries.

SOUND THERAPY TOOLBOX SUMMARY

Sound therapy is a useful coping tool for people who can hear enough to use it. If the person can hear in both ears, then they must listen to sound therapy in both ears, even if the person only has tinnitus in 1 ear. That's because the sound therapy target is central hearing system hyperactivity in the brain.

It can take at least 3 to 6 months of regular consistent daily sound to notice benefit, e.g. managing and coping better. The length of time needed for hyperacusis sound therapy depends on how severe it was to start with, and how the person tolerates using sound therapy.

For tinnitus, it depends on the individual and the cause. The longer you've had tinnitus, the longer it can take. Certain causes might not show improvement until up to 18 months after the injury date, e.g. acoustic trauma, head injury, brain injury. Don't give up on using daily sound therapy too early.

Sound therapy results are similar no matter what approach is used. For most people the main benefit is making tinnitus less noticeable. People stop focussing on their tinnitus, even if the tinnitus characteristics don't change. If the tinnitus disappears when sound is turned on, it's residual inhibition. The tinnitus is still there when the sound is turned off. Most people don't get residual inhibition.

About 5 to 10% of people notice slightly worse tinnitus after they start using sound therapy. This can be a sign the hearing system is responding to treatment. If sound makes your tinnitus seem worse, lower the volume to a softer loudness. Talk to your care provider for guidance.

If tinnitus changes from using sound therapy, the first change noticed is a drop in tinnitus pitch. Less high frequency; less annoying. With ongoing sound therapy, there can be a drop in tinnitus loudness, typically about 50% softer. These benefits will go away if the person stops using sound therapy right after the improvement. Continuing daily sound therapy for 3 months after improvement—or as recommended by your care provider—helps permanently reset the hearing system. Once this happens, the improvement often lasts even if you stop using daily sound therapy.

Identify situations where you need sound enrichment or therapy, e.g. concentrating, relaxing. Pick the device or aid that plays the sound(s) that best suit your needs. Choose devices you'll use and/or wear regularly. Choose devices that fit your budget and lifestyle.

Most people with hyper ears end up with different devices they use at different times for ambient, personal listening, and/or wearable sound therapy tools. Use tool combinations when possible, e.g. personal music library for reading at same time as ambient coloured noise to fill in quiet gaps.

Guidelines

- Use sound therapy consistently for at least 3 months.
- Choose pleasant, comfortable relaxation sounds.
- Choose pleasant, interesting distraction sounds.
- Never use loud sound.
- Use soft to medium volume sound, usually mixing loudness or softer.
- Always use <50% volume for personal listening.
- Some sound, no matter how soft, is better than no sound.
- Set and forget the volume.
- Use sound as recommended or as needed, awake and/or asleep.
- Consider using devices for ambient soundscapes, personal listening, or try hearing aids with or without built-in sound generators.

2

AMBIENT SOUNDSCAPES

The three great elemental sounds in nature are the sound of rain, the sound of wind in a primeval wood, and the sound of outer ocean on a beach.

- Henry Beston -

People with hyper ears often need to create their own soundscape by using sound generating machines or devices. Ambient sound comes from a person's environment. This is where stand-alone devices are useful for any quiet place a person with hyper ears spends time. The goal is to build up sound in the space surrounding you. Avoid silence.

What sound can you turn on so there's less silence? I've described a few options below. Keep in mind that depending on the sound type, ambient sound often changes in volume, and can have occasional quiet periods.

For people with more severe hyper ears distress, ambient sound types might not have constant enough volume. Combine them with a more constant sound. For example, sometimes when I listen to music, I have coloured noise playing to fill in any silent gaps. Tool combo: 2 sound types at the same time.

Air Appliances

Fans, air conditioners, and air purifiers make a white type noise. There might be different power settings, with volume changing for each setting, e.g. louder on high. Appliances don't let you adjust the volume in small steps like audio or media devices. People with hyperacusis must be able to adjust volume. Consider this option if the sound quality and sound loudness made by an appliance is comfortable and not annoying. Try something you own if you can.

Audio or Media Devices

Choices keep getting better with improvements in audio, media, and communication technology. People usually own at least one audio and/or media device including mobile phone, radio, home stereo, record player, car stereo, TV, tablet, computer, gaming system.

Dock a phone or personal audio system with a speaker for ambient sound from your own music or audio library. Devices offer a huge variety of sounds including music, nature sounds, coloured noise, news, shows, movies, videos, podcasts, audiobooks, gaming system soundtracks. This is a good way to start sound therapy without spending extra money.

For example, hyperacusisfocus.org has download options for different length tracks of white noise, brown noise, pink noise, and softer pink noise.

Dr. Ir. S. Pigeon in Brussels is a signal processing engineer who developed myNoise®: a noise generator that takes people's hearing thresholds into account. The website myNoise.net gives you control of every sound in a soundscape mix with pre-set sliders. For example, for the

Japanese Garden soundscape, you can adjust the volume of water, wind, leaves, birds, and wind chimes to personalize the mix. There are many different soundscape options for concentration and relaxation.

Tabletop Sound Machines
Sound Type—Coloured noise, nature sounds.
Duration—Asleep and/or Awake.
Cost <$250.

These are also called Bedside Sound Generators. They're available through hearing or tinnitus or decreased sound tolerance clinics, retail stores, or online. Sound therapy machines help different situations, e.g. reading, concentrating, sleep.

Each sound therapy machine relaxation sound type is an audio clip of a set length that depends on the manufacturer. When the machine reaches the end of the audio clip, it loops back to the start and plays it over again. The longer the audio clip used for the loop, the better. For example, a 1 hour track is better than a 5 minute track.

Our brain recognizes the pattern if the loop repeats too soon. This puts the brain's focus and attention on the sound instead of helping relaxation. Popular models like Sound Oasis and Marsona cost more because they use a longer loop of sound than lower cost products.

When considering a tabletop sound machine, look for these features:

- Variety of sound types including coloured noise, e.g. white, pink, or brown .
- Volume control.
- No automatic shut-off; machine should run constantly until turned off.
- Input jack (optional) to use with a sound pillow that some people use for sleep sound therapy.

It's possible to use a computer to take a shorter track of helpful sound and convert or loop it into a longer playing track. With current tech, it's easy to load custom sound or other sound types on a device you own, e.g. phone or personal music player. Dock it to an audio or speaker system and you have a "tabletop sound machine" with sound types customized for you. Play on repeat for continuous sound therapy.

Manufacturers, like Sound Oasis, have developed sound therapy apps, including Tinnitus Sound Therapy Pro app ($6) and free Tinnitus Therapy Lite app.

Tinnitus Suppressor System
2011 To Date.
Manufacturer—Audio Bionics.
Sound Type—Processed nature sounds.
Duration—Awake, Falling asleep.
Device—Tabletop sound machine and MP3.
Cost <$1000.

Also called Dynamic Tinnitus Mitigation System. The Tinnitus Suppressor System has 12 different processed nature sounds. The manufacturer reports regular use of this system helps suppress tinnitus and promote relaxation. It's very hard to find pricing info; websites suggest it costs less than $1000. The manufacturer did not answer my emails requesting price info.

The Tinnitus Suppressor System includes a 3 month habituation training program; habituation trains people not to focus on their tinnitus. Once habituated, people can tune out tinnitus like we tune out the sound of breathing unless we pay attention to it. Dr. P.J. Jastreboff, the developer of Tinnitus Retraining Therapy, introduced the concept of habituation.

Jan's View

I was skeptical, but I gave these sound types a try back in the 1990s when Petroff Audio Technologies sold it as the Dynamic Tinnitus Mitigation system. None of the sounds suppressed my tinnitus just by listening to them. So I picked the sound most like my tinnitus, and made myself listen to it for 15 minutes, 3 times a day. It shocked me when my tinnitus loudness dropped a little and the pitch shifted to less annoying. My tinnitus stayed that way even after I stopped using the system. This proved to me that sound therapy can help. If using the Tinnitus Suppressor System, follow the manufacturer's instructions.

Water Sound Devices

Many people find water sound types helpful. This can include fish tanks or fountains. Fountains give a soothing relaxing water sound effect. Small tabletop indoor fountains are now available, but protect tabletops from water splashes. Various stores and garden centres sell outdoor water features, e.g. stand-alone fountains.

PERSONAL LISTENING

Without music, life would be a mistake.

- Friedrich Nietzsche -

Personal listening devices or audio systems make sound and music portable. It's one of the most convenient ways to do sound therapy outside of wearable aids.

With personal listening, only the person with hyper ears hears the sound therapy through earbuds or headphones. Advantages include good sound quality, personal music and sounds, and hours of listening time.

Options for personal listening get better and better every year with improvements in audio and communication tech. The internet arrived in the 1990s. Manufacturers sold the first portable digital cell phones, smartphones, and MP3 players, with constant improvements to date. Wireless connections became available for transferring data between devices. Manufactures sold the first cell phone with digital music capability in the 2000s. First generation iPod and iTunes arrived.

The headphones or earbuds people use make a difference to sound quality and volume needed for listening. Some styles are better for listening at a softer volume than others.

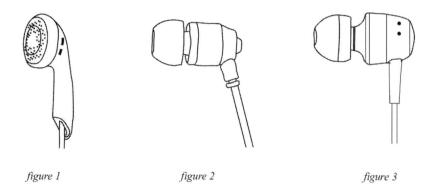

figure 1   figure 2   figure 3

Stock earbuds (figure 1) don't fit as tightly in the ear canal or isolate the listener from outside sounds. People usually listen at a much louder volume if in background noise. Isolating canal earbuds that fit a bit deeper (figure 2) seal off the ear canal better, but can still let in outside sound or noise. The deepest fit earbuds (figure 3) are called noise reduction or noise isolating. They screen out environmental sound or noise best, because they fit deeper and seal off the ear canals best. People like these earbuds, because the volume doesn't have to be as loud for personal listening in background noise situations.

Headphones also come in different styles including sitting on the ears (supra-aural) and sitting around the ears (circum-aural). Headphones that fit snugly around the ears will cut more outside sound so volume doesn't have to be as loud.

Warning:
Using personal audio systems >50% volume increases risk of permanent progressive hearing health damage including sound or music distortion,

impaired speech understanding, tinnitus, hyperacusis, and noise-induced hearing loss.

Experts now recommend listening < 50% volume for safer personal listening using earbuds or headphones. Otherwise, personal listening is a risk for noise damage to hearing health. It's higher risk than some other types of noise, because the sound goes from the headphones or earbuds straight down the ear canals like a high pressure firehose of sound.

In the European Union and Switzerland, manufacturers must include warnings on device packaging: To prevent possible hearing damage, do not listen at high volume levels for long periods. In my opinion, this is a weak warning.

Earbud and Headphone Volumes

Noise cancellation uses a second sound to cancel out unwanted sound. Devices make the exact opposite pitch and loudness of a sound wave and play both together. The sound wave and its opposite cancel each other out. For example, noise cancellation headphones for people travelling by airplane cancel out the steady drone of the airplane's engines. This lowers the volume of background noise. If only we could cancel tinnitus in the same way.

Passive noise cancellation doesn't use electronics. Active noise cancellation uses electronics with battery power. Products get labelled as noise cancellation or that they noise cancel speech when they don't.

Noise cancellation doesn't work for speech, because speech sound waves are too complex. It works for steady constant low frequency noise made up of similar sound waves. It works best for personally worn devices and smaller enclosed spaces.

Scientists have studied personal listening with different headphones and iPod earbuds finding:

- Higher risk for stock earbuds due to loose fit.
- No big differences between canal earbuds or headphones in hearing damage risk.
- The safest are any earbuds/headphones with noise cancelling or noise isolating feature, because users can keep the volume lower but not hear much environmental sound.
- Headphones <50% volume = no listening time limit.
- Canal earbuds: <50% volume = no listening time limit.
- Stock earbuds <50% volume = no listening time limit.
- Noise isolating or cancelling earbuds <50% volume = no listening time limit.

Personal Listening Loudness Limits
There are other ways to limit volume, depending on the device. These are some of the options. Under parental control settings or music settings, you can limit maximum volumes for mobile phones or tablets. If using headphones or earbuds to listen to computer audio, in PC computer control panels, you can go to mixer or volume mixer settings to adjust system volume. It's harder to limit volume on a Mac, but some people set the volume and then lock the keyboard so hitting volume keys can't accidentally change the volume. In Google Chrome, you can make a supervised user account and set up parental controls including max volume.

Loudness Limiting Headphones
These headphones are usually sold for children. Many manufacturers are making false claims about "safe" headphones don't limit loudness.

The website thewirecutter.com shared test results on 50 models of loudness limiting headphones for kids. 20 brands were so bad they weren't even worth testing. For the rest, design flaws let kids bypass loudness limit settings. And 50% of so called "loudness limiting" headphones advertised as safe for kids went well over 85 dB when scientists tested them at full volume. Noise trauma. Permanent hidden painless damage to hearing nerves and inner ears.

Every year, thewirecutter.com regularly reports lists of wired and wireless kids loudness limiting headphones that work. What if this was air bags in cars? What if 50% of car manufacturers didn't install air bags that worked? So scientists had to share a list on the internet of car models with air bags that worked as advertised. Would society put up with that? Why is it ok for personal listening headphones?

Education & Training
When my kids were little, I didn't let them do personal listening. They had to wait until they were 12 to 13 years old. I figured that was old enough for the responsibility. We talked about all the people I've known who cried when talking about dealing with their hearing loss. About their support people who came to appointments with them that cried about dealing with communication breakdowns. Nobody wants to get hearing loss if they can avoid it.

There were no loudness limiting headphones then, so I taught my kids over 50% volume isn't safe with earbuds or headphones. We set the parental controls and device loudness limits together. This is a good teaching moment for young children on noise damage and protecting their hearing health.

When loudness limiting headphones came out, I planned to buy them for my kids. But in a local store, there was one product advertising 85 dB loudness limit for younger kids and a different pair from the same manufacturer with 95 dB loudness limit for "older kids." If the manufacturer doesn't know over 85 dB is not safe for anyone of any age, do they know anything about safe loudness limiting or the tech needed? When all the science on unsafe "loudness limiting" headphones came out, I knew I'd been right to worry.

If ears bled from noise damage, I'm sure manufacturers would be selling headphones and earbuds with a safe engineered loudness limit.

Volume Limiter Apps

Android devices don't have a built-in volume limit, so developers are making apps that say they limit volume. If there is independent science proving an app works as claimed, and noise limits meet public health guidelines, then apps could be useful. Otherwise, there could be the same problem with loudness limiting apps that don't work as loudness limiting headphones that don't work. Be cautious about using these types of apps, especially if you're assuming it will protect your hearing at volume >50%.

Personal Music or Audio Library
Many people already have a phone or personal music player they can use for comfortable pleasant sound therapy. People can use the same sound types as ambient sound therapy for personal listening. Some personal listening sound types like music can fluctuate in volume and have silent breaks. For people with more severe hyper ears distress, this might not be constant enough sound for the best benefit.

Relaxation Sound Apps
There are different apps and MP3s that play different sound types for ambient sound or personal listening. Usually tinnitus-decreased sound tolerance scientists haven't independently tested benefit. But this is an area where digital tech can really help people with hyper ears.

There are a wide range of sound types, depending on the app, including coloured noise, nature sounds, birds, wind, rain, streams, ocean waves, cat purring, campfire sounds, etc. Some have unexpected sound types like vacuums, city noise, or thunder storms that could still be helpful depending on the individual.

Several apps let you record your own sounds. You can do custom sound mixing on some by combining more than 1 sound type together. This is an excellent tool combo. Some apps also let you loop sound types for continuous play or set timers for how long you want the sound to play.

Free apps are available on iOS and Android. Look for apps with positive reviews on multiple websites and high user ratings. Be careful about sound quality, because some apps are better than others.

Warning: Be careful when checking out sound therapy options. Start at minimum volume. Be ready to stop playing sound if you don't like it.

Jan's Case

I made the mistake of having the volume on an app too loud at first. My hyperacusis wasn't too happy after I blasted myself with a clap of thunder from a stormy sound type.

Some highly rated free options include myNoise® app (myNoise.net) with sliders to customize soundscapes, and Free Relaxing Nature Sounds and Spa Music app with 25 nature sounds and a sound board with 35 sounds to mix your own sound. Another app called White Noise has 40 pre-recorded coloured noise, nature, and environmental sounds. You can record your own sounds, mix your own sound combos, and it has loop samples, or you can loop your favourite sound.

Hearing aid manufacturers are also offering free sound therapy apps, including The Beltone Tinnitus Calmer, Oticon Tinnitus Sound app, Resound Tinnitus ReliefTM app, and Starkey Relax app. Some include brown noise and choices of other relaxing coloured noise or nature sounds you can use alone or mix and customize, depending on the app. The Beltone app also has other helpful tinnitus management features including daily plans, goals, and relaxation exercises. These apps will have more features and options with future updates.

Relaxation Music Apps
There are different apps that play relaxation music with no vocals. Again, tinnitus and decreased sound tolerance scientists haven't inde-

pendently tested benefit. Most of this music is no percussion or low percussion. It sounds very different from regular music.

The melodies are soothing and repetitive. Volume stays constant from start to finish. There shouldn't be big fluctuations in loudness, although some apps aren't as good about this as others. Music has different instruments and sound effects depending on who composed the music for the app.

You can find free relax music apps on iOS and Android. Look for apps with positive reviews on multiple websites and high user ratings. Sound quality is better on some apps than others. Be careful when listening to the music to see what you like. Start at minimum volume when checking music to see if it's relaxing for you.

Jan's Case

I like different music options on several apps. On the app Calm, I like 4 of the relax piano music options by composer Michael Denny. I also like some of the relax music on iAwake and Sleep Pillow.

I use these for rest and refuel breaks. When I can—if I'm feeling tired or having trouble concentrating—I get comfortable in a quiet place, close my eyes, and try to zone out listening to the relaxation music on my phone with earbuds, or docked for ambient music soundscape. The music selections run for different times from about 15 minutes to 1 hour, but you can also set a timer based on how much time you have.

Personal listening tech has completely changed over my time with hyper ears. When the Sony Walkman came out, I wasn't interested. Lots of people loved having portable music; I hated the static and analog sound quality.

In the 1990s, I had to get tested for cancer. I sat in the waiting room. Everybody there was fidgeting with nerves.

"Just try the Sony Walkman," said my partner.

"No. I don't like analog."

"It'll help distract you. Make you feel more relaxed."

"I won't like how it sounds."

"Just try it. You don't know unless you try."

I tried it. Ripping the headphones off my ears as soon as the music turned on. No way. I was never using a Sony Walkman to listen to music. Analog was not in my toolbox.

When digital personal music players came out, everybody raved about the sound quality. Eventually I ended up getting an iPod. It was fantastic. Clear, crisp sound. My personal music and audio library to listen to. A digital personal music player was in my coping toolbox.

Phone tech got better. When I got a mobile phone that I could load with my personal music library and sound or relax music apps, my phone replaced my iPod as my portable sound therapy device.

One of my long time difficult coping situations is sitting in the car alone, e.g. waiting for an appointment or to pick somebody up. I don't leave the car running with the stereo on, because it's bad for the environment and drains the car battery. I sit in silence. All I can hear is my tinnitus. No matter how hard I try not to listen to it.

Now when I have to wait in a quiet car, I listen to my music. It takes the focus off my tinnitus, pushing it into the background where it belongs. Often I combine this with reading or playing games on my phone. Mental distraction plus relaxation sound therapy. A double tool combo that helps me tune out my tinnitus.

The great thing about personal listening is being able to customize your own sounds. One of my most helpful relaxation sounds is listening to my cat purring. My anxiety and hyper ears were flaring up in 2017, so I taped the purring on my new cell phone so I could listen to it anywhere, anytime. Nobody has ever recommended I use cat purring as a sound type.

I figured it out myself.

PERSONAL LISTENING THERAPY APPROACHES

Beyond Tinnitus Therapy Program
2008 To Date.
For tinnitus.
Normal hearing or hearing loss.
Developed by—Mindset Technologies.
Sound Type—Processed music.
Duration—Awake.
Loudness—Mixing to slight masking.
Device—Internet-based software; personal MP3 player and headphones.
Cost—$400 6 month standard membership.
$700 6 month premium membership.

ENTs Dr. J. McGuire and Dr. H. Djalilian developed this online therapy program. Consumers complete an online Tinnitus Matching Program (pitch/ loudness). The company uses the tinnitus match to generate custom processing files for the consumer. The files process audio or music from the person's personal music library. They say this processed sound lowers hearing system hyperactivity.

The company website states the processed music is like Neuromonics, but their product costs less and you can use the therapy with any of your own MP3 music. People can also listen to the processed music through hearing aids.

The company sells the product over-the-counter direct to consumers at beyondtinnitus.com. Subscriptions include 6 months of unlimited sound and music therapy, unlimited pitch adjusting, and email support. The premium membership includes phone or remote support.

Often the first sign of lower hearing system hyperactivity is a change in pitch, e.g. changes to a lower frequency. People say their tinnitus sounds less piercing.

Free Tinnitus Notch Therapy
2016 To Date.
For tonal tinnitus.
Normal hearing or hearing loss.
Developed by—Kraken Labs, LLC.
Sound Type—Notched white noise.
Duration—Awake.
Loudness—Mixing loudness or less.
Device—Online, Android, or Chrome app.
Cost—Free or by donation.

The first step is a tinnitus pitch match at tinnitusnotch.com. The website calls this finding your tinnitus frequency. Start with volume on minimum and slowly turn it up. After you pick the frequency that sounds the closest to your tinnitus, the program adjusts the notched white noise sound for you. People listen one hour a day and retune before listening each day. In the future, they could develop an iOS version of the app.

There are testimonials on the website from people who had tinnitus changes, including softer, even when not listening to the notched sound therapy. Some people reported it took a year of daily listening before their tinnitus changed.

Jan's Case

In 2018, I found tinnitusnotch.com and used the website to find my tinnitus pitch match or frequency. My tinnitus is a mix of sounds, so I matched to my tinnitus's highest pitch squeal. Most of the frequencies sounded super annoying when trying to find my match.

I started with the volume on minimum and turned it up to mixing loudness to listen to my notched white noise. My tinnitus almost disappeared like with residual inhibition; I could barely hear my tinnitus over the notched white noise.

My tinnitus volume returned as usual when I turned off the sound. It dropped deeper in pitch from 10,200 Hz to 9,400 Hz. I've been listening while writing on my computer to see if anything else changes. Turns out this sound type helps my concentration. It's not distracting like other sound types I've tried.

Neuromonics Tinnitus Alleviator App
2001 To Date.
For tinnitus and/or hyperacusis.
Normal hearing or hearing loss.
Developed by—Neuromonics The Tinnitus Company.
Sound Type—Processed music with embedded acoustic neural stimulus.
Duration—Awake.
Loudness—As instructed.
Device—iOS or Android mobile devices .
Cost—Subscription program from about $10 per week to about $150 for unlimited use.

Neuromonics is an Australian company. The sound types are 4 tracks of processed relaxation music plus embedded acoustic neural stimulus. People use the music at key distress times, for at least two hours a day to start.

Sound Relief Tinnitus Sound Therapy App
2009 To Date.
For tinnitus.
Normal hearing or hearing loss.
Developed by—Restored Hearing.
Sound Type—Low frequency sound combination.
Duration—Awake.
Device—iPhone, iPad, iPod.
Cost—Subscription options of $30 for 1 month or $80 for 3 months of unlimited use plus customer support.

This Irish manufacturer recommends listening to the sound therapy 5 minutes a day with headphones. This seems a short time to reset hearing system hyperactivity. The low frequency sound could be more comfortable for some people to use, and easier to hear for people with hearing loss.

The app comes with a free Monthly Tracker and Daily Diary. As long as it doesn't add stress, people could use them to record how often they're doing things that help with coping, e.g. goals, deep breathing, exercise routine. The goal of reducing hyperactivity is not to pay attention to tinnitus.

Tinnitus Pro Music Therapy App
2011 To Date.
For tonal tinnitus.
Normal hearing or hearing loss <35 dB
Developed by—Okamoto et al. (2010).
Sound Type—Notched personal music.
Duration—Awake.
Loudness—Mixing loudness or less.

Device—iOS app.
Cost—$10.

Scientists at the Institute for Biomagnetism and Biosignalanalysis and
the Department of Otorhinolaryngology in Muenster, Germany developed Tinnitus Pro Music Therapy. People use the app to find their
tinnitus pitch match using a tinnitus profiler. The website calls this
finding your tinnitus frequency.

The app saves the frequency. When you play your iTunes, the app
notches the music. You can adjust the filtering or notch shape on the
app. People must listen to the notched music therapy with noise
cancelling or in-ear headphones to block out environmental sounds.

At promedicalaudio.com, they recommend listening spread out over
the day. For week 1, people should check their tinnitus profile daily,
and listen 1.5-3 hours/day. For week 2-4, check tinnitus profile once a
week, and listen 3 hours/ day. Week 4 to 6 months, check profile every
2 weeks, and listen 2 hours/ day. The website states after 1 year of
using notched personal music, people reported significantly softer
tinnitus compared to people with tinnitus listening to music with
random frequencies notched out.

Widex Zen Tinnitus Management App
2012 To Date.
For tinnitus and/or hyperacusis.
Normal hearing or hearing loss.
Developed by—Widex.
Sound Type—Fractal music.
Duration—Awake.
Loudness—As comfortable.
Device—iOS or Android mobile devices.
Cost—Free.

People can use this app on its own or as part of the Widex Zen Therapy treatment plan. The app includes 4 fractal music options only found on the app, tinnitus info, and exercises for relaxation and sleep.

PERSONAL LISTENING GUIDELINES

- Personal listening could include personal devices, personal music player, mobile phone, personal music or audio library, MP3s, myNoise® (myNoise.net), gaming systems, or apps such as Beyond Tinnitus, Free Tinnitus Notch Therapy app, Tinnitus Pro Music Therapy app, Widex Zen Tinnitus Management app.
- Always listen ≤50% volume.
- Don't use default earbuds in noisy environments; use isolating canal earbuds or headphone styles.
- Only buy loudness limiting headphones independently proven to protect at public health recommended noise limits.
- Only trust volume limiter apps independently proven to work.
- Set and lock maximum internal volume on device settings, if possible.
- Turn device sound equalization on, if possible. This keeps volume an even loudness when your personal listening library comes from different sources, e.g. downloaded from music store, uploaded CD.
- Only use good sound quality tracks without static, distortion, or unexpected bursts of loud sound.
- Overall loudness is softer if you hum or sing along.
- Enjoy the music or sounds you're using. That's the whole point of personal listening.

4

PROFESSIONAL SOUND THERAPY

Healing is a matter of time, but it is sometimes also a matter of opportunity.

- Hippocrates -

People with higher distress more likely need professional sound therapy. Audiologists fit sound therapy hearing aids or devices and offer in-depth counselling. Counselling can be telehealth, one-on-one, or group sessions depending on the therapy provider.

Experts recommend Shared Treatment Decision Making. With Shared Treatment Decision Making, audiologists and patients decide on treatment together. This helps make sure the treatment plan meets the person's goals and preferences.

Over the decades, different sound therapies have come and gone. There are only so many sound types. When some fade away, years later they're brought back as "new" after consumers have forgotten they've been tried before.

Proprietary sound therapy approaches from companies or clinics are common. Sometimes audiologists are authorized sales distributors.

Independent science proves some sound therapies work. These approaches have stood the test of time with hyper ears consumers. Others haven't been around long enough for there to be independent science on treatment benefit. There is no brain imaging to support many manufacturer claims about lowering brain hyperactivity.

Many professional sound therapy approaches use wearable aids. The advantage is customized sound therapy in your ears that goes wherever you go. Sound enrichment is always available. Making it easy to avoid silence. The volume is controlled in small, precise steps so sound is always a comfortable loudness.

Most professional approaches recommend wearable aids plus counselling therapy, especially for people with more severe hyper ears distress.

For people with hearing loss and hyperacusis, sound therapy to improve hyperacusis needs to happen first before using hearing aid amplification. Professional care providers can give guidance and support on this process.

Some professional sound therapy approaches are described below from the oldest to the newest, including when they became available and details on devices and how sound is used. People can't use some approaches if they have too much hearing loss, or if they have conductive hearing loss.

I don't recommend or endorse any particular approach. This chapter is an information summary comparing treatment details so people can make informed decisions.

Tinnitus Masking Therapy
Available since 1980s.
For tinnitus.
Developed by—Dr. J. Vernon, research psychologist.
Sound Type—White/pink noise.
Duration—Awake.
Loudness—Complete Masking .
Device—Analog in-ear sound generators or combination devices.
Treatment no longer used.

This approach arrived in the US in the 1980s. Dr. Charles Unice was visiting Dr. Jack Vernon in Portland Oregon, when they happened to walk by a water fountain. Dr. Unice had distressing tinnitus and noticed he couldn't hear it when standing by the fountain. He couldn't stay near the fountain all day. He and Dr. Vernon decided the answer was wearable sound therapy. They became co-founders of the American Tinnitus Association.

Audiologists provided Masking Therapy. It used white or pink noise set to complete masking loudness. Loud enough to cover up the tinnitus. People used analog tinnitus instruments or combination devices. There was counselling, but sound was the main treatment.

Masking Therapy helped some people cope better. But most people can't completely mask their tinnitus. Either because of their tinnitus loudness or because the masking noise is uncomfortably loud before any masking effect. Masking loudness also made tinnitus worse for many people.

Clinics stopped using Tinnitus Masking Therapy fast. People still talk of masking as if it's a current tinnitus treatment. But they usually mean sound therapy in general, at partial to mixing loudness. Not the original approach that tried to use complete masking loudness.

Jan's' Case

In 2018, for the first time, I found an app sound that completely masked my tinnitus: crickets. I was so excited. I masked my tinnitus with crickets for 30 minutes. After, my tinnitus blared. It took several days to settle down again. I did a cost-benefit analysis. Was a short period without hearing tinnitus worth much worse tinnitus afterwards? Not for me.

Tomatis Method Sound Therapy
Since 1989 To Date.
For tinnitus and/or hyperacusis.
Normal hearing or hearing loss.
Also for imbalance, vertigo, Meniere's.
Developed by—Dr. A. Tomatis, ear specialist.
Manufactured by—Sound Therapy International.
Sound Type—Processed music.
Duration—Awake.
Loudness—As directed.
Device—Electronic Ear digital music player.
Provider—Tomatis® Practitioner or Consultant.
Outcome Measure—Tinnitus Handicap Inventory.
Cost—Package fee for professional therapy.
Free ebook: How to become your own sound therapist.
New Listener's Program $650-$1700.
Ear Brain Connection Program $600.
Audio Activation Program $600.
Bone Conduction Program $250.
Other Listening Programs also available.

French ear specialist Dr. A. Tomatis developed the Tomatis® Method
of sound therapy for children and adults. He based it on what he called
loops between the voice, ear, and brain. He pioneered theories on brain
plasticity and neuroscience as well as the paired middle ear muscles
that scientists still don't completely understand today.

Tomatis® uses processed or filtered classical music to exercise middle
ear muscles, stimulate the inner ear hearing and balance systems, and
repair hearing system pathways in the brain. The website states Toma-
tis® Sound Therapy Programs help central auditory processing disorders, head or brain injury, speech-in-noise performance, and middle
ear problems, e.g. Eustachian tube or sinus problems and ear
infections.

According to the website, programs help dizziness and Meniere's,
improve hearing, lower tinnitus-hyperacusis hearing system hyperactivity, and improve learning, concentration, attention, and memory. The
Tomatis Method is also said to make people more relaxed and improve
sleep.

Dr. Tomatis believed the key to treatment was processed high
frequency sound like Mozart, low frequency relaxing sound like
Gregorian chants, and interactions between air and bone conducted
sound. He also believed in psychological approaches along with
hearing disorder treatment.

Tomatis won the Gold Medal for scientific research in 1958 when he
presented the first Electronic Ear at the Universal Exhibition in Brussels. His work was considered unorthodox and controversial. After
becoming tired of critics, he left France in the 1970s to travel the
world, introducing the Tomatis® Method to centres in Europe, Canada,
US, South Africa, and Japan.

In the 1980s, Tomatis® treatment in Montreal helped Canadian writer
Patricia Joudry so much she adapted the program to use with cassette

tapes, headphones, and an analog Sony Walkman. It was the first portable personal listening sound therapy.

Patricia's daughter Rafaele established Sound Therapy International in Australia in 1989, writing several books, improving the listening programs, and updating to digital tech for devices.

Books include Triumph Over Tinnitus ($25) and Sound Therapy: Music to Recharge 12th edition ($25). Trained hearing healthcare professionals offer the Tomatis® Method. People can also use guided self-help Listening Programs, selected based on each individual person's needs. Coaching tools that come with the listening device and pre-loaded listening programs include a Tomatis® book, workbook, online videos, telephone support, and 3 months of email support.

Dr. Tomatis' theories would be considered less radical today. This method of sound therapy is one of the few for conductive hearing problems and inner ear balance disorders. The bone conduction approach is interesting and unique. People can listen to the sound therapy by air conduction or bone conduction regardless of hearing loss type. They can use the sound therapy with or without hearing aids. The Method is said to help about 80% of people with hyper ears.

There isn't much science on this method for hearing disorders. A 2015 study looked at one subject. Independent scientists want to see more studies on the Tomatis® Method. Brain imaging results are important to identify any brain activity changes from treatment.

Tinnitus Retraining Therapy (TRT)
1990 To Date.
For tinnitus and decreased sound tolerance.
Normal hearing or hearing loss.
Developed by—Dr. P.J. Jastreboff, neurophysiologist.
Provided by—Audiologist: TRT Training Course.
Sound Type—As preferred/recommended.

Duration—Awake and Asleep.

Loudness—Mixing or less.

Device—As preferred/recommended.

Outcome Measure—Tinnitus Handicap Inventory.

Cost—Hourly rate and/or package fee plus cost of devices .

Trained audiologists, ear specialists, and psychologists offer Tinnitus Retraining Therapy (TRT). Tinnitus Retraining Therapy for people with hyperacusis is sometimes called Hyperacusis Retraining Therapy. TRT is one of the only approaches to include treatment for misophonia (including phonophobia). More info is at tinnitus-pjj.com.

Dr. P.J. Jastreboff developed the neurophysiological model of tinnitus-decreased sound tolerance and the concept of habituation. He was awarded the 1993 Robert W. Hocks award for his tinnitus-decreased sound tolerance work as well as the 2014 Award for Clinical Excellence from the international tinnitus community. Over 25 years of independent international science supports Jastreboff's neurophysiological model and tinnitus retraining therapy effectiveness.

Ear specialist Dr. J. Hazell helped develop the TRT clinic protocol. TRT treatment is much shorter now than when it was first introduced over 25 years ago. The TRT goal is to treat tinnitus-hyperacusis hearing and emotion system hyperactivity and treat misophonia-phonophobia emotion system hyperactivity.

Sound therapy to both ears day and night is an important part of tinnitus-hyperacusis treatment. People use sleep sound to habituate and sleep better. The sound type is more important than the device. Providers often recommend combination hearing aids and tabletop sound machines people can use while awake or asleep. TRT was the first approach to use mixing loudness.

Directive counselling protocols are a key part of TRT. The specialized counselling teaches people how to habituate to tinnitus and how to desensitize for hyperacusis to lower hearing system hyperactivity. This lowers any related emotion system hyperactivity.

Approximately 80% of people with tinnitus-hyperacusis cope better within 3 months of TRT, with some seeing improvement after one month. This typically includes a drop in tinnitus loudness along with habituation. People can tune out tinnitus like they do the sound of a refrigerator in the background.

For misophonia (including phonophobia), directive counselling helps desensitize the emotion system and lower hyperactivity for the disliked or feared sounds. TRT has an 85% success rate with misophonia.

Experts recommend 9 months of treatment to prevent relapses, but it could take longer for people with severe distress. After finishing TRT, people might not use sound 24/7, although regular 24/7 sound therapy can prevent tinnitus-hyperacusis flare-ups. People with less severe distress often find a TRT evaluation and directive counselling appointment—approx. 2 hours long—is enough to help them understand tinnitus-decreased sound tolerance and learn coping strategies with no extra therapy needed.

In a 2015 American Tinnitus Association interview, Jastreboff warns if people are taking medications like benzodiazepines (>1.5 mg per day), habituation doesn't happen because the drugs stop brain activity from getting less hyperactive. These drugs include Xanax® (alprazolam), Ativan® (lorazepam), Klonopin® (clonazepam), and Valium® (diazepam). If you're on these drugs, don't stop taking them without medical guidance, and wean off very slowly to prevent withdrawal symptoms.

Jan's Case

When I was most distressed by my tinnitus, my doctor prescribed

Ativan. I didn't know there was no hope of less brain
hyperactivity or tinnitus improvement while I was taking Ativan.

Neuromonics Tinnitus Treatment (NTT)
2001 To Date.
For tinnitus and/or hyperacusis.
Normal hearing or hearing loss.
Manufactured by—Neuromonics The Tinnitus Company.
Provided by—Audiologist: authorized distributor.
Sound Type—Processed music with embedded acoustic neural
stimulus.
Duration—Awake.
Loudness—As recommended.
Device—NTT device and custom earbuds.
Outcome Measure—Tinnitus Reaction Questionnaire.
Cost—$5000.

An Australian company developed Neuromonics Tinnitus Treatment
(NTT). It's available from audiologists authorized to distribute NTT.
The sound types are tracks of processed relaxation music plus
embedded acoustic neural stimulus.

The audiologist custom sets NTT based on people's hearing ability and
tinnitus characteristics. The customized music can mask tinnitus at a
low comfortable listening level. This isn't always possible to do with
regular music, especially for people with hearing loss and tinnitus.

The device looks like a small MP3 or personal music player. Different
device models are available depending on tinnitus severity. It's used
while awake over 6 months of treatment. People use the music in a
quiet calm location at key distress times, about 2 hours a day to start.

The company reports an 83% NTT success rate on their website. It
states NTT can decrease tinnitus awareness by 40 to 50%.

Neuromonics is being used to treat hyperacusis, although independent science on success rates is limited. A past review in 2013 reported problems with NTT science, including weak study methods and clinical trial researchers with financial links to the Neuromonics company.

NTT uses the Tinnitus Reaction Questionnaire (TRQ) to measure treatment results. TRQ results can't be compared to Tinnitus Handicap Inventory (THI) results used by other professional treatments to see which works best. It's unknown why Neuromonics didn't use the THI —used for 11 years before NTT came on the market—so it could be directly compared to TRT or other approaches using the THI.

An independent study using the THI to compare NTT with combination hearing aids found both helped tinnitus about the same amount, even after 6 months. Combination hearing aids could be more cost-effective, especially for people with hearing loss, but consumers also considered their sound preferences and lifestyle when deciding.

Progressive Tinnitus Management (PTM)
2005 To Date.
For tinnitus and hyperacusis.
Normal hearing or hearing loss.
Developed by—Dr. J. Henry, research scientist.
Provided by—Audiologist: PTM Approach.
Sound Type—As preferred/recommended.
Duration—Awake and/or Asleep.
Loudness—Mixing or less.
Device—As preferred/recommended .
Outcome Measure—Tinnitus Handicap Inventory.
Cost—Hourly rate and/or package fee plus cost of devices
$80 How to Manage Your Tinnitus workbook, CDs, DVDs.

Dr. J. Henry and a team of doctors, ear specialists, audiologists, and psychologists at the US Department of Veterans Affairs developed Progressive Tinnitus Management (PTM) for managing tinnitus and decreased sound tolerance. In the 1990s, Dr. Henry used a progressive style approach for treatment. In 2005, the American Journal of Audiology published PTM clinical guidelines. In 2016, the Veterans Affairs Rehabilitation Research and Development Service awarded Dr. Henry their highest honour with the Paul B. Magnuson Award.

PTM is progressive because treatment is based on distress level. As little or as much treatment as needed, depending on each individual person. People with the lowest distress might only need education and counselling. Different people with more distress might manage better using self-help tools, guided self-help, hearing aids, combination hearing aids, one-on-one, or group counselling. People with the highest distress might manage best with specialized professional therapy or counselling therapy with a psychologist. The goal is to guide people to cope better by managing their hyper ears without spending more effort, time, or money than necessary.

Sound therapy for tinnitus and decreased sound tolerance is flexible, and used while awake and/or asleep. Various sound types are used for ambient sound, personal listening, or wearable aids depending on the person. People listen at mixing loudness or softer. The sound therapy plan adjusts as needed over time.

People like a PTM approach since it doesn't involve the cost, waitlists, time, or travel commitments common with other professional therapy approaches. Hearing clinics are widely available, and local audiologists can provide PTM. Even if an audiologist hasn't used PTM before, audiologists offering tinnitus and decreased sound tolerance management services could work with interested people using the step by step workbook and provider materials.

Plural Publishing sells the materials. People can use the step by step workbook on their own or with professional guidance. Providers use a 3 book PTM bundle: PTM Clinician Handbook, PTM Counselling

Guide, and the client How to Manage Your Tinnitus workbook with CDs and closed captioned DVDs.

The Tinnitus Handicap Inventory is the usual distress or treatment result measure, same as Tinnitus Retraining Therapy. Evidence-based science shows about 80% of people cope better using the PTM approach. PTM uses Shared Treatment Decision Making, so providers take the client's goals and preferences into consideration.

Tinnitus Activities Treatment (TAT)
2006 To Date.
For tinnitus and hyperacusis.
Normal hearing or hearing loss.
Developed by—Dr. R.S. Tyler, audiologist.
Provided by—Audiologist: TAT Approach.
Sound Type—As preferred/recommended.
Duration—Awake and Asleep.
Loudness—Partial Masking.
Device—As preferred/recommended.
Outcome Measure—Tinnitus Handicap Questionnaire.
Cost—Hourly rate and/or package fee plus cost of devices.

TAT and Hyperacusis Activities Treatment (HAT) were developed by Dr. R.S. Tyler at The University of Iowa. He has a background in clinical audiology and psychoacoustics, and has authored several books including The Consumer Handbook on Tinnitus. Dr. Tyler is associated with Signia, a manufacturer of combination HAs with notched sound therapy.

Unlike many approaches, TAT uses open-ended questionnaires, developed by Dr. Tyler, so people can describe and rank difficulties they're having. These include Tinnitus Reaction, Tinnitus Problems, and Iowa Tinnitus Activities Questionnaires. Dr. Tyler does not recommend the Tinnitus Functional Index, because it focuses on quality of life more

than specific tinnitus-hyperacusis problems to work on during
treatment.

TAT and HAT focus on four main distress factors including thoughts
and emotions, hearing and communication, sleep, and concentration.
Providers use one-on-one counselling or group sessions using a
picture-based program along with homework activities and strategies.
The programs usually take 3 to 5 sessions depending on the person's
individual needs.

Sound therapy uses partial masking at the softest volume that gives the
most relief, although some people prefer complete masking loudness.
For hyperacusis treatment, some people use recordings of problem
sounds to help slowly desensitize their hearing system.

Strategies to focus attention away from tinnitus, lower stress, and
improve relaxation are important, along with Shared Treatment Decision Making. The end goal is for people to self-manage their hyper
ears. More info is at medicine.uiowa. edu/oto/research/tinnitus-and-
hyperacusis.

Levo Tinnitus System
2010 To Date.
For tinnitus.
Normal hearing or hearing loss ≤70 dB thresholds.
Manufactured by—Otoharmonics.
Provided by—Audiologist: authorized distributor.
Sound Type—Pitch match.
Duration—Asleep.
Loudness—As recommended.
Device—Apple devices + custom earbuds.
Outcome Measure—Tinnitus Functional Index.
Cost—$5,000.

Levo Tinnitus System cost may be less if you own the required Apple device. The Levo sound is a tinnitus pitch match, so it's not an option for people who only have hyperacusis. For some people, a pitch matched sound is less comfortable to listen to than coloured noise.

Audiologists authorized as distributors load the Levo app on the device and custom set the sound therapy. People listen to sound therapy with an in-ear sound generator during sleep for 3 months so the brain can learn to habituate or tune out the tinnitus sound. Habituation is based on Dr. P.J. Jastreboff's neurophysiological model of tinnitus.

The treatment outcome measure is the Tinnitus Functional Index (TFI). It's unknown why Levo wouldn't use the Tinnitus Handicap Inventory, already widely used to measure Tinnitus Retraining Therapy and Progressive Tinnitus Management treatment outcomes. Because it uses a different outcome measure, Levo can't be compared to TRT, PTM, or Neuromonics to see which works best.

A $5000 tinnitus pitch match CD sold by hearing clinics around 2008 didn't catch on with consumers. That suggests a pitch match sound type isn't necessarily better than other sound types. The Levo cost seems high for digital audio tech.

In 2017, Levo won Gold at the Medical Design Excellence Awards. Combined published science by Levo employees/associates at the time was on a subject pool of 23 people, who also received psychological counselling as part of the clinical trials. There was no independent science using treatment outcome measures that allow direct comparison of Levo benefit to existing tinnitus therapies. In my opinion, this product didn't deserve an award based on the available science.

Widex Zen Therapy
2012 To Date.
For tinnitus and hyperacusis.
Normal hearing or hearing loss pure tone average ≤70 dB.
Manufactured by—Widex.

Provided by—Audiologist.
Sound Type—Fractal music.
Duration—Awake.
Loudness—As recommended.
Device—Combination hearing aids.
Outcome Measures—Tinnitus Handicap Inventory.
Cost—Hourly rate or package fee + cost of hearing aids.

Science shows fractal music helps people relax and lowers fight-or-flight stress responses. ENT Dr. R. Sweetow, with expertise in hearing aids, tinnitus, and cognitive behavioural counselling, helped develop Widex Zen Therapy. It uses habituation based counselling, combination hearing aids with fractal music sound generators, and exercises for relaxation and sleep management.

Fractal music sounds like wind chimes; there are different music choices as well as white noise and filtered white noise. Studies specifically on Widex Zen Therapy for tinnitus have found about 75% of people show significant improvement in tinnitus distress within 2 months of starting treatment. This therapy could help people with hyperacusis.

Cognitive Behavioural Intervention (CBI) is available for more distressed people. This is cognitive behaviour therapy style counselling, described in the chapter Mind Therapy Tools. For an explanation by Dr. Sweetow, see YouTube CBI video by Widex Academy from April 2016. For more details on combination hearing aids, see chapter Personal Amplifiers & Hearing Aids.

Heidelberg Neuro-Music Therapy
2005 To Date.
For sudden onset tinnitus or tonal tinnitus.
Normal hearing or hearing loss.
Developed by—German Centre for Music Therapy Research Heidelberg.

Provided by—Heidelberg Neuro-Music Therapist.
Sound Type—Notched music.
Duration—Awake.
Loudness—As recommended.
Device—As recommended.
Outcome Measures—Tinnitus Questionnaire; Tinnitus Impairment
Questionnaire.
Cost—Package fee.

The German Centre for Music Therapy developed Heidelberg Neuro-Music Therapy to treat sudden onset or chronic tonal tinnitus. This therapy is also used for cochlear implant users to help with early speech. Music therapists or other providers must take advanced training courses in Heidelberg Neuro-Music Therapy. Therapy is customized for each individual. If the person has hearing loss, hearing aids must be used during the music therapy.

Neuro-Music Therapy for Tinnitus is reported to work by changing brain activity that shifts attention away from tinnitus. It divides the brain's attention so tinnitus isn't a focus. A compact treatment version takes nine 50 minute sessions over one week. The person does visual attention tasks, listens to music, and makes music with music therapist guidance. Therapy includes habituation based counselling and stress management.

Scientists report about an 80% success rate. People report softer tinnitus and less Ttinnitus distress. Brain imaging shows changes in brain activity before and after therapy. Improvements lasted when measured 6 months after treatment ended. The control group given a placebo music procedure showed some improvement, but less than the active treatment.

Most of the science was done by the same group of scientists although it is a specialized therapy. They're using the Tinnitus Questionnaire and Tinnitus Improvement Questionnaire as a treatment outcome measure, so their results can't be compared to most other longstanding tinnitus therapies.

Sound Options
2016 To Date
For tonal tinnitus.
Normal hearing or hearing loss.
Manufactured by—Sound Options Tinnitus Treatments.
Provided by—Hearing Healthcare Professional: authorized distributor.
Sound Type—Notched music.
Duration—Awake.
Loudness—As recommended.
Device—Sound therapy files used on personal device(s).
Outcome Measure—Tinnitus Handicap Inventory.
Cost—$400-$500 depending on time/counselling needed.

In 2016, a Canadian team of scientists at McMaster University studied notched classical music therapy to lower hearing system hyperactivity causing tinnitus. There were only 34 participants; the music therapy significantly lowered tinnitus loudness and tinnitus distress over 12 months of treatment. Most people saw changes within the first 3 months of therapy, and benefit lasted by the 12-month follow-up appointment.

Some of these scientists founded Sound Options Tinnitus Treatments and developed the Sound Options product. With this system, the hearing healthcare provider evaluates each person's hearing and tinnitus. Results are sent to the manufacturer. They individually customize the notched music therapy and return the individual sound therapy files to the clinic within about 48 hours. People listen to the files on their own device(s) with earbuds or headphones.

AudioNotch Tinnitus Treatment
2012 To Date.
For tonal tinnitus.

Normal hearing or hearing loss ≤55 dB thresholds.
Manufactured by—AudioNotch.
Provided by—Audiologist: clinic partners with audionotch.com.
Sound Type—if tinnitus frequency ≤8 kHz =Notched personal music or white noise.
If tinnitus frequency ≥8 kHz =Notched white noise.
Duration—Awake.
Loudness—Mixing or softer.
Device—iOS/Android mobile app; MP3 files on personal devices.
Cost—2 month Trial Program subscription = $40.
6 month Starter Program subscription = $80.
12 month Full Program subscription = $100.

Mr. Adrian Green developed AudioNotch. His education and experience is in Electrical and Computer Engineering, focusing on biomedical systems. AudioNotch is online software that creates custom sound therapy to treat tonal tinnitus. If people have more than one tinnitus tone, AudioNotch recommends people use the therapy on one tinnitus tone at a time.

The first step is a tinnitus pitch match. The website calls this finding your tinnitus frequency. People can do this at audionotch.com or at a clinic participating in AudioNotch's Audiologists Partnership Program. At a clinic, audiologists do a tinnitus evaluation including frequency or pitch match. The suggested fee is $75 for a 30 minute appointment, but clinics can charge what they want. The therapy doesn't work if the notch isn't at the right frequency for the person's tinnitus.

Based on the pitch match, AudioNotch creates custom notched sound therapy using pre-set sounds or your own music notched for you. They recommend listening to the sound therapy for 1 hour a day, increasing up to 3 hours a day in more than one session, e.g. morning, noon, night. The more people listen in a day and the longer they use the software daily, the better the results. Headphones are used, or earbuds as long as they block outside sound.

AudioNotch recommends people re-check their tinnitus pitch once a week to make sure the notch frequency is still best for their tinnitus. The subscription cost includes unlimited tinnitus frequency re-adjustment with an app tuner, unlimited notched sound therapy, email support, and Web and mobile app access. When the subscription expires, people can keep the sound therapy on their personal devices. You'd have to pay again if you needed to retune the notch frequency.

Tinnitus & Decreased Sound Tolerance Management Services
1990 To Date.
For tinnitus and decreased sound tolerance.
Normal hearing or hearing loss.
Developed by—International tinnitus and decreased sound tolerance research community.
Provided by—Audiologist.
Sound Type—As preferred/recommended.
Duration—Awake and/or Asleep.
Loudness—Mixing loudness or less.
Device—As preferred/recommended.
Outcome Measures—Tinnitus Handicap Inventory most common.
Cost—Hourly rate for counselling and/or package fee plus devices.

Tinnitus and decreased sound tolerance management services were a challenge for audiologists. Decades ago, nothing much could be done. It was an awful feeling as an audiologist telling people there was no cure and no particular options, especially knowing what it was like from having tinnitus distress myself. Over time, more and more coping tools became available.

Many international experts have spent their careers doing tinnitus and decreased sound tolerance research and clinical work, adding to the evidence-base for best clinical practice. This includes Dr. D. Baguley, British Tinnitus Association president and Professor in Hearing Sciences, who won the 2018 Royal Society of Medicine Section of Otology Norman Gamble Prize. This award was based on Dr. Baguley's original published otology papers, including promoting a multi-disciplinary approach for hearing research between audiology, otology, psychology, and neurology.

Audiologist education and continuing education programs cover tinnitus and decreased sound tolerance management including evaluation, sound therapy, and counselling. Some audiologists specialize, and take extra tinnitus and decreased sound tolerance management training, advanced courses, or certification available in different countries. Other trained professionals can also offer tinnitus and decreased sound tolerance management, e.g. ear specialists, psychologists.

Evidence-based science proves benefit of tinnitus and decreased sound tolerance management. Audiologists can offer different levels of service as needed, from guided self-help to in-depth counselling and sound therapy for people with hyper ears. Some offer Tinnitus Retraining Therapy or other sound therapy approaches, e.g. Neuromonics® or Levo®. The tinnitus or decreased sound tolerance management approach typically uses Shared Treatment Decision Making, so the client's input is important for putting together a treatment plan.

NEW SOUND THERAPY APPROACHES

Most approaches like tinnitus and decreased sound tolerance management, Tinnitus Retraining Therapy, and Progressive Tinnitus Management are updated over time based on evidence-based science. The latest therapy version will be offered at clinics. But what about other sound therapy aids and devices for people with tinnitus or hyperacusis?

In business, when companies go after a specific consumer target market, they're called pursuers. There are many pursuing tinnitus consumers. One day, they might pursue hyperacusis consumers too. Either way, they see millions of possible customers; they've done the math. They see dollar signs.

So there are lots of products for sale online with fantastic names and fantastic claims. If they're not backed by independent evidence-based science, it's a problem. What will manufacturers come up with next? The Super Suppressor, T-errifier, Hyperacusis Helper? Hopefully, the facts and info in this chapter will help you check if something sounds too good to be true (no pun intended).

Consider these questions when deciding if a sound therapy approach or tool might be useful to help you cope better:

- Who developed it? Do they have skills or experience in tinnitus and decreased sound tolerance science?
- What reputation or experience does the manufacturer have in producing reliable, good sound quality audio products?
- What type of sound generating device or aid is it?
- What sound type(s) does it offer?
- When and how is it used?
- Is there independent science proving the product works?
- Is there a trial period? Trial periods may be shorter than length of time needed to see any benefit, e.g. 3 months of sound therapy.
- Are there counselling or fitting fees?
- What is the cost, including any return fees?
- What type of reviews does it have from the hyper ears community?
- Is the cost worth the potential benefit of coping better?

PROFESSIONAL SOUND THERAPY SUMMARY

Distress or treatment outcome measures should show improvement or better coping. If treatments really lower hearing system hyperactivity, there will be brain activity changes on brain imaging tests during clinical trials.

If you're getting professional therapy or treatment, it's best to get hearing aids or combination hearing aids recommended by the same care provider.

Guided Self-Help

- Tomatis® Method Sound Therapy Programs and/or books (Triumph Over Tinnitus, Sound Therapy: Music to Recharge).
- Progressive Tinnitus Management How to Manage Your Tinnitus Workbook (includes CD, closed captioned DVDs).
- Audiologist: Progressive Tinnitus Management, Tinnitus Activities Treatment, Tinnitus and Decreased Sound Tolerance Management.

Professional Treatment

- Hearing Healthcare Professional: hearing aids or combination hearing aids fitting.
- Audiologist: Progressive Tinnitus Management, Tinnitus Activities Treatment, Hyperacusis Activities Treatment, Tinnitus Retraining Therapy, Hyperacusis Retraining Therapy, Tinnitus and Decreased Sound Tolerance Management.
- Audiologist (authorized distributor or partner): Neuromonics®, Levo®, Sound Options, AudioNotch.
- Tomatis® Method Practitioner or Consultant.

Sound therapy works best when any negative emotional reaction is treated. For misophonia, mind therapy is the key to lowering negative emotional reactions to disliked or feared sound. See section on Mind Therapy Tools for more detailed info.

PART II

HEARING AID TOOLS

5

COMBINATION HEARING AIDS

It is far preferable to listen to clear speech in clear noise than distorted speech in distorted noise."

- Mead Killion -

Hearing aids are not just for people with normal hearing. They offer sound therapy at your ears that goes wherever you go. Often with built-in personal listening or personal sound therapy depending on the manufacturer. Speech communication is easier with aided hearing.

Using hearing aids makes it easy to avoid silence. The volume is controlled in small, precise steps so sound is always a comfortable loudness. Wearable aids are most helpful combined with counselling therapy, especially for people with more severe hyper ears distress.

Combination hearing aids are the most recommended wearable sound therapy device for people with tinnitus or hyperacusis. They help people with normal hearing or hearing loss. This wearable sound

therapy combines hearing aids and in-ear sound generators. The
hearing aid part can turn on or off. The sound generator part can turn
on or off.

This makes combination hearing aids helpful for people who want
wearable sound generators but don't need amplification. It also makes
them very flexible for people with decreased sound tolerance who
can't tolerate amplification early on in the treatment process whether
they have normal hearing or hearing loss. Professional care providers
can give guidance and support on this process.

Some people with hyper ears and hearing loss don't need or want built-
in sound generators. They cope well with regular hearing aids for
amplification, sound enrichment, and easier communication.

HISTORY OF WEARABLE SOUND GENERATORS

Analog In-Ear Sound Generators
Also called Tinnitus Instruments, these were used from the 1990s to
2000s. Sound was white or pink noise. These wearable aids were
helpful for people with tinnitus and hyperacusis and normal hearing.
Many people with hyper ears couldn't use these because they couldn't
stand the analog sound quality with high static.

Analog Combination Devices
These were used from the 1990s to 2000s. These were a combination
hearing aid plus white or pink noise sound generator for people with
tinnitus or hyperacusis and hearing loss. Sound generator analog sound
quality was much worse than digital tech. The hearing aid tech had
more limited features than digital hearing aids. Many people couldn't
use these devices because they couldn't stand the analog sound quality.

Manufacturers have sold digital hearing aids since the 1980s, but
people with tinnitus and hyperacusis were stuck with analog amplifica-

tion tech until about 2005. This is partly because tech needed wasn't available for wearable sound therapy. It's also because most hearing aid manufacturers ignored hyper ears as a target consumer market.

It got to where audiologists prescribed digital hearing aids so people with tinnitus and hearing loss could have hearing aids with good sound quality and the latest tech for improving communication. This helped lower stress and improve coping more than using out-of-date analog combination devices.

Digital Hearing Aids
These are often recommended for people with hearing loss and tinnitus. Manufacturers introduced digital hearing aids in the 1980s, with tech and features rapidly improving since then.

Hearing aids help restore hearing and reduce straining to hear which is always helpful for tinnitus and hyperacusis. Hearing aids give sound enrichment by boosting relaxation or distraction sounds around you. Sometimes people only need hearing aids and basic tinnitus counselling to cope better.

Digital Combination Hearing Aids
These are hearing aids plus sound generators. Hearing aid manufacturers introduced this product around 2005. It's wearable digital sound therapy to use while awake.

These aids are called different names including combination instruments and combination devices. I use combination hearing aids in this book, because I think it's easiest to understand and is clearly hearing health related.

Often people listen to the sound generators constantly for early treatment, plus amplification if needed. The sound generator can be phased out, and only turned on as needed for flare-ups, once coping has improved.

PRESCRIPTION HEARING AID MANUFACTURERS

Prescription hearing aids and combination hearing aids are classified as medical devices. There is manufacturing quality control and industry oversight to make sure devices meet required sound quality and performance standards. Manufacturers must meet national and/or international regulations.

People of all ages from newborns to adults can use prescription hearing aids. They're prescribed by hearing healthcare professionals: audiologists licensed to fit hearing aids or licensed hearing aid professionals. Licensing requires 1 to 2 years of theory and practical work as well as written and oral exams.

Professional hearing healthcare starts with hearing testing including tinnitus and decreased sound tolerance evaluation. There must be medical clearance before going ahead with prescribing and fitting aids. Fittings start with professional recommendations for aids that are best for each individual person's hearing loss, speech-in-noise loss, tinnitus and decreased sound tolerance needs, and lifestyle.

Prescription hearing aids are individually programmed, and objective testing is done to verify performance. There's professional counselling and follow-up, including warranty services, maintenance, and repairs.

Reputation is everything with hearing aid manufacturers. There are 6 hearing aid manufacturers—sometimes called The Big Six—that experts include on best-of lists for having the highest reputations internationally for manufacturing good quality hearing aid and combination hearing aid. Over 90% of hearing aid sold around the world are manufactured by these 6 companies: GN Store Nord (Resound brand), Sivantos (Siemens, Signia brands), Sonova (Phonak, Unitron brands), Starkey Technologies (Starkey brand), Widex (Widex brand), and William Demant (Oticon brand).

These companies have good reputations because they've spent decades researching, designing, and manufacturing reliable quality product. Improving hearing aid tech along with advances in audio and communications tech. Prescription hearing aids meet acoustic, engineering, and manufacturing regulatory standards, and hearing aid performance is based on current hearing health and hearing aid science.

Consumers around the world like the state-of-the-art tech from these manufacturers. They become repeat customers, and often loyal customers for life, like with car brands. Hearing aids all amplify, but manufacturers have their own proprietary sound processing. So customers typically stick with a hearing aid brand since they get used to the sound quality of a particular manufacturer's amplification.

PRESCRIPTION COMBINATION HEARING AIDS

The Big Six prescription hearing aid manufacturers make combination hearing aids with amplification and/or sound generators with specific sound types and features. Most have settings controlled by compatible apps, e.g. on a mobile phone or other personal device.

Combination hearing aids typically let the person fine-tune sound types, set custom sound combinations, and have a library of custom sounds for different listening situations. Some include extra features like deep breathing or guided meditation exercises.

Since combination hearing aids are wireless and compatible with Bluetooth enabled devices, people can download relax sound or relax music apps, personal music library, or other favourite relaxation sounds.

Model names change over time when old models are phased out and new are phased in, just like with car model names. These are the combination hearing aid makes, models, and sound types as of 2019. In alphabetical order:

Oticon: Tinnitus SoundSupport

- Manufacturer: William Demant (1904 – date).
- Coloured noise including white, pink, and brown.
- Ocean themed sounds.
- Personal music library.
- Oticon Tinnitus Sound app (free) includes coloured noise and nature sounds.

Phonak: Tinnitus Balance Portfolio

- Manufacturer: Sonova (1947 – date).
- Coloured noise including white.
- Other default sound types.
- Personal music library.
- Phonak Tinnitus Balance app (used with Phonak hearing aids).

Resound: Resound Relief

- Manufacturer: GN Store Nord (1943 – date).
- Sound types include nature sounds and music.
- Resound Tinnitus Relief app (free).

Starkey: Multiflex Tinnitus Technology

- Manufacturer: Starkey Technologies (1976 – date).
- Coloured noise including white.
- Starkey relief sound.
- Starkey Relax app (free).

Siemens/Signia: Tinnitus Solutions

- Manufacturer: Sivantos (1878 – date).
- Notched sound therapy.
- Coloured noise including white and pink.
- Ocean sounds.
- touchControl app (used with Signia hearing aids).

Unitron: Tinnitus Masker

- Manufacturer: Sonova (1947 – date).
- Coloured noise including white and pink.
- Unitron uControl app (used with Unitron hearing aids).

Widex: Zen Tinnitus Management

- Manufacturer: Widex (1956 – date).
- Fractal music.
- Coloured noise including white and pink.
- Widex Zen app (free).

Notice how none of the model names include hyperacusis? Even though analog in-ear sound generators and combination devices were used—for decades—for people with hyperacusis prescribed wearable aids for sound therapy. Maybe one day combination hearing aid manufacturers will name their models to reflect the actual consumer target market. Wearable aids for tinnitus-hyperacusis sound therapy. Not just tinnitus.

Since combination hearing aids are new to the consumer marketplace, options and features will change over time. Some of the sound types or options offered by one manufacturer now might end up being offered by more than one manufacturer in future. For example, at first one car manufacturer had back-up cameras; now they're standard in most cars.

Which manufacturer has the best combination hearing? It depends on what sound type(s) and features you want. Talk to your hearing health-care professional. Check the different manufacturer websites. See what they're offering. There are always updates to products and apps used. What best meets your individual needs and preferred sound types to listen to while awake?

The Shared Treatment Decision Making model of treatment is impor-tant if your care provider prescribed combination hearing aids. Were you involved in the decision making on what best suits your needs? You're the one who has to wear the aids. Your input is valuable. Don't just accept a recommendation without knowing what you're getting. People involved in making decisions do better coping over time than people who get what they're told.

NO PRESCRIPTION COMBINATION HEARING AIDS

No prescription over-the-counter combination hearing aids are also for sale at retail stores, including online. These hearing aids are usually classified as consumer electronic devices, not medical devices. So they are not covered by quality control regulations or manufacturing standards.

I bet there will be a lot more manufacturers targeting people with tinnitus with unregulated electronic devices being advertised as hearing aids whether they are classified as a medical device or not. People with hyperacusis are ignored since manufacturers don't know what it is for now.

When independently tested, most no prescription hearing aids and personal sound amplification products (PSAP) don't pass basic sound quality standards and important features for speech understanding don't work as advertised. For example, one product made people's speech understanding in noise over 10% worse when they used it.

Lloyds Hearing Aids and Hansaton are manufacturers currently selling no prescription combination hearing aids. Some manufacturers still have their no prescription hearing aids classified as a medical product based on international standards, e.g. Hansaton. It's not surprising Hansaton made the only no prescription hearing aids that passed all sound quality standards when independently tested.

Hansaton: Tinnitus Solutions

- Manufacturer: Hansaton (1957 – date).
- White noise.
- Meets International Organization for Standardization ISO 13485 certification for manufacturing medical products that meet product safety and quality assurance standards.
- In 2015, Hansaton entered a partnership with Sonova, manufacturer of Phonak and Unitron prescription hearing aids.

HEARING AID STYLES

Hearing aid style shouldn't depend on cosmetic appearance or visibility. The size or style of hearing aid depends on ear canal size, pattern of hearing loss, and technology features needed. Larger hearing aid have more advanced tech because there's room to fit in more features like sound generators. Hearing healthcare professionals recommend the style best for each person's individual needs.

The smallest hearing aid styles are invisible hearing aids worn inside the ear canals. Larger aids include Completely-In-Canal, In-The-Canal, or In-The-Ear. The in-canal styles fit in the ear canals, and are harder to see than bigger styles. The In-The-Ear hearing aid style sits in the ear canal openings. These smaller styles can be ready-to-wear or custom molded.

Ready-to-wear costs less because there's no need for custom ear impressions used for shaping custom molded hearing aids. Ear canals come in all shapes and sizes, so ready to wear will only fit average sized and shaped ears.

The problem with these styles is the ear canals are blocked off by the hearing aids. This causes the occlusion effect. The occlusion effect muffles sound, a person's own voice can sound strange or loud, and tinnitus is louder when the hearing aids are worn.

There can still be some occlusion even if these hearing aids have venting or air holes running through the hearing aid shells. Other disadvantages of smaller styles include more frequent repairs, less powerful amplification, higher finger dexterity needed to insert hearing aids, and fewer high tech features.

Open Fittings

Open fittings are recommended for people with hyper ears. That means the ear canals should be left as open or un-occluded as possible. People with tinnitus-hyperacusis find open fittings more comfortable, pleasant, and natural sounding. Combination hearing aids have open fittings as much as possible.

Behind-The-Ear (BTE) style hearing aids sit behind the ears and have custom earmolds attached that sit in the ear canal openings. This is the lowest cost style, because the hearing aids don't have to be custom molded.

One BTE style is called Receiver-In-Canal or open fit. These are small BTE hearing aids with thin tubes, wires, or very small earpieces, pre-sized ear domes, or custom earmolds that feed sound from hearing aids into the ear canals.

Open fit BTE hearing aids are most recommended for people with hyper ears since it's the most open style of all the options available. This is the style used by Prince Philip, The Duke of Edinburgh. Combination hearing aids are typically BTE or open fit BTE style.

Open fittings aren't possible for people with a lot of low frequency hearing loss or severe to profound hearing loss . The greater the hearing loss , the more likely there will be feedback or squealing if sound leaks out the ear canal and gets re-amplified by the hearing aids. BTE hearing aids with a snug custom earmold are a better choice in these cases. The care provider can make the fitting as open as possible with earmold airflow vents if feedback isn't a problem.

Colours & Patterns
Hearing aid style isn't just about the size of hearing aid. There are many ways people can personalize their BTE or open BTE hearing aids to make them stand out instead of hiding them. Hearing healthcare advocates recommend this to help fight the stigma of hearing loss . If people can see you wear hearing aids, it helps open up discussion about hearing loss and hyper ears.

Colour is the most obvious style choice. Manufacturers offer different colours, mainly in the beige to brown range for adults. Some come in pure white, black, or grey options. In the past people have often chosen the colour of hearing aids based on their skin or hair colour. Nobody picks eyeglasses based on skin or hair colour.

Eyeglass colours and patterns trend with fashion. It's not a long-term commitment. Eyeglasses, like hearing aids, last about 5 years. When it's time for replacement, people usually pick something new or different than the colour or pattern they picked in the past. It should be the same for hearing aids. When choosing hearing aids, does the care provider show you colour or pattern options to choose from?

Jan's View

When I fit hearing aids in the 1980s, there was a great range of colours and patterns. Bright red, blue, green, yellow, zebra print, and more. There was even an option to get a clear plastic casing so you could see all the parts inside the BTE hearing aids. Very steampunk. I would show the options to people getting hearing aids.

Children would get so excited, jumping up and down in front of their parents.

"Can I get the green one?" they would beg. "Please?"

Other children begged for the clear casing. "Please? Please? I can show it to my friends at school. It's so cool."

I never saw any child allowed to get hearing aids in any colour or pattern except matchy matchy skin or hair.

I only saw adults pick matchy matchy skin or hair.

People sometimes complain that hearing aid manufacturers don't offer a range of colours or pattern options. The problem is that manufacturers supply what consumers demand. There hasn't been enough demand for personal hearing aid style. So manufacturers stopped offering a range of bright or fun options, especially for adults. There are many colourful options for children who like picking bright colours.

Earmolds & Decorations

Style can be fun for earmolds too. Earmolds for children come in more than 1000 colour combinations. There are also options like swirls of colour or sparkles. These should be available to adults too.

Hearing aid decoration shops sell jewellery, charms, coloured earmold tubes or tube decorations, storage pouches, hats, headbands and safety clips, as well as other stylish accessories depending on the shop.

Some people use nail stickers, or other stickers, to customize their BTE casings. Stickers can be small and used alone or as a combination of stickers. Bigger stickers can be cut to shape. If using stickers, make sure you don't stick them over any important hearing aid part like a microphone. Check with your audiologist or hearing healthcare professional first.

Some people choose short hairstyles or special braiding that keep the hair away from ears so that hearing aids are most visible. Will people notice you're wearing them? Will people react? What will they think?

In 2017, Angie Aspinall blogged at hearinglikeme.com that the first time she went to the supermarket with hearing aids "nothing happened." Why should strangers or anybody else care? People don't notice or react if you wear eyeglasses. Obviously they're used for vision loss. How are hearing aids for hearing loss or hyper ears any different?

Maybe hearing aid stigma is partly because people know so little about hyper ears and hearing loss. Barely anybody knows what tinnitus is. And what is that other thing? Hyper what? Until people with hyper ears start raising awareness, the situation will never get better.

Wearing hearing aids or combination hearing aids visibly can open conversations. Give curious people the chance to ask why you're wearing them. Give you the chance to explain. Share information about hyper ears and hearing aids or combination hearing aids. Start getting people to realize that hearing aids are not just for hearing loss any more. And hyper ears can happen to anybody at any age.

6
_____

HEARING AID FEATURES

---

*A hearing aid is an ultra-miniature electro-acoustical device that
is always too large.*

- Samuel Lybarger -

A hearing aid digital processing system is like a car engine. Engines
have certain basic parts. Hearing aid processing systems have certain
basic parts.

Basic sound quality depends on how well the hearing aid works to give
low static, low distortion, directionality, proper gain for person's
hearing loss, and proper output for person's loudness discomfort levels.

In addition to sound quality, hearing aids also have standard or optional
features to improve hearing and make speech communication easier.

SOUND QUALITY

Paired hearing gives nice natural sound quality for music, speech, and daily life. If people can be aided in both ears, paired hearing aids or combination hearing aid are really important for tinnitus-hyperacusis sound therapy.

Sound input from hearing aid amplification and hearing aid sound generators is as natural as possible when the brain gets aided info from both ears. Because wearable sound therapy targets the brain's central processing system, if you can hear in both ears, you'll need a pair of hearing aids or combination hearing aids even if you only have tinnitus-hyperacusis in one ear.

People with misophonia often have normal hearing and don't need hearing aids. If they do need hearing aids, the hearing aids are to cope better with hearing loss. Relaxation or distraction sound therapy from hearing aids or combination hearing aids might help with coping, but it's not going to make misophonia better by lowering negative emotional reactions like hate or fear.

People switched to eyeglasses from monocles in the 1800s, except as a fashion statement. Eyeglasses give visual depth perception and different magnification can be prescribed for each eye as needed. Hearing aids give auditory depth perception and different amplification can be prescribed for each ear as needed. Pair of eyeglasses. Pair of hearing aids.

People who only need one hearing aid or get the most tinnitus relief from one hearing aid are the exception, not the rule. If a person has hearing loss in both ears, but the person only gets one hearing aid, it causes auditory deprivation. The unaided ear loses its ability to process or understand speech. If the person gets a hearing aid for that ear later, speech understanding is never as good as what it would have been if they got two hearing aids in the first place.

I've never met a person with tinnitus-hyperacusis who didn't have high sound quality standards. Hearing aids or combination hearing aids must have good sound quality or they won't help the person with hyper ears cope better. Sound quality specifications are based on nationally and internationally recognized standards, e.g. ANSI S3.22 (American National Standards Institute).

Good sound quality comes down to good manufacturing. The result is well-made product with low static, low distortion, sound amplified as needed for hearing loss, and aided sound isn't too loud.

No manufacturer has a 0% defect rate. Sometimes a product is manufactured that doesn't work as advertised. In North America, these are called lemons. Reputable manufacturers do quality control testing to keep their defect rates as low as possible. If a prescription hearing aid or combination hearing aid is a lemon, the hearing healthcare professional returns it to the manufacturer who exchanges it for a hearing aid that works.

Static
This is crackling or hissing noise just from turning an audio device on. It's internal noise from the electronics. If there's more static or internal noise than there should be when an amplifier is turned on, the sound quality is bad.

Distortion
This should be low for good sound quality. If there's too much distortion, speech and music will be unclear or blurry. Like blurry distorted eyeglass lenses. Too much distortion causes difficult communication and bad sound quality for music.

Directionality

This restores the outer ears effect closer to normal hearing. For ambient sound, there are 3 dB volume differences between the front and back of your head, and between the left ear and right ears.

The brain uses these volume differences to tell where sounds are coming from. That's really important for safety. If something is coming at you but you can't tell where it's coming from, you won't be able to react properly.

Directionality helps people communicate and understand speech-in-noise better. With directionality, speech from the front— from the person(s) you're facing and talking to—will be louder than speech sound waves coming from the back and sides of the head. Directionality is the only thing that helps people understand speech better in background noise. Ask anybody who can only hear in one ear; it's extremely difficult to understand speech in difficult listening situations.

Gain or Target Amplification
This is the amount and pattern of boost or gain that happens when the hearing aid amplifies sound. The gain should fit a person's amount and pattern of hearing loss. Like how eyeglass magnification is fit for a person's vision loss.

Prescription hearing aid manufacturers have different models with amplification ranging from mild to moderate gain up to high gain hearing aids for severe to profound hearing loss. Prescription hearing aids can fit any pattern of hearing loss including flat, gently to steeply sloping, ski slope, reverse slope, cookie bite, and left corner audiograms.

Reserve gain is important. Hearing aids last about 5 years. Hearing loss is usually slowly progressive, changing from age or other causes. It's expensive if you have to replace hearing aids after 2 or 3 years because hearing thresholds got worse, and the hearing aids didn't have enough reserve gain to still fit the loss. They could be working fine, but they won't help speech understanding if they can't be re-programmed to fit at least mild hearing changes. Hearing healthcare professionals select hearing aid with reserve gain as needed by each individual based on factors like their hearing loss, style of hearing aid, and user experience with hearing aids.

After selection, prescription hearing aid gain is programmed so each individual has the best speech understanding possible in quiet and difficult listening situations. Programming gain is more complicated than people think. Unlike eyeglasses that just need to make things larger and more visible, hearing aids have to process soft, moderate, and loud sounds across a wide frequency range. Different volume levels of incoming sound waves, made up of different frequency combinations, should only be amplified as needed to be heard comfortably. The catch is the amplified sound needs to fit the hearing loss as well as fall within a person's dynamic range.

That means soft sounds are amplified enough to hear at frequencies needed. Loud sounds aren't amplified higher than a person's loudness discomfort levels at each frequency. Sometimes gain is programmed softer only at certain frequencies, making sound softer so it's heard comfortably.

This is really important for people with tinnitus-hyperacusis who typically have lower loudness discomfort levels than average. This is a big part of why hyperacusis is treated first to increase the person's dynamic range before amplification is used for any hearing loss.

Frequency compression, also called frequency shifting or frequency lowering, is something different. With this advanced tech, if a person has very severe to profound hearing loss or cochlear dead zones at certain frequencies, Prescription hearing aids can be programmed to shift incoming sound in that frequency range to a lower frequency range where it can be heard.

Many people assume hearing loss is hearing loss. And any hearing aid works for anyone. One family of parents and children who all had sensorineural hearing loss used to take their hearing aids out at night and put them in a bowl by the front door. At the start of the next day, each person would grab a couple of hearing aids out of the bowl to wear. They were counselled over and over again on how they all had different hearing loss—amount, pattern, cochlear dead zones, word recognition in quiet, speech-in-noise loss, loudness discomfort levels, dynamic ranges—with individual hearing aid needs. They needed to wear their own prescribed custom programmed hearing aids. Hearing aids with the wrong amplification gain are bad for communication and bad for hearing health.

Output or Max Loudness
This is the loudest sound that can come through the amplifier. If the max loudness possible at any frequency is higher than a person's loudness discomfort level for that frequency, sound will be too loud and the aid will be too uncomfortable to use.

PROTECTIVE COATING

Protective coating is put on hearing aids to help protect the delicate electronics from dirt, dust, earwax, skin oils, and moisture.

Prescription hearing aids have high quality protective coatings and offer the option of completely waterproof hearing aids with nano-coating. This can be very useful for people at risk of having their hearing aids exposed to a lot of moisture, e.g. very sweaty, outdoor activities in the rain, boating or water sports, etc. IP68 certified is a basic international Ingress Protection standard for plasma coated hearing aids.

SOUND PROCESSING SYSTEM

Basic hearing aid "engine" or processing system features include built-in components that help people hear and communicate more easily. These include compression, frequency channels, feedback reduction, and noise reduction.

Compression
This raises the volume for soft sounds a person can't hear and lowers the volume for loud sounds a person can hear so amplified sound waves fall within a person's dynamic range for useable hearing. This type of compression happens to the sound input to the amplifier. Prescription hearing aids have different compression features depending on the model, including basic input compression to advanced programmable compression.

Frequency Channels
Back in the 1980s, hearing aids had one channel for processing different volumes of sound across the low, mid, and high frequency range. Over time, prescription hearing aid manufacturers began designing hearing aids with more than one channel. The more channels there are, the more accurately the hearing aids can be programmed to fit the individual's hearing loss and loudness discomfort levels.

For example, a three channel hearing aid can amplify differently for low, mid, and high frequency sounds. Some prescription hearing aids have 15 or more frequency channels that are programmed by the hearing healthcare professional.

This is really helpful when people have more difficult patterns of hearing loss to fit or different loudness discomfort levels across the frequency range. Amplified hearing aid output level could be set for hearing comfort in the mid frequency channel, and set to a different level for hearing comfort in the high frequency channel.

Feedback Reduction or Cancellation

This should be part of any hearing aid processing system. It helps stop hearing aid whistling. This happens when amplified sound leaks out the ear canal and gets re-amplified by the hearing aid. With feedback reduction, the feedback noise is automatically cancelled out. Feedback is mainly a problem with higher gain aids where the hearing aid fitting is too open, airflow vents are too big, or earmolds don't fit snugly.

In the past, people used to check if hearing aids were turned on by putting their hand against the microphone and making the hearing aid squeal. Feedback also happened if anything or anyone came too close to the hearing aid, e.g. during a hug, wearing a hat or turban. That doesn't happen with modern prescription hearing aid tech.

Noise Reduction

This should be part of any hearing aid processing system. It's not what it sounds like. Noise reduction doesn't help with clarity, communication, or with understanding speech in noisy situations. When people talk about problems hearing in noise, they usually mean problems hearing a person talking when there is other background speech happening.

But current tech can't reduce the loudness of one voice among other voices. Noise reduction doesn't work for speech. That's why directional microphones are the must-have feature for better aided speech understanding in difficult listening situations.

Noise reduction processing helps lower internal noise from hearing aid electronics. In more advanced amplifiers, it also makes soft environmental sounds softer, e.g. hum of refrigerator screened out. But this low level background sound is useful for people with hyper ears for sound enrichment. It helps people with hyper ears avoid silence. Hearing healthcare providers often turn noise reduction off in certain prescription hearing aid listening programs for people with hyper ears.

In some cases, hearing healthcare professionals can program a different type of noise reduction in prescription hearing aids with multiple frequency channels. If a particular noise is uncomfortable, e.g. cars keys dropping on table, amplification could be reduced in that frequency channel so that particular noise isn't bothersome any more. This type of noise reduction can be helpful for people with hyper ears. It's never used if it will make speech understanding worse.

HEARING & COMMUNICATION FEATURES

Hearing aid features are standard or optional depending on the manufacturer, model, and clinic. Features also depend on the cost of the aid, with less features in basic economy hearing aids, more features in midlevel hearing aids, and high-end models fully loaded with the latest tech.

The most important hearing aid features make hearing and communication easier, especially by improving understanding for speech in noisy or difficult listening situations. Some features are must-have.

Some features depend on individual preference or lifestyle. Prescription hearing aids have the most advanced tech and state of the art features currently available to consumers.

Volume Control-Adjustable

Prescription hearing aids have high tech volume control options including remote controlled depending on the manufacturer. Many hearing aids adjust volume automatically depending on the listening environment so people don't have to fiddle with the volume all the time like in the olden days of analog hearing aids. Remote controls can work wirelessly, e.g. operated from a separate device, compatible watch, or compatible mobile phone app.

Directional Microphones

These are a must-have feature for safety, more natural sound quality, and best hearing and communication possible in daily listening environments. Directional microphones are the only feature to help locate where sounds are coming from, and to understand speech better in noisy or difficult listening situations.

With basic directional microphones, there is a front facing microphone and a rear facing microphone. Sound from the front is boosted compared to softer sound from the rear. This helps restore directionality and improve understanding for speech-in-noise.

The microphones must be spaced properly for best directional benefit. There are some limitations for picking up low frequency sound. Because of the microphone size needed, usually only larger style hearing aids like Behind-The-Ear or open fit BTE have space for directional microphones.

With more advanced directional multiple microphone tech, hearing aids process the wearer's 360 degree sound environment in more detail. Between ear volume differences are maintained for aided hearing, so the brain gets the most natural input possible. High-end prescription hearing aids have wireless paired multiple microphone arrays to sync sound input the most naturally for locating sounds and for the best speech understanding in difficult listening situations.

Omni-directional Microphones
Omni-directional microphones do not help with understanding speech in background noise. On this setting, the amplifier picks up sound evenly around a person instead of boosting sound from the front. Don't get any amplifier that only has omni-directional microphones.

Prescription hearing aids typically have both directional and omni-directional microphones. Usually directional microphones are the default, but the hearing aid wearer can switch between directional and omni-directional depending on their listening environment. This is a handy feature.

Wireless and Bluetooth Compatible
Many hearing aids now connect without wires to each other and other devices. It's a good feature to have. Bluetooth compatibility is an important hearing aid feature given its widespread use in audio and communications.

Bluetooth tech allows safe wireless data transfer between electronic devices. It needs more power to run than hearing aid batteries can supply. Wireless hearing aids use a separate streamer to connect compatible hearing aids with Bluetooth enabled devices. People wear the small streamer around their neck or have it in a pocket.

The streamed signal is amplified based on the hearing aid programming. More than one device can be connected to the hearing aids at the same time, e.g. stream a movie from another device while still being able to take phone calls. Bluetooth streaming lets the hearing aids work as hands-free wireless earbuds, e.g. for music, telephone calls.

Bluetooth streaming can connect to one or both hearing aids. People can have phone calls go to both hearing aids or only one hearing aid, letting the other hearing aid still pick up environmental sounds or voices. It depends on personal preference and what works best for different listening situations.

Apple has patented a Bluetooth connection system that works between compatible hearing aids and Apple products like iPhones or iPads. This system has less battery drain and also works with compatible cochlear implants.

Telecoil (T-Coil or Hearing Loop Switch)
This tech has been available for decades, and should be a must-have low cost feature. Originally hearing aids with telecoils were used with

land line telephones. The telecoil picks up a magnetic signal from the phone directly, so the person with hearing loss only hears the person talking on the phone without picking up or amplifying any background noise nearby during the call. Telecoils now work with compatible mobile phones.

Telecoils also work with looped spaces. Hearing loops are an important type of Assistive Listening Device (ALD). ALDs improve communication and access especially in difficult listening situations. Loop technology is not expensive compared to other types of ALDs. Internationally, various rooms or buildings have hearing loops installed. When using the telecoil to access a loop system, people set the volume on their hearing aid.

Looped spaces have a cable or loop placed around a specific area, giving off a magnetic field that fills the looped area. A wireless sound signal from the loop is sent directly to the connected hearing aid so target voices or messages are heard clearly without any interference from other noise going on inside the looped space. Hearing loops are used for movie theatre soundtracks, public address system announcements for government buildings, train stations or airports, and places with microphone linked to loop for speaker to talk into, e.g. auditoriums; places of worship, courtrooms, and some meeting rooms.

North America is far behind other countries, especially the UK and EU, for installing hearing loops to make accessibility better for people with hearing loss. When locations do have loop systems, they're often not working or have never been taken out of the box. In London, even taxis have loops in the backseat for passengers with hearing aid telecoils to hear the driver speaking into a loop mic.

People around the world are working on getting more hearing loops installed, in various public spaces, wherever possible. Imagine if a bus was looped, and everyone could hear the next stop announcement without background noise interference. Same for subways or airplanes.

Shouldn't everyone have equal access to public address systems and other important announcements?

Multiple Listening Programs

Some hearing aids have controls or remote controls so people can switch between listening programs. These work like changing stations on a stereo. For example, the hearing aid user can change from standard amplification to telecoil, or directional to omni-directional microphones.

With prescription hearing aids, hearing healthcare professionals program different listening programs based on the person's hearing loss, hyper ears, needs, preferences, and lifestyle. For example, a person might have a regular amplification program, background noise program to hear better in difficult listening situations, a program for listening to music, and program for sound generators or sound therapy.

ASSISTIVE LISTENING DEVICES

Assistive Listening Devices (ALDs) can be used with compatible hearing aids to help a person hear and understand speech better in difficult listening situations than with hearing aids alone. The whole point of ALDs is to help make the speech of people talking louder than any background noise. ALDs are sometimes described as "binoculars for the ears." When selecting hearing aids, people should consider compatibility with ALDs, especially if they have speech-in-noise loss.

Assistive listening devices help speech-understanding in noise, communication, and quality of life. This can lower fatigue and stress so people cope better with hearing loss and tinnitus-hyperacusis. If you're getting hearing aids, assistive listening device compatibility is a very important feature. Especially if you have more severe hearing loss or any speech-in-noise loss.

Remote Microphone

Remote directional microphones are a very helpful assistive listening device for communication. The microphone is separate from hearing aids. These products are like the microphones used by Jerry Springer or Jimmy Kimmel when getting comments from audience members.

The remote microphone needs to be within 1 meter or 3 feet of the speaker(s). People can point the microphone or have it on a table or counter top pointing in the speaker(s) direction. The wireless microphone boosts speaker voices over background noise, sending the sound directly to compatible hearing aids or cochlear implants for easier speech understanding. This helps in different listening situations like in the car, at the pharmacy counter, at a meeting table or restaurant. Some remote directional microphones have wireless connectivity to other devices, including Bluetooth enabled devices.

Prescription hearing aid manufacturers sell remote microphones compatible with their hearing aids. The remote microphone often look like a small remote control, about the size of a mobile phone or smaller. Phonak has designed a remote directional microphone that looks like a pen. Marketing materials say Phonak's Roger Pen increases speech understanding in noise by about 62%. The Roger Pen has won international awards for design excellence and outstanding product design.

Apple has developed wireless earbuds called AirPods with a new feature called Live Listen. It uses the iPhone as a remote microphone wirelessly connected to the AirPods and helps people hear conversations better in noisy settings. With Live Listen, iPhones can also be used as a remote microphone with Apple compatible hearing aids. AirPods are not recommended as a replacement for hearing aids, because the sound and features can't be customized or programmed for people's hearing loss.

A wide variety of other personal or group devices and systems are available. Some group systems are installed in public places to work for anyone with compatible hearing aids or a rented receiver. Group systems are more common in Europe than North America. Newer tech includes special captioning or subtitle apps or glasses at plays or theatre events.

Besides speech, assistive listening devices can help with other important sounds, e.g. alarm clock, telephone, television, doorbells, smoke detectors, etc. These usually work with other senses. For example, alarm clocks vibrate to wake a person up. Lights flash when the doorbell is pressed. Bellman & Symfon sell a range of this type of assistive listening devices. Associations or organizations for people with hearing loss usually have assistive listening devices info and resources. Your hearing healthcare professional should also be a good resource.

FM System
Frequency Modulated (FM) systems used alone or with hearing aids can be very helpful in many work, school, and social situations. FM Systems are a technology that uses a separate microphone worn by the target speaker. Voice signals entering the microphone are sent wirelessly to the hearing aid receiver. These systems make the speaker's voice heard as if the hearing aid were as close to the speaker's mouth as the FM microphone. This helps cut out any background room noise. FM Systems make voices sound closer, louder, and clearer.

Different microphone or microphone settings are available. Some let you pick up the sound of a speaker from one direction; some let you pick up the voices of several people, e.g. sitting around a table. For example, the microphone can be pointed toward someone speaking in a car, placed in the centre of a dinner or conference table, clipped on a shirt collar near the mouth of a teacher or worship leader, etc.

Too often there are news stories about educators or other people who refuse to wear FM microphones when asked by students or anyone with hearing loss. It's discrimination; it prevents access for people with hearing disabilities. It's like no wheelchair ramps for people who need to use wheelchairs for access.

There are other news stories about people with more severe hearing loss and Deaf people on teams getting an unfair advantage by using FM systems. In 2017, there was a story about a team of players on a soccer team with severe to profound hearing loss and Deafness who were using FM systems to communicate during play. Because that's what team members do. They talk to each other giving directions or support during the game no matter what sport it is. Other teams and the league wanted to ban their FM systems. It's discrimination preventing access to sports for people with hearing disabilities.

Jan's View

Back in the 1980s, I was on a curling team. There was a team of Deaf people in the league. I wasn't surprised when they started using FM systems at the rink.

Curling is the worst possible listening environment. Hard ice, ceilings, walls. Multiple people talking, yelling, and sweeping brooms all at the same time, all around the curling rink. With curling you need to hear the skip or team leader for directions. Where should you aim the rock? How hard should you push it? Sweep? Don't sweep? All key spoken information when trying to win at curling. It's hard for normal hearing people to catch what their skip is saying, let alone people with hearing loss.

One day, some skips were complaining about the Deaf team and their FM system. They wanted to get the FM system banned. I thought they were joking. They weren't, so I explained the discrimination situation. Without the FM system, there's no way they can understand what their skip is saying. With the FM system, it's easier. But they're still going to have communication problems, because they have severe to profound hearing loss and

Deafness. The FM system gave them access to curling. It still wouldn't let the Deaf team hear and communicate better than any other team. There was no more talk of banning FM systems.

BATTERIES & MAINTENANCE

Rechargeable batteries are a very important feature. Millions of disposable hearing aid batteries end up in landfills every year, contaminating the environment. The hearing healthcare industry is working hard to stop this. Experts recommend lithium rechargeable batteries for quality and environmental reasons.

Rechargeable Hearing Aids
Some hearing aid manufacturers sell overnight charging stations to use with their hearing aids. There is also a ZPower rechargeable battery system on sale that's compatible with some hearing aid models.

With these systems, the pair of hearing aids get docked overnight in the charging station. No taking batteries in and out. This makes charging batteries easy to do, especially for people with finger dexterity problems who find it hard to change small batteries. The charge lasts up to 24 hours, and the batteries last about 300 days before they need replacing. Replacement batteries are expensive.

Scientists are working on 6 year batteries. Currently Phonak is the only hearing aid manufacturer with a 6 year rechargeable battery option.

Using battery recharging stations is not the same as using other battery types like zinc-air. Experts recommend people always charge hearing aid on the charging station when sleeping or not using hearing aid. When hearing aids are in the charger, it must be plugged in with power on or batteries will drain.

Drying System

Some charging stations include an active drying system to get moisture out of hearing aids. Moisture is bad for electronic devices. You don't want moisture getting into your computer, tablet, or phone. You don't want moisture in your hearing aids.

Disinfection

Some charging stations use UV or ultraviolet light to disinfect hearing aids by killing any micro-organisms. There are also separate dry aid kits or combination dry aid sanitizer boxes big enough to hold a pair of hearing aids. Only use a recharging station, active drying system, or UV light system approved for your make/model of hearing aids.

Talk to your hearing healthcare professional about options for charging, active drying, and disinfection. For the future, manufacturers are developing solar powered hearing aids and charging stations.

7

HEARING AID FITTING

---

*Damn it Jim...why do they call the speaker a receiver? It
confuses me.*

- Captain James T. Kirk -

Prescription hearing aids and combination hearing aids should be
custom fit by the hearing healthcare professional who prescribed them.
This includes checking hearing aid sound quality, programming, objective verification of hearing aid performance, and more fine-tuning and
follow-up at appointments over the fitting and trial period. Overall,
professional hearing aid fitting takes about 2 to 3 hours over multiple
appointments.

In a 2017 healthyhearing.com survey, 94% of people said it was very
or absolutely important to have a professional hearing evaluation and
have a professional select, fit, and program prescription aids for their
individual needs. A MarkeTrak IX (MT9) survey showed prescription

hearing aid owners rated satisfaction with their hearing healthcare professionals at 93%.

Hearing Instrument Test Box

The Hearing Instrument Test or HIT Box is an electroacoustic analyzer. It measures if sound quality and amplification meets manufacturer specifications and required standards for static, distortion, gain, and output. The HIT Box simulates how the hearing aid performs in the ear canal of an average adult.

At the hearing healthcare clinic, hearing aids are hooked up inside the HIT Box. The HIT Box tests different sound types at a range of intensities across the amplification frequency range. If a hearing aid doesn't pass this electroacoustic testing, it gets returned to the manufacturer and exchanged.

This is an extra level of quality control when people get hearing aids from hearing healthcare professionals. In the rare case a hearing aid with manufacturing defects slips past the prescription hearing aid manufacturer quality control process, it will get picked up at the hearing healthcare clinic. Any defective hearing aids are not sold to the consumer.

Programming

After the person chooses from recommended hearing aids, audiologists or hearing aid professionals program hearing aid settings, features, and listening programs so each individual has the best speech understanding possible in quiet and difficult listening situations. Digital tech has made this a much more complex process than adjusting hearing aid performance with a screwdriver like in the early days of hearing aids.

Hearing healthcare providers use science-based prescriptive fitting formulas to custom program gain. They choose the fitting formula that is best for each individual client, depending on factors like age and experience with hearing aids. Prescriptive formulas include the latest version of NAL (National Acoustic Laboratories) or DSL (Desired Sensation Level) mainly used for children's hearing aid fittings. Prescription hearing aid manufacturers also have their own proprietary fitting formulas.

Sometimes people online argue over which fitting formula they want used for their hearing aid fitting. This is wrong for two reasons. Would you tell your vision healthcare professional how to prescribe the magnification for your eyeglasses? No. So why would anyone want to tell their hearing healthcare professional how to prescribe hearing aid amplification? Hearing aid professionals have advanced education, specialized training, licensing, and the experience required to prescribe and properly fit hearing aids.

Also, fitting formulas only give a first fit for programming based on a person's hearing test results on paper. Programming for gain, output, listening programs, and other features is adjusted or fine-tuned based on objective real ear measures and the person's real life experiences during the trial period.

Self-Learning
Prescription hearing aids adjust programming themselves over a period of days or weeks after the fitting. One reason is because new hearing aid wearers often find sound too loud when they first start using hearing aids. If they're left to choose a comfortable volume, they under-fit their hearing loss. They don't turn the volume up enough to get the gain needed for best speech understanding.

Prescription hearing aid programming starts with comfortable volume. Then over time the hearing aids gradually increase the gain until it reaches best fit for the person's hearing loss. Because it happens very slowly and amplified sound is still comfortable, people usually don't even notice it's happening.

Another type of self-learning is when prescription hearing aids learn your preferences for volume in different listening programs. For example, if you always listen to the music program at half volume, the hearing aids will learn to start at half volume for that program. If you're at a noisy restaurant, the hearing aids will learn to automatically switch to the program and volume that you like to use.

Data Logging

Hearing aid fittings happen over more than one appointment, so the hearing healthcare professional can do more programming adjustments or fine-tuning based on the person's real world experiences with their hearing aids. Data logging helps with this. This feature tracks data like how much the person has to change volume over time, how many hours a day the person is using their hearing aids, and when different listening programs are used. This info is very helpful for follow-up counselling.

Real Ear Measures (REM)

This testing shows how the hearing aid performs in the ear canal of the specific hearing aid wearer. It is best practice to use for all hearing aid fittings. Ear canals come in different shapes and sizes. A person's ear canal changes outside sound energy, including boosting sound at certain frequencies. Hearing aids can over-amplify or over-fit the hearing loss with too much gain if there's too much natural boost added to amplification. The hearing aid can under-fit the hearing loss with too little gain if the ear canal changes sound energy enough to cancel out hearing aid amplification at certain frequencies.

For REM, the provider places a thin flexible probe-tube in the ear canal along with the hearing aid. Testing uses soft, moderate, and loud sounds to see how the hearing aid performs in the person's real ear. REM objectively confirms the person is getting the best gain possible for their hearing loss and confirms output is not louder than each individual's loudness discomfort levels across frequencies.

REM does speech mapping to check how much speech is audible with amplification. This is useful to know for realistic expectations. Sometimes all speech falls into the person's dynamic hearing range with amplification. Sometimes when the person has more severe hearing loss, parts of speech are still missing even with properly programmed amplification. People will hear better aided than unaided; but hearing aids can't make hearing normal.

Speech-in-Noise Testing
Best practice for hearing aid fitting includes unaided and aided speech-in-noise testing. There should be significant improvement when aided with amplification. Results show how much speech-in-noise loss a person has while using their hearing aids compared to no hearing aids. Again, this is helpful for realistic expectations so people know how much impact difficult listening situations will have on aided speech understanding. It also helps show if a person is a good candidate for Assistive Listening Devices.

REALISTIC EXPECTATIONS

Most people have no idea sensorineural hearing loss can cause added processing distortion from speech-in-noise loss. The impact is greater for people who also have tinnitus or hyperacusis. It makes a big difference to how well a person will do with hearing aids.

The most important part of a stereo system is the source sound. A clear crisp sound from a digital music file should still sound clear and crisp after being played through a good quality stereo system. Clear crisp music should still sound clear and crisp after getting processed through a hearing system that's working properly. With speech-in-noise loss, clear crisp music will get distorted during hearing system processing. It will be heard distorted even though the source sound was clear. Same for speech.

There's not a lot hearing aids can do about that. The sound quality entering the ear canals can be fine, and the hearing aid can be working fine. But once the sound leaves the hearing aid it has to travel through the inner ears and up the hearing nerves. Getting processed through the hearing system to be heard and understood if possible. Hearing aids can't remove processing distortion added after amplified sound is sent down the ear canals.

People getting hearing aids fall into 3 main categories:

1. Good to normal word recognition in quiet—No speech-in-noise loss.People will communicate better with hearing aids in quiet or difficult listening situations.
2. Good to normal word recognition in quiet—Speech-in-noise loss. People will communicate better with hearing aids in quiet, but will have more problems understanding speech in difficult listening situations than someone with the aided hearing loss but no processing distortion.
3. Fair to very poor word recognition in quiet—Speech-in-noise loss. With hearing aids, people will have much more problems understanding speech in quiet and difficult listening situations than someone with the same aided hearing loss but no processing distortion.

People often get hearing aids that "don't work", because they still can't understand what people are saying, especially in background noise. But if the person has speech-in-noise loss, the problem isn't the hearing aids. It's the person's built-in hearing system processing distortion.

Providers can counsel people with speech-in-noise loss on realistic expectations for how well they'll do with hearing aids in different listening situations. It's important to choose hearing aid features that help the most in background noise. People can consider options like hearing aid compatible assistive listening devices and communication strategies.

TRIAL PERIOD

Hearing healthcare clinics usually offer a 2 to 3 month trial period
although it can be longer in complicated cases if the manufacturer
agrees. The trial period gives people time to get used to hearing with
hearing aids.

Most people struggle with hearing loss for many years before getting
help. The brain adjusts to incomplete info coming through the hearing
system. Hearing aids suddenly bring back all those missing and incomplete sounds. Everything sounds strange and different. This might
include the sound of your own voice, burps, water running, telephone
ringtone, sound of clothes rustling as you walk, sound of appliances or
devices, etc. Your brain will not instantly adapt to the new sounds. It
takes time and practice for your brain to adjust to hearing and start
better processing the sounds coming through the hearing aids.

Acclimatization is better speech understanding that happens after
hearing aid fitting. It takes about 2 to 3 months of wearing hearing aids
daily for acclimatization to happen. Once it happens, people notice
they understand speech better than when their hearing aids were
first fit.

Sometimes before acclimatization happens, people stop wearing their
new hearing aids or don't wear them regularly because they still can't
understand words and they think things sound strange. Other people think
it is ok to wear their hearing aids "just when they need them." Wearing
hearing aids or combination hearing aids consistently while awake is the
only way for your brain to get used to processing a full range of sound
again. It's the only way to get the most benefit from sound therapy.

Think about where to first try using hearing aids. Quiet situations are
going to be easier to practice in than difficult listening situations. Try

hearing aids at home first, walking around and seeing what things sound like through the hearing aids, e.g. fridge hum, outdoor sounds. Get used to communicating with one person in quiet. After some practice, try talking with a radio or TV on in the background.

Gradually increase the number of people you talk with. Try having conversations in small groups, e.g. 3 or 4 people, instead of one-on-one. Gradually increase the number of situations where you use your hearing aids. After you've adjusted fairly well in your own home to background sounds and to conversation with several people at once, if possible, you'll be ready to try your hearing aids in different spaces like work, stores, coffee shops, places of worship, and other public places.

The trial period lets the hearing aids fitting be fine-tuned even more. The wearer can try the hearing aids in their daily life and report back on any difficulties or concerns they're having. Shared Treatment Decision Making is important. Best results happen when the consumer and hearing healthcare professional work together over time to get the best fit and best communication possible. When you've practiced and adjusted to hearing aids:

- Hearing aids should feel comfortable.
- The sound of your voice should be acceptable.
- You should hear average speech at a comfortable level.
- Loud speech should be loud but not uncomfortable.
- In quiet, you should hear better with hearing aids than without.
- In noisy situations, you should hear better with hearing aids than without .
- Communication in difficult listening situations will be harder than in quiet.
- Hearing aids won't make hearing as good as you remember it to be.

- Hearing aids won't make hearing normal. Hearing aids will help you hear better, but not perfectly.
- Sound generators should sound comfortable and help with coping better.

In most cases, people notice benefit during their trial period. If not, hearing aids or combination hearing aids should be returned or exchanged. Returns are not accepted after the trial period ends. It's a good idea to get written details on the trial period including the specified time the aids may be returned for a refund or credit, and whether any non-refundable charges apply.

8

HEARING AID COST

---

*When someone in the family has a hearing loss, the entire family
has a hearing problem.*

- Mark Ross -

Cost depends on how good the hearing aid engine or processing system
is and what low to high tech features are included. The most powerful
high tech engines and latest features are going to be in the most expensive cars. The most advanced state of the art processing systems and
latest features are going to be in the most expensive prescription
hearing aids.

Cost is based on two hearing aids if your hearing can be aided in both
ears. People need good sound quality amplification with basic amplifier features that help make communication easier in quiet and difficult
listening situations. Basic expected processing features include noise
reduction and feedback cancellation. For people with hearing loss

and/or tinnitus-hyperacusis, hearing healthcare and communication
benefit is best with:

- Pair of hearing aids.
- Open fit Behind-The-Ear styles or as open fitting as possible.
- Volume control, adjustable.
- Directional microphones.
- Telecoil.
- Multiple listening programs.
- Wireless and connectivity with Bluetooth enabled devices .
- Lithium rechargeable batteries and overnight charging station.
- Connectivity with assistive listening devices like remote
  microphone (if needed).
- Sound generators (if combination hearing aids needed).

BUNDLED PRICING

Bundled pricing is when hearing healthcare clinics combine costs and
fees under one price. It makes billing simpler, especially for third party
providers. For example, healthcare, worker's compensation systems,
and Department of Veterans Affairs have billing codes that cover
different bundled products and services.

Different costs and fees are bundled for billing. For example, a hearing
exam includes set tests and counselling at the end. But the biggest issue
is prescription hearing aids cost and fitting fees bundled together. Some
people talk about unbundling hearing aid services, separating the
hearing aids cost from the fitting fee. But there will be people who
want to skip the fitting and fitting fees.

Prescription hearing aids and combination hearing aids are medical
devices. Overall, professional HA fitting takes about 2 to 3 hours over
multiple appointments. No professional will sell a person a pair of
prescription hearing aids that haven't been individually programmed

based on their hearing-tinnitus-decreased sound tolerance evaluation. It takes time to use best practice fitting standards including verification using Real Ear Measures and speech-in-noise testing.

Counselling is a key part of prescription hearing aid fitting, especially for combination hearing aids. Realistic expectations are important, especially when people have poor word understanding or speech-in-noise loss. It takes time for follow-up appointments.

The fitting fee covers the time the hearing healthcare professional spends to make sure people's hearing aids are giving them the best communication possible. Prescription hearing aids plus fitting fee will always be sold together as a package.

Even with bundled pricing, people can comparison shop. Watch for local sales. Clinics are starting to offer BOGO (buy one get one free) sales for pairs of hearing aids. Clinics might offer sales like car dealerships, e.g. seasonal, showroom samples, last year's models, or lightly used loaner hearing aids. If there's a package deal for any products or services, it should be clear what's included.

A new popular bundled option is rental hearing aids. Some hearing healthcare clinics in Canada use a program by Hearing Aid Rental Canada. The consumer gets a 3 year rental including evaluation, hearing aids, all accessories needed (e.g. remote control), fitting, telehealth follow-up, maintenance services, full warranty, and free loss and major damage replacement. At the end of 3 years, the hearing aids are refurbished and donated to hearing loss related charities. If interested, check with your local clinic to see if this is an option.

BUILD A PRICE

Bundled pricing makes it hard for consumers to see what's included. With changing tech and no prescription products easily available, many

consumers want unbundled pricing. Hearing healthcare clinics are
going to have to look at new ways to handle pricing and billing.

This is similar to car dealerships. In the past, people were quoted a
cost, and that was the price of the car. Now, many car manufacturers
use a build-a-price model. Consumers pick the features they want, and
don't pay for features they don't want.

Hearing healthcare clinics could use a build-a-price model for selling
hearing aids, or at least 3 different pricing options. Prescription hearing
aid manufacturers typically offer economy, mid-level, and high-end
models at 3 different price points. Combined with fitting fees, clinics
could show consumers what hearing aid features are included at each
price level. Consumers could choose the amplification that meets their
needs without paying extra for features they don't want.

A survey of hearing aid professionals found about 19% of people get
basic economy, 44% get mid-level, and 37% get high-end model
hearing aids.

PRESCRIPTION HEARING AID COST

Despite what you might read in the media, basic economy prescription
hearing aids start around $1,000/pair. Directional microphones and
telecoils are not expensive tech, and are usually standard features or an
available option. Other important basic to high tech communication
features are available on prescription hearing aids and combination
hearing aids. Some prescription hearing aid manufacturers sell lower
cost no prescription hearing aids internationally. These are usually sold
under different brand names than their prescription hearing aids.

NO PRESCRIPTION HEARING AID COST

No prescription amplifiers or hearing aids classified as consumer electronic devices can be bought over-the-counter at retail stores, online, or by mail-order. These are supposed to be the hearing healthcare version of reading glasses. They're for adults who think they have mild to moderate high frequency hearing loss. No need for a hearing test, professional hearing healthcare evaluation, prescription, programming, or fitting of aids.

No prescription amplifiers include hearing aid apps, personal amplifiers or Personal Sound Amplification Products (PSAP), Behind-The-Ear open fit PSAP, and no prescription hearing aids. These products have been sold internationally for years.

These products are a one size fits all mild high frequency amplifier. They have a volume control and sometimes have on/off switches for features, bass/ treble "programming" adjustments, or settings for different listening environments.

Independent testing has found the majority of no prescription hearing aids don't work as advertised. Testing in 2016 found sound quality problems with almost all of the popular over-the-counter brands tested including Etymotic Bean, amplifier apps, Williams Sound Pocketalker Ultra, Woodland Whisper, Cyberscience Amplifier, and MD Hearing Aid Pro.

Directionality didn't work at all in 83%. For products costing less than $150, 100% didn't amplify as advertised. For products costing up to $1,000, 66% didn't amplify as advertised. Amplifier problems included high static, high distortion, unwanted low frequency gain, no high frequency gain, and output or max loudness was much too loud.

In 2000, 2008, and 2015, other independent scientists objectively tested no prescription hearing aids. They found serious sound quality problems, including faulty volume controls, high static, high distortion, too high output/max loudness, and unwanted low frequency gain with little to no gain in the high frequencies where needed. Chan and McPherson (2015) concluded, "*The low-cost over-the-counter devices were generally not suitable for the main consumers of these products, and there has been little improvement in the appropriateness of these devices over the past decade.*"

On July 12, 2017, the American government passed *The Over-The-Counter Hearing Aid Act of 2017*. It deregulated the hearing aid manufacturing industry so hearing aids don't need to be classified as medical devices. As part of deregulation, this Hearing Aid Act states that within 3 years of July 12, 2017, hearing aids will be defined as anything a manufacturer claims, markets, advertises, or sells as a hearing aid. Buyer beware!

If considering a no prescription hearing aid, cost-benefit analysis must include the possibility that low cost often means poorly manufactured or missing therapy features—including output too high for loudness discomfort levels--needed to cope best with hyper ears.

I don't endorse or recommend any particular hearing aid company so am sharing estimated costs for a few popular manufacturers for information only.

No prescription open fit Behind-The-Ear style hearing aids and combination hearing aids manufactured by Hansaton cost about $1000 a pair. This includes recommended basic features including telecoil, directional microphones, wireless and connectivity to Bluetooth enabled devices, multiple listening programs, app to control volume and features, compatible with assistive listening devices including Hansaton remote microphone., lithium rechargeable batteries and charging station, and sound generators on combination hearing aids.

A pair of no prescription open fit Behind-The-Ear styles sold by Lloyd's Hearing Aids for hearing aids or combination hearing aids cost about $1600 a pair, but batteries are not rechargeable. It costs extra for wireless or Bluetooth connectivity (about $2,000 a pair), and it's about $3500 a pair for an added sound generator (nature sounds). This is more than some prescription hearing aids fit by a professional.

Hearables

Hearables are usually wireless in-the-ear Bluetooth style earphones for listening to music, with extra features like fitness activity trackers. They have an equalizer, so the listener can change the pitch or frequency emphasis of incoming audio signals and environmental sounds.

Tech insiders want to add amplification to hearables for an all-in-one no prescription hearing aid for people with mild hearing loss. It's unlikely they've considered how complex hearing loss is including loudness discomfort levels. Without quality control or independent testing, there's no reason to think hearables will meet sound quality or amplification standards any better than most other no prescription products.

Hearables are a problem for people with hyper ears because they block off the ear canal. No open fitting for natural sound quality. Since hearables are usually worn in only one ear, there are no paired hearing benefits.

The equalizer is a concern. Changing how a person normally hears in one or both ears for extended periods of time could have unknown effects on hearing health. With good quality hearing aids, amplification doesn't change the sound frequencies so it's different from normal. Between the single-sided closed fitting, equalizer, loud output risk, and unknown amplifier quality, hearables are not recommended for people with tinnitus-hyperacusis.

OTC PSAP or HA	Rx HA
» consumer electronic device	» medical device
» 40% consumer satisfaction	» 90% consumer satisfaction
» adults with mild hearing problems	» newborns to adults; any type, amount, or pattern of HL
» no hearing test	» hearing evaluation or T-DST evaluation
	» medical red flag referrals
» self-selected amplifier	» self-selected, guided by professional recommendations
» economy models	» economy, mid-level, high-end models
» basic tech	» advanced tech
» limited features	» state of the art features
» no programming or bass/treble adjustments	» professional programming of processing system and communication features based on person's HL, hyper ears, needs, and lifestyle
	» professional verification that aids are programmed best for T-H and communication
	» professional counselling including HL and T-DST management
» return period	» trial period and fine-tuning fitting (usually 60-90 days)
» warranty	» 1 year warranty
» high rates of breakdowns; repairs may not be possible	» low rate of breakdowns; repair and follow-up services through hearing healthcare clinic and manufacturer

CLINIC SERVICES

Depending on whether they're an audiologist or hearing aid professional, care providers could bill for more specific services including pro-rated hourly rates where possible. Services might even be offered to people who've bought an over-the-counter product somewhere else. For example:

- Prescription hearing aid or combination hearing aid fitting.
- Hearing aid rental programs.
- Tinnitus-decreased sound tolerance counselling, e.g. face-to-face; telehealth; eHealth.
- Custom molded hearing protection fitting.
- Assistive Listening Devices fitting.
- Hearing loss or tinnitus-decreased sound tolerance management or therapy programs.
- Hearing loss or tinnitus-decreased sound tolerance auditory brain training programs
- Over-the-counter hearing aid Hit Box testing.

Over-The-Counter Sales and Services

There are products receptionists or other clinic staff could sell directly to the consumer. Hearing healthcare clinics might consider selling personal sound amplification products (PSAP), no prescription hearing aids, and no prescription combination hearing aids.

The selling point is the product would be quality assured. The clinic could stick with reputable manufacturers and products with required communication features, e.g. telecoil, directional microphones, rechargeable batteries and charging station, sound generators.

Clinics could give a guarantee. The consumer wouldn't have to worry about the sound quality or performance. No professional evaluation or fitting needed.

More product lines could be added to make clinics more of a one stop hearing healthcare shop, including self-help hearing healthcare and tinnitus-decreased sound tolerance workbooks and books.

Experts say treatment success depends mainly on your relationship with the care provider. People need a hearing healthcare clinic that offers a variety of products and trusted professionals offering a range of hearing loss and tinnitus-decreased sound tolerance evaluation and management services. In the end it comes down to professionalism, knowledge, variety and quality of services, and level of empathy. Your care providers should make you feel hope that they can work together with you. To help you cope better and have a better quality of life.

WAITING ROOM SHOWROOM

If hearing healthcare clinics add to their product lines or services, waiting rooms could be more like showrooms. This could include displays with samples of different hearing aid styles and colours along with info on features included for economy, mid-level, and high-end pricing. There could be samples of different hearing aid accessories as well as table top sound machines.

There could be samples of different colour options for custom molded earplugs. Samples of social hearing protection are nice for people to try, especially electronic earmuffs with safe built-in amplification.

It's nice when clinics have samples and info on popular assistive listening devices for people to see what options are possible. It's helpful if the hearing healthcare clinic has a looped space so people can test their hearing aid telecoil. If there's a TV to watch, it should have sound off and subtitles on.

UNIVERSAL HEARING HEALTHCARE

As of 2017-2018, the World Health Organization estimated 253 million people around the world have vision loss and 466 million people have hearing loss that makes communication difficult. In many countries, it's common to have vision healthcare coverage including annual vision exams, prescription eyeglasses or contacts, and prescription sunglasses.

Even though over 200 million more people have hearing loss, hearing healthcare coverage is limited even for children. Too many people don't get baseline hearing exams to compare hearing changes over time. Too many adults with hearing loss don't have coverage and can't afford hearing aids. People can't prevent noise-induced hearing loss if they can't afford hearing protection.

Unprotected hearing raises the number of people with noise-induced hearing loss. Unaided hearing loss raises healthcare costs for high blood pressure, heart disease, anxiety, depression, diabetes, and some cases of dementia.

Some countries like the UK already have basic universal hearing aid coverage. Other countries don't, including North America. Universal hearing healthcare should cover:

- Universal newborn infant hearing screening.
- Universal child hearing screening.
- Annual hearing exams, or as professionally recommended.
- Prescription hearing aids or combination hearing aids with basic hearing and communication features.
- Prescription hearing protection.

Coverage should be for everyone, no matter how old. Hearing exams sometimes need to be more often, especially for progressive hearing loss, ototoxic monitoring, or more complicated cases.

Hearing aids, or implantable devices like cochlear implants, should be properly fit and adjusted for mild or greater hearing loss in one or both ears. Pairs of hearing aids should be standard for coverage if both ears are aidable. There needs to be replacement coverage, e.g. earmolds, significant hearing changes, wear and tear.

Ferguson et al. (2017) state, "hearing aids are effective at improving hearing-specific health-related quality of life, general health-related quality of life and listening ability...The evidence is compatible with the widespread provision of hearing aids as the first-line clinical management."

There should be coverage for suitable hearing protection, prescribed as needed, e.g. earmuffs for younger children or professionally fit custom molded hearing protection.

Universal hearing healthcare would identify people with hearing loss earlier, get them aided sooner, and give everyone access to hearing protection. In the long run, this would significantly cut high healthcare costs for serious health problems linked to unaided hearing loss and unprotected hearing.

People who can afford more expensive or advanced hearing aids could still pay more than provided under basic coverage. But universal hearing healthcare would give at least basic access to hearing aids and hearing protection for everyone who needs it.

PART III

MIND THERAPY TOOLS

9

BRAIN TRAINING

Sitting on your shoulders is the most complicated object in the known universe.

- Michio Kaku -

The main hearing problem people with hyper ears report is speech seems muffled or unclear. It's from different causes including divided attention and differences in how our hearing systems process incoming sound. The end result for people with tinnitus or hyperacusis is that it's harder to understand conversations, especially when there's background noise.

Emotion system hyperactivity increases from feeling frustrated, angry, or sad at communication breakdowns and social isolation. Hearing system hyperactivity also increases when people strain to listen. It's also tiring which is not good for coping better with tinnitus or hyperacusis.

People with tinnitus and hyperacusis have a harder time communicating, even if their hearing thresholds seem normal.

People with hearing loss will also have some distortion and different amounts of speech communication problems depending on the type, degree, and pattern of loss. In general, people with conductive hearing loss can understand speech once the voice is loud enough, in quiet listening situations. Speech is still unclear in quiet places for people with sensorineural hearing loss, even for loud or shouted speech. Background noise is a problem for anyone with hearing loss.

The easiest speech sounds to hear are vowels [a, e, i, o, u, y] and louder low frequency consonant sounds [m, n, b, d, g]. The hardest sounds to hear are soft high frequency consonants [s, sh, p, t, k, f].

With hearing system distortion, all the speech sounds are harder to hear. The hearing system adds the extra distortion during processing through the inner ears and up the hearing nerves. Common causes are recreational or work-related noise damage and noise-induced hearing loss. One of the earliest signs of noise-induced hidden hearing loss is impaired understanding of speech-in-noise. Speech-in-noise loss is also caused by genetics, age-related hearing loss, head injury, brain injury, and central auditory processing disorders.

BRAIN TRAINING

There are different auditory training or hearing rehab courses to help people learn to discriminate speech sounds better, using hearing aids if needed for hearing loss. Some focus on improving hearing in difficult listening situations, e.g. having less severe speech-in-noise loss after training than before.

Hearing healthcare professionals have info on auditory brain training options, e.g. clEAR from clearworks4ears.com.

Listening and Communication Enhancement (LACE®)

One online program is called LACE® (Listening and Communication Enhancement). It runs on different platforms including computers, iOS and Android devices. Independent science shows people have a 30% improvement understanding speech in difficult listening situations after completing the LACE® training.

It takes around 20 minutes a day over 11 sessions, with people doing practice sessions when convenient. If done through an audiologist or hearing healthcare clinic, it costs about $100. The audiologist gives guidance, monitors how the person is doing, and gives feedback and support as needed.

I knew a man who had severe hearing loss, severe speech-in-noise loss, and high stress from communication breakdowns even with well fit hearing aids. He completed the LACE® program using his hearing aids, and improved to a moderate speech-in-noise loss, doing much better in difficult listening situations. His only complaint was that he couldn't repeat the program to practice more. Once he finished the sessions, the program was no longer open to him. Months later, his aided communication ability stayed improved.

Brain Fitness Program-Tinnitus

The Washington University School of Medicine looked at computer-based cognitive training to help the attention problems seen in people with tinnitus. Participants had to do a Brain Fitness Program-Tinnitus (BFP-T) online, 1 hour a day, 5 days a week for 8 weeks. It included training exercises using sound and speech signals.

After BFP-T, 50% of participants didn't notice their tinnitus as much, and had better memory, attention, and concentration than the control group. The BFP-T group also showed neuroimaging changes. The authors believe this shows the brain's neuroplasticity or ability to re-organize and reset itself with cognitive training. More research was recommended to confirm findings and make the program more effective.

Cognitive training rehab could be an important tool for maintaining and improving brain health in adults with tinnitus. Similar cognitive training rehab should likely be helpful for people with hyperacusis.

BrainHQ

The Brain Fitness Program-Tinnitus study used the Brain Fitness Program-Auditory developed by Posit Science to "sharpen" the auditory system, and improve communication, hearing, and memory. The Brain Fitness Program-Auditory is available by subscribing to BrainHQ for about $15/month. The subscription gives online access to train on any computer, and additional brain training exercises including for vision, thinking, attention.

People with significant hearing loss or in the Deaf community could focus on brain training exercises that aren't sound based. Other brain training programs by other developers are available.

Cognitive Fitness

This is a $40 online course from Harvard Health Publishing, developed by experts at Harvard Medical School. It covers a practical 6 step plan for better brain health and mental sharpness with aging. It includes interactive learning tools, worksheets, games, and puzzles. The course never expires. People can view it as many times as they want on any device.

Brain Games

Different websites and apps have selections of brain or mind games to help with attention, memory, concentration, and thinking. These can be distraction and relaxation tools as well as brain training.

Proprofs.com has free Brain Training Games Online under their

Puzzles category. Their Puzzles category includes Daily Games with new games loaded daily. This website also has Family Fun games. They offer over 100,000 brain games in over 70 languages.

Many other free or paid brain game apps are also available for different devices.

10

COMMUNICATION STRATEGIES

Much unhappiness has come into the world because of bewilderment and things left unsaid.

- Fyodor Dostoevsky -

People with tinnitus and hyperacusis cope better when using communication tools or strategies. Communication strategies help when having divided attention from hyper ears makes communication harder. They help people with hearing loss communicate more easily even if they're using hearing aids.

Hyper ears get worse when people strain to hear whether it's from hearing loss and/or being in difficult listening situations.

Signs of communication problems include:

- Can't hear in background noise, e.g. family dinner, in a restaurant, in car.

- Can't understand people when they talk from a distance or from another room.
- Can't hear women's or children's higher pitch voices.
- Can't understand people speaking from within 1 metre (3 feet).
- People need to repeat what they said.
- People mumble.
- People accuse you of not listening.
- People say "Never mind," or walk away from conversations because you can't hear them.

Jan's View

I have communication problems more often than in the past. I was chatting about science with a friend.

"We're studying moths," I heard her tell me.

I thought a moment. "Will you find out why they fly to the light?"

"What?" Very puzzled look.

"Will you find out why moths fly into lights?"

Laughing before answer. "Moss. We're studying moss."

Many people ignore hearing problems. Some smile and nod, pretending they can hear conversations when they can't. This means mistakes. Communication breakdowns.

For example, you agreed you'd pick me up after dinner. Why did you buy French bread instead of red thread?

Sometimes faking it doesn't matter too much. Sometimes faking is a problem. Hearing problems are invisible. If people don't know you have hearing problems, they might think you're stupid or don't care as you smile and nod even though you haven't understood them.

This happened to a man I knew. He was at a restaurant with his wife. An old friend who he hadn't seen in a long time stopped by their table to chat. The man had trouble communicating with the background music and voices in the restaurant. At one point the friend said something and stopped talking.

The man didn't catch the words, but he smiled anyway and commented, "That's nice."

The friend said goodbye and left abruptly. The man's wife asked what was wrong with him. It turned out his friend had told him his wife of 40 years had just died after a long illness.

Faking it is bad. When communication strategies aren't enough, hearing aids help people stop faking it. Other hearing aid benefits include good mental and physical health, and better quality of life.

Unaided Hearing Loss

Communication keeps our minds healthy. Use your brain or lose it. People with hearing loss who don't use hearing aids have worse health than people who use hearing aids. If you can't communicate with people, it's stressful. Trying to pretend your hearing is fine—when it's not—is stressful.

If the hearing system in the brain hears less sound and speech because of unaided hearing loss, there's a 10% higher risk of dementia. That's 1 in 10 people with dementia that hearing aids might prevent.

Does this mean people in the Deaf community are at higher risk of dementia and health problems? No. Deaf people communicate mainly with sign language. As long as they can communicate, they're not at risk like people using hearing to communicate who can't.

Stress triggers fight-or-flight chemicals that cause chronic health problems like anxiety, depression, high blood pressure, and heart disease. People with hyper ears don't need any extra fight-or-flight chemicals.

When people use hearing aids, they have the same risk of mental and physical health problems as people with normal hearing. Easier communication keeps the mind active and lowers stress. People with aided hearing loss are healthier. Overall hearing aid benefits include:

- Better coping with hearing loss and hyper ears.
- Better mental and physical health.
- Better quality of life.
- Less depression and anxiety.
- Lower risk of dementia and cognitive problems.
- Less tired from straining to hear.
- Better hearing for speech in noisy or difficult listening situations.
- Better memory for words or conversations.
- Faster thinking for decision making.
- Fewer accidents.
- Less time spent in hospital.

DIFFICULT LISTENING SITUATIONS

It's obvious people will need to use more communication strategies in difficult listening environments where there's background noise or speech. Turn off interfering background sound (e.g. from TV, radio, music) so it doesn't cause communication breakdowns when talking. It makes hearing and understanding easier. The person with tinnitus, hyperacusis, and/or hearing loss will communicate better and be less tired after chatting in quiet than chatting in noise.

Understanding is based on knowing the context or info behind the conversation. Is this a topic you've chatted about before with a friend or family member? Are you talking to a stranger and don't know the topic? That makes it harder.

High echo makes communication difficult. In enclosed rooms or spaces, sound waves echo by reflecting off surfaces and travelling in new directions. Soft materials and surfaces absorb sound wave energy, leaving less of the sound to reflect, making sound waves get smaller and softer. But hard walls and surfaces make sound waves hit and reflect without losing much energy or loudness.

It will be easier to hear in rooms with more soft surfaces and less echo. It's easier to talk in a living room, with more soft surfaces, than in a kitchen. At restaurants or coffee shops, booths are easier than chairs out in the open. The more soft surfaces around, the better for communication, e.g. booths, upholstered seating, carpets, curtains.

Hopefully more architects will design interior spaces with quiet acoustics in mind. It helps everyone with quiet communication needs.

The way a person speaks makes a difference. Higher pitched voices of children or females are often harder to understand. It's harder to understand people with accented speech or facial hair that stops you from seeing their lip movements for speech reading.

There are good speakers, average ones, and poor ones. People who hear well don't notice these differences. People with hearing loss or hyper ears do. It depends on the speaker's loudness of voice and speed of talking. Soft speech will be hard to understand. But shouted speech doesn't help. Shouting distorts speech, making the words less distinct and harder to understand.

Speaking fast hurts speech understanding since vowels and consonants run together.

For example, one gorilla = wangrilla.

Did you eat yet = Jeetyet?

How old are you = Haulryu?

Speakers need to speak slow. Pause between phrases and sentences to give the listener more time to process and understand the message. Sometimes this means talking like William Shatner. Each. Word. A. Sentence.

This is important for people age 65 and older. Science shows that even with normal hearing, it takes older hearing systems slightly longer to process sound than for middle aged and younger adults with normal hearing.

Speakers should be within a 1 meter or 3 foot range and get the attention of the person with communication problems before talking. Some people don't get this no matter how many times they're reminded.

Jan's View

My family walk up behind me, talking to me, when I have no idea they're even there. No matter how many times I tell them, "I can't understand you if you don't get my attention first."

They talk from another room to me, "Mumble mumble mumbldy dum."

I used to tell them, "I can't hear you if you talk from another room."

Louder, "Mumble mumble mumbldy dum."

Not helpful.

Now I'm trying to train them like the famous Pavlov's dog experiment. Pavlov studied how reinforcement changed behaviour. He found positive reinforcement kept the behaviour happening. In real life, if people talk to me from a distance and I answer, they'll keep talking to me from a distance.

Intermittent reinforcement works best at maintaining a behaviour, e.g. if sometimes I answer and sometimes I don't, people will be even more likely to keep talking from a distance.

Negative reinforcement stops the behaviour. If I never answer when people talk from a distance, eventually they should stop talking to me from a distance. I don't even try to listen or strain to hear my family anymore if they're not near me when they talk. Even if I catch what they said, I don't respond. This experiment is still in progress.

In background noise or difficult listening situations, you don't have to hear every word of the target sentence perfectly. Even people with totally normal hearing don't catch every word. Our brain fills in the blanks when it can use clues from the topic.

If a person has problems understanding, the speaker should rephrase the message instead of repeating the original words. There is nothing more frustrating than getting the same difficult-to-hear message over and over again.

Jan's View

I try to let the speaker know which words I missed. But even that doesn't always help.

They say, "Can you get the mumble from the mumble?"

"The what from the what?"

Again. "Can you get the mumble from the mumble?"

"Just tell me the what from the what!"

"Chives. Garden."

Key words help. Understanding single words, in quiet or background noise, is going to be easier than running speech.

Harder to understand: "We're buying a new truck from Big Bob's."

Easier to understand: "Truck. Buying. Bob's."

If necessary, write the message down. Especially addresses or phone numbers. Use words examples for letters like the military or people sharing information over the phone, e.g. B as in Bravo, S as in Sam.

Central Auditory Processing Disorders

Some children and adults have normal hearing for standard testing, but still have mild to severe hearing problems because their brain doesn't process sounds properly. There are different causes of tinnitus and hyperacusis where the person can also have a central auditory processing disorder (CAPD). This includes genetics, chronic ear infections, head injury or concussions, and brain injury (strokes, epilepsy, tumours).

Experts estimate 5% of school aged kids and 55% of people with head injuries have CAPD.

Signs of CAPD include problems hearing in background noise, trouble listening or paying attention to spoken or auditory info, problems remembering heard info, not being able to distinguish different sounds or words, and not understanding conversations or spoken instructions. CAPD can be very frustrating and upsetting.

In kids, CAPD can be confused with depression, learning disabilities, and Attention Deficit Hyperactivity Disorder. Audiologists can do CAPD testing, if children are over age 7 to 8.

Treatment includes coping strategies like lowering background noise as much as possible, moving to quiet low distraction areas to listen, writing down info, organization and scheduling aids, computerized brain training games for attention, memory and concentration, speech language therapy, and assistive listening devices to hear better in background noise if needed.

QUIET LOCATIONS

Piped in music or muzak in public spaces (e.g. shops, stores, bars, restaurants, hotels, libraries, hospitals) is a problem for communication and listening comfort. Especially for people with tinnitus and hyperacusis or hearing loss. Other people need low noise due to quiet communication needs, including the elderly or people with autism, cognitive delays, head or brain injury, and central auditory processing disorders.

Piped in music hasn't been around forever. When it arrived, consumers and customers didn't ask for it. It is only based on perceived or expected sales. The idea that background music makes consumers buy more. Financial experts say many retail stores and malls are closing because there aren't enough customers; they blame millennials who do more shopping online. Maybe there aren't enough customers because too many people with impaired hearing health or quiet communication needs have to avoid noisy public environments playing loud muzak.

Pipedown.org.uk, an international campaign that started in the UK, states "there is no genuine evidence to show that such music increases sales by one penny." In the UK, music is getting turned off at big retail chains, national bookstores, airports, and banks or credit unions. Pipedown is campaigning to get canned music turned off in hospitals and doctor's offices where accurate communication is essential. Pipedown chapters have opened in Australia and the US.

Quiet Location Apps

Mobile apps help people measure and map noise levels and find quiet locations near home or when travelling. These are helpful to find accessible public spaces. There's nothing worse than going out for a nice meal or a quiet drink and not being able to talk because it's too noisy.

SoundPrint, described as Yelp for noise, is an app with noise data submitted from North America and other countries around the world. It includes sound levels for different locations like restaurants, pubs, nightclubs, cinemas, gyms, and more. Soundprint.co have a blog, and share The Monthly SoundPrint newsletter and Quiet Spot lists of participating restaurants.

Some cities have their own maps or residents or visitors, e.g. Quiet City Maps for New York City at quietcitymap.com. Other apps include iHEARu; it has info on public spaces with assistive listening options.

Apps usually have a noise colour code, e.g. green for easy conversation, yellow for tolerable but sometimes you have to raise your voice to talk, and red for avoid because it's impossible to communicate without raised voices. Noise can depend on time of day and other factors. Green will have the lowest background noise levels and red will have the worst.

SPEECH READING

Speech reading or watching the speaker's face and body movements definitely helps to understand speech better. We all do it subconsciously. We know what the hockey players are saying when they get sent to the penalty box or if the football players don't like a call.

Consider that feeling of annoyance if you're in the audience listening to a speaker and then somebody moves in front of you and blocks your view. Or you're at a movie or show and worry that a big head or big hat person will sit in front of your carefully chosen seat.

On TV, you can hear the announcer facing you as they read the news, but you don't catch comments in a movie when the speaker's face is out of sight. Or when the soundtrack volume is louder than the dialogue.

People usually have a harder time communicating on the telephone when they can't see the speaker. Losing visual cues from a speaker's face, mouth, or body language can interfere with communication, making it harder to understand.

Speech reading can help with speech clarity, and can help separate one voice out—the person you're talking to—from among other speakers or background noise. It's not about staring at a person's mouth. It's about watching a person's mouth, face, and expressions to get the most info possible about what they're talking about.

The problem with speech reading is that very few speech sounds are clearly visible except those made near the front of the mouth. Fortunately, many sounds that are difficult to hear tend to be visible on a person's face.

More visible sounds include: f/v, th/sh, p/b/m, r, o/oo.

Most sounds are formed too far back in the mouth and are too fast to be visible. Nobody can completely speech read a conversation despite what you may have seen on TV or in movies.

Sign Language Alphabet
Learning the alphabet in sign language can be helpful for communicating with people who have hearing loss or tinnitus-hyperacusis. Sometimes they're stuck on a word. Having their communication partner sign the letters of the word, or the letter for a missed sound, can

make communication much easier, especially in difficult listening situations.

Jan's View

I was telling an elderly neighbour about my cat Jake who had secretly snuck a ride outside in a backpack.

"What type of cake?" she asked.

"Jake. Jake the cat."

"Chocolate?"

"Not cake. Jake!"

It took several minutes before I could clear up the confusion. If she knew the alphabet, I could have signed the letter 'j' or 'c-a-t', and she'd have understood sooner.

Communication partners have to want to learn and use sign language alphabets. The letters used the most to help with communication break-downs will be consonants like c, f, h, k, p, s, t. Different books and websites have info on learning sign language alphabets.

It would be nice if more people learned to communicate in the full sign language used in their country, e.g. British Sign Language in UK, American Sign Language in North America. I think part of the problem is there's no way to practice if you don't know anybody who signs. It's too bad, because there are so many advantages to knowing sign language.

People can lose their voice or hearing, temporarily or permanently, for different reasons. Knowing sign language means they can still communicate. Making it easier to cope.

Science shows people who have strokes in the right side of the brain can still communicate with sign language. Making it easier to cope for people who can't speak clearly enough to understand.

The more people learn sign language from a young age, the better. Many people think all children should learn sign language, starting with baby sign language and then having classes in elementary and high school. Children learn languages much easier than adults. Kids love signing across distances or when they don't want people to over-hear. It's a good skill to have that would carry through as adults.

Cued Speech
Most people who communicate by speaking and using hearing don't usually know sign language. A different option is to learn simple hand signs along with your most frequent communication partners to help make speech reading easier. Cued speech is a hand positioning system that helps make the speech sounds more visible for people with hearing loss or problems understanding speech in difficult listening situations.

The system includes 8 hand shapes used in 4 different positions. The person talking uses the hand shapes near their face or mouth. This helps the listener see the difference between speech sounds, especially consonants that are hard to hear. For example, if a listener thought the speaker said, "pat" when they said "cat", the speaker could use the hand shape for "c" while speaking to make it easier to distinguish.

The listener and their most frequent conversational partners need to learn cued speech and practice regularly to get good at it. Cued speech has been adapted for 60 languages and dialects and is mainly used by people who communicate through speech and hearing. Different books and websites have info on Cued Speech.

SPEECH RECOGNITION-TEXT

Newer technology takes people's speech and converts it to text for reading instead of hearing. Some options include a relay service where speech goes to the service, is converted to text, and then delivered.

You don't have to be Deaf or hearing impaired to use this type of tech. Anyone who has difficulty understanding speech could consider this options. A couple of options are described below.

SpeakSee

This is a new speech recognition-to-text tech that works in quiet and background noise for group conversations. SpeakSee was created in the Netherlands and uses individual clip-on microphones and specialized directional microphone tech to isolate specific people's speech and filter out any background noise.

It's recommended for people with moderate to total hearing loss. It costs about $700 for a set of 3 microphones and charging dock. The set can be expanded to 9 microphones. It's available at speak-see.com in more than 120 languages and dialects. It also lets users enter their own words into the app, e.g. names, jargon, technical words.

Speakers clip the microphones on their shirts to pick up their voice. Conversations are turned into script-like-transcripts where different speakers are highlighted in different colours. These can be read like subtitles on personal devices like smartphones or tablets. SpeakSee also works with conference calling systems and TVs.

MyEar App

The MyEar app was designed by a graduate from the University of Rochester. It's called closed captioning for personal conversations. The person opens the app, speaks into the phone, and the app translates the words into text. The app goal is to help Deaf and hard of hearing people communicate more easily with anyone using speech communication.

COMMUNICATION STRATEGIES SUMMARY

Communication strategies or coping tools are mainly self-help, since each person has to do them or use them regularly. It's great if communication partners can learn suggestions and use strategies to help have smooth conversations.

In every situation, the lower the background noise compared to loudness of people talking, the easier it will be to communicate.

- Be close to speaker so their face is easily visible.
- Let speaker know if they need to speak louder, stop shouting, or slow down their speech so it's easier to understand.
- Speakers should get the listener's attention before beginning to speak.
- Rephrasing and key words can be helpful along with using a clear message.
- Turn off background sounds or music when talking, if possible.
- Choose locations with more soft surfaces and less echo for easier communication.
- Move to a quieter or less busy location to talk, especially for important conversations.
- Choose quiet locations to shop, eat, drink, or spend time; use apps to locate quiet locations and map them for others, e.g. SoundPrint, iHEARu.
- Consider signing tools to help with speech reading, e.g. sign language alphabet, cued speech.
- Consider speech recognition to text technology or apps, e.g. SpeakSee, MyEar app.

11

MIND THERAPY BASICS

Men are disturbed not by things, but by views which they take of them.

- Epicetus -

Science shows people have up to 50,000 thoughts per day, and mental chatter—that voice in the back of our mind—is up to 70% negative. That's for people in general. People who don't have hyper ears distress.

Science shows people with hyper ears distress think more negatively than people who don't have hyper ears anxiety or depression. This causes a cycle of anxiety, stress, sadness, anger, and difficulty coping.

Distress makes our bodies release fight-or-flight chemicals. Working on changing thought patterns helps lower people's distress levels so their body isn't always in fight-or-flight mode. This helps people feel better mentally and physically.

Hyper ears distress isn't related to tinnitus pitch or loudness, amount of hearing loss, or having hyperacusis. The primary distress factor is how severely a person reacts to having hyper ears. How often they have negative thoughts about it. The more negative thinking, the more hyperactive your emotion system gets. The more noticeable the hyper ears get. Hyperactivity keeps on, maybe getting worse. And so the distress cycle carries on in a downward spiral.

Mind therapy techniques lower emotion system hyperactivity. Brain imaging shows significant changes between people's brains before and after mind therapy. These changes can mean softer tinnitus, less hyperacusis, better sleep, and less anxiety, depression, anger, negative thinking, and negative what if thinking about the future.

Sound therapy tools don't help misophonia, including phonophobia, but mind therapy tools do target the negative emotional dislike or fear reaction. The goal is to find and use specific tools that help when triggers happen.

The more emotion system hyperactivity settles down, the better a person copes. The end result is better mental health and better quality of life. Science shows even people who don't have hyper ears have better mental health after using mind therapy techniques.

Mind therapy is psychology based. So it doesn't rely on hearing. Anyone with hyper ears from the Deaf, hearing loss, or normal hearing communities can use it. With or without added sound therapy. These are proven techniques. They take practice. The more a person uses them, the better they work over time. Most hyper ears websites don't even mention them as coping tools.

Tinnitus-Hyperacusis Sound is treated with Sound Therapy.

Tinnitus-Decreased Sound Tolerance Negative Reaction is treated with Mind Therapy.

Hyper ears are often compared to chronic pain because they have a lot in common: they are invisible and long lasting. Many people have chronic pain and hyper ears. Pain and hyper ears also get better and worse, up and down, for no reason. They can change from hour to hour or from day-to-day. This is the normal nature of the beast. It can also lead to similar distress. It's why most, if not all, mind therapy now used for hyper ears was first used to help people with chronic pain or other chronic conditions.

Often people are told by well-meaning folks (friends, families, health-care providers) to "just stop thinking about it", "stop worrying" or "cheer up, it could be worse."

Jan's View

One doctor told me, "If hearing loss is like having no feet, then tinnitus is like having no shoes." In other words, it might be uncomfortable, but it's not that bad.

This advice did nothing to help stop my negative reaction to my non-stop screeching with no end in sight. I kept thinking the worst. I wasn't given any coping tools to help me change my negative, anxious, and depressed thinking.

Many people successfully use sound therapy to cope better with hyper ears. But social media is full of stories from people who say they've tried everything. Nothing helped. But they were focusing on listening to sound. Never dealing with their hyper ears distress.

Why are people still distressed when using sound? Most people still hear their tinnitus when using sound therapy. This is because sound is set at a soft to moderate comfortable mixing loudness that doesn't completely cover up the tinnitus. Sound therapy takes time for people with hyperacusis or decreased sound tolerance. Improvement doesn't happen overnight.

The bigger reason for distress? It's really hard to stop reacting negatively to a chronic condition. Sound therapy or sound enrichment is a helpful tool for coping better with the sounds of silence. Mind therapy or mental techniques are a helpful tool for coping better with the emotional side of hyper ears distress.

Hyper ears can cause a mix of emotions including sadness, depression, anger, anxiety, fear, annoyance, irritability, and guilt. This causes what I call mind spin. Agonizing. Overthinking, thinking, thinking, thinking about hyper ears and future what ifs. When your inner voice only focuses on upsetting, negative, or bothersome hyper ears thoughts, mind therapy is the answer.

SELF-HELP

Many people do self-help mind therapy on their own after their tinnitus-decreased sound tolerance evaluation and medical clearance. There are different options people can try. Most have been available for years, and can be used by anybody.

Once you learn a technique, it takes regular practice to see results. You can't try something once or twice and then quit. It takes time. At least 3 months of adding technique(s) into your daily routine.

Think about mind therapy tool combos. It's hard to use more than one mind therapy tool at the same time. But a person could use more than one mind therapy technique within the same 24-hour period. Or combine mind therapy techniques with sound therapy or other tools as needed. Either at the same time or over a 24-hour period.

The more you divide your brain's attention by using a mind therapy tool and as many senses as possible, the less the brain can focus on hyper ears. Mind therapy focuses on the thinking 6th sense. Depending on the coping tool, looking, touching, smelling, or tasting can be added, as well as hearing if possible. For example, when doing a relaxation exercise, some people turn on some relaxation music or light a scented candle to get a multiple senses tool combo.

Self-Help Books or Workbooks
Reading self-help books or workbooks on learning to cope better is called bibliotherapy. A coping tool to use anywhere. Anytime. People who read self-help books cope better than people who don't. This book lists different tinnitus and decreased sound tolerance related self-help books and workbooks, e.g. *Living with Tinnitus and Hyperacusis* by McKenna, Baguley, and McFerran. Other books on managing hearing loss, sleep, anxiety, depression, hypersensitivity, and chronic pain can be helpful too.

Different studies prove reading self-help books helps lower hyper ears distress. One often recommended book is *Tinnitus: A Self-Management Guide for the Ringing in Your Ears* by Henry and Wilson.

Compared to people put on a wait-list, people using tinnitus self-help book techniques had less tinnitus distress and less general distress even a year after receiving the book. Australian scientists Malouff et al. (2010) say self-help books *"can provide inexpensive treatment that is not bound by time or place."*

There are lots of books and workbooks from libraries or bookstores that cover coping tools and techniques for distress, whether the cause is tinnitus, hyperacusis, misophonia, or something else. Helpful reading includes self-help books on coping better with stress, anxiety, depression, insomnia, chronic pain, or high sensitivity.

I've read many self-help books. A lot of the tool ideas are the same across books. But each author includes different ideas. At least one

new tool I'm interesting in trying. I either put it in my toolbox for
future use or use the technique and see what happens. What if it's more
helpful than a tool I'm using now? What if it's a good tool for
flare-ups?

Books
People have read fiction and non-fiction (not self-help) for centuries to
help heal or cope better. Reading is relaxing, distracting, cheers people
up, or helps them work through problems or distress along with characters. For example, therapists often prescribed Jane Austen novels for
British soldiers returning from WWII to help them cope with anxiety,
depression, and post-traumatic stress disorder.

In *The Novel Cure: An A-Z of Literary Remedies*, bibliotherapists
Berthoud and Elderkin (2013) recommend specific books depending
on your brain or body pain. For example, they suggest *The Shining* by
Stephen King for alcoholism. They've also written *The Story Cure* for
children. See thenovelcure.com for more info.

Art Therapy Books
Art therapy books are easy to use for self-help relaxation and distraction. These are adult colouring books. Glenn Schweitzer who wrote
Rewiring Tinnitus also sells *Rewiring Tinnitus: Tinnitus Art Therapy*
books with butterfly and flower themes.

There are other art therapy books with different design choices in
stores and in apps including mandalas, cats, gardens, and zombies.
Some books have pictures double-sided so whatever you colour can
bleed through to the back side. Other books are blank or black on the
back side of pages. Some sets come with relaxation music CDs to
listen to while colouring.

Jan's View

I was given an adult colouring book as a gift. It's very relaxing. Much more than I expected. Choosing what colour to use. Smelling the crayons or felt pens. Feeling my hand moving across the paper, touching the crayon. How easy it is to colour without worrying about going outside the lines. I think it took me back to a simpler time when I was little and didn't have anything more to worry about than smelling crayons and colouring.

Mind Therapy Apps

There are many mind therapy apps for coping better with stress, anxiety, and depression. Benefit for most has never been studied scientifically, e.g. in a clinical trial or compared to proven programs. Most mental health apps weren't developed for people with hyper ears, but apps can help people cope better no matter what is causing emotional distress.

Scientists and experts gathered input from the tinnitus-decreased sound tolerance community, and are working on developing specific tinnitus-decreased sound tolerance apps. Some hearing aid manufacturers already have mind therapy and sound therapy included in their combination hearing aid apps.

There are apps on iOS and Android for children, teens, and adults. Many apps have been translated into different languages. Some apps are free. Some are free with extra features or upgrades to buy. Some are available on a monthly, yearly, or lifetime subscription basis. Watch out for apps that automatically renew subscriptions on the expiry date.

People can use apps on different multimedia devices like phones, tablets, or personal music players, depending on the app. I loaded self-help mind therapy apps on my mobile phone for my daily routine, and they're handy in case of anxiety or panic attacks.

Fully accessible apps can be used by the normal hearing, hearing loss, and Deaf communities. There are visual indicators, text, and/or open captioning for spoken audio content. It's open captioning because subtitles are automatically turned on; it doesn't have to be turned on like closed captioning.

Some apps have no visual indicators, text, or open captioning, and are only accessible to people able to hear the audio enough to understand it. Some speakers giving instructions in apps are very difficult to understand because they talk in soft, high pitched, running speech or have accents. The opposite of what's needed for people with hearing difficulties.

It takes trial and error to find which apps are accessible and which aren't. There's no reason developers can't make these apps accessible, e.g. adding open captioning to existing content, using trained speakers talking at a comfortable volume, low pitched, slow paced speech with pauses.

The apps mentioned in this book aren't the only options. If you're considering a self-help app, consider your preferences, science behind it, accessibility, features, positive reviews on multiple websites, and high user ratings when deciding which apps you'd like to try. Keep an eye out for tinnitus-decreased sound tolerance scientist developed apps coming around 2020.

The best accessible apps will likely have:

- Habituation or cognitive behaviour therapy style education.
- Deep breathing exercise with visual indicator.
- Cognitive techniques for negative thinking.
- Relaxation, meditation, mindful meditation, and/or guided imagery exercises .
- Trained speaker for audio with deep, clear, slow paced speech.
- Content that is text based or audio with open captioning.
- Relaxation sound types.

- No percussion relaxation music.

eHealth – Telehealth

Computerized eHealth programs, including tinnitus-hyperacusis mind therapy options, are available online. For example, the British Tinnitus Association has an online course called Take on Tinnitus (takeontinnitus.co.uk). Some programs are more self-help like the Tinnitus First Aid Kit (tinnituskit.com).

Some e-Health programs include peer support online. Others include face-to-face guidance from a trained therapist. Sometimes professionals offer telehealth, guiding the person through a program with regular phone call appointments instead of office visits. Telehealth can be done by Skype or other ways of communication.

PROFESSIONAL GUIDANCE

Counselling helps people with hyper ears distress. People with mild distress often just need basic education and reassurance counselling by an audiologist after the tinnitus-decreased sound tolerance evaluation to ease any worry, concern or negative thoughts.

People with moderate to severe distress often need more counselling therapy from their audiologist or psychologist. This can be in individual or group sessions, face-to-face, or by telehealth.

Self-help workbooks can be a useful way to learn techniques guided by specific approaches. These could include the Progressive Tinnitus Management *How to Manage Your Tinnitus* workbook, *The Highly Sensitive Person's Workbook*, or other workbooks on mind therapy techniques.

Audiologists

Audiologists offer tinnitus-decreased sound tolerance management educational counselling. Some offer the counselling used with their specific sound therapy treatment approach. This could include directive counselling, habituation training, and/or cognitive behaviour therapy style counselling.

Psychologists

Psychologists study people's minds, emotions, and behaviours. They test for any issues, and offer different mind therapy approaches, depending on their specialty. This could includes professional mind therapy approaches like cognitive behaviour therapy (CBT), hypnotherapy, mindfulness based therapies, and more. Counselling therapy can be individual or in groups, face-to-face, or telehealth. It usually takes a series of sessions. The more severe the distress, the more likely mind therapy from a psychologist will help.

Psychologists are more widely available, so local therapy could be possible where there are no audiologists. Since most psychologists don't specialize in hyper ears, look for psychologists who specialize in helping people cope with chronic pain or chronic conditions.

A 2018 British Tinnitus Association survey found 2% of people with hyper ears distress are referred to psychologists for therapy, even though mind therapy techniques are proven to lower distress and help people cope better. People may need to self-advocate and request these referrals from their family doctor.

There are options now for online counselling or therapy sessions with licensed therapists through websites or apps, e.g. Talkspace app.

Directive Counselling

This specialized counselling is used in Tinnitus Retraining Therapy in combination with sound therapy as needed. The directive counselling is based on each individual's tinnitus-decreased sound tolerance evaluation results and includes specific customized counselling protocols to help lower distress.

The idea is for a person to stop having negative emotional reactions. To habituate to tinnitus. Get used to tinnitus so that even though people might notice their tinnitus if they stop to think about it, they aren't bothered anymore.

Specialized directive counselling helps lower decreased sound tolerance, including hyperacusis, misophonia, and phonophobia. Dr. J. Hazell, who helped Jastreboff develop Tinnitus Retraining Therapy clinic protocols, shares guidelines and exercises at The London Tinnitus and Hyperacusis Centre (tinnitus.org). People aren't supposed to use other therapies while doing Tinnitus Retraining Therapy.

Habituation Training
Some treatment approaches use educational counselling to help clients habituate as first described by Jastreboff in his neurophysiological model of tinnitus. Approaches using habituation training include the Levo Tinnitus System and Widex Zen Therapy. Tinnitus or Hyperacusis Activities Treatment uses a combination of habituation and cognitive behaviour therapy based counselling.

NEW MIND THERAPY TOOLS

Professional tinnitus-decreased sound tolerance counselling and mental health counselling approaches like cognitive behaviour therapy (CBT) or mindfulness therapies are updated over time based on evidence-based science. Clinics provide the latest therapy version.

For new coping tools, I look at the science and the source for current techniques to help relaxation, stress, chronic pain, anxiety, or depression. In the media, recommendations from experts on overall wellness are often helpful. For example, I read an article that eating ice cream cones makes people feel less depressed. It's because almost everyone associates ice cream cones with happy, fun times. If that's true for you, it's an easy coping tool to use as a pick-me-up.

When looking for new coping tools, try to find ones that use multiple senses if possible. Coping tools to consider adding to your regular daily routine should help distract you or relax you and make you feel better when you're done. The best and safest options are science-based and developed by professionals like tinnitus-decreased sound tolerance experts, audiologists, ear specialists, and psychologists. Look past the fancy names used for marketing to what the product or treatment is. The most important question is whether the cost is worth the potential benefit of coping better.

MIND THERAPY TOOLBOX SUMMARY

When looking at mind therapy options, consider science-based approaches, including apps and programs developed by scientists with a background in tinnitus-decreased sound tolerance treatments.

For example, a tinnitus clinic in Calgary, Canada, is using TART: Tinnitus Activities Retraining Therapy. It's something their audiologists came up with, combining Tinnitus Activities Treatment and Tinnitus Retraining Therapy. Although there's no science on TART, there is for Tinnitus Activities Treatment and Tinnitus Retraining Therapy. Knowing that, consumers can make an informed decision.

On the other hand, I've seen tinnitus products with fancy names developed by yoga instructors. They have no background in tinnitus-decreased sound tolerance management or psychology science. Again it's about looking past the program or product names to make informed decisions about possible coping tools.

In addition to professional mind therapy approaches, there are many toolbox options that include mind therapy techniques. They include, but aren't limited to:

- Self-help books or workbooks including: tinnitus, hyperacusis, anxiety, depression, chronic pain, stress reduction, art therapy, highly sensitive person, mindfulness based stress reduction, self-hypnosis.

- eHealth or e-learning, e.g. Take on Tinnitus (British Tinnitus Association).
- Tinnitus Retraining Therapy guidelines and exercises, e.g. tinnitus.org.
- Tinnitus Retraining Therapy (habituation; directive counselling protocols).
- Tinnitus-decreased sound tolerance management (habituation and/or cognitive behaviour therapy based), Tinnitus Activities Treatment or Hyperacusis Activities Treatment.
- Cognitive Behaviour Therapy based counselling (e.g. Progressive Tinnitus Management, Neuromonics).
- Habituation based counselling (e.g. Levo Tinnitus System, Widex Zen Therapy).
- Licensed therapists on apps or websites, e.g. Talkspace.
- Other mind therapy coping tools described in this book including professional mind therapy approaches and cognitive, distraction, relaxation, and guided imagery techniques.

Mind therapy or mind enrichment does not get rid of the tinnitus sound, or the decreased sound tolerance painful, disliked, or feared sound. This type of treatment helps change how you react to the sound. There is no single mind therapy technique that will work best for everyone.

For self-help, tool combos work better than one tool alone. Combining as many senses as possible (sight, taste, touch, smell, hearing, thinking 6th sense) helps distract the brain away from hyper ears.

Mind therapy techniques are coping skills that need to be practiced and used in daily life to be most helpful. Often cognitive techniques work best when people are having negative thoughts. Distraction techniques work best when tinnitus-decreased sound tolerance is grabbing people's attention. Relaxation techniques work best when people are feeling tense or anxious. And guided imagery techniques work best to relax or calm the mind.

Practice helps people know what works best for them in different situations. For example, during the day, a person might use cognitive or distraction techniques, and then use relaxation or guided imagery techniques before falling asleep.

The idea of fighting stress, depression, or anxiety is not to drown yourself in busy work. Don't schedule every second of your life. Do schedule some time for coping techniques and tools without overloading or stressing yourself out.

Mind therapy techniques help lower the amount of time spent focusing on hyper ears. It takes persistence and hard work. By changing our thoughts or thought patterns—by retraining our brains—it's possible to lower or stop any negative emotional reaction. This can help people feel more in control. It can also help the emotional centre of the brain reset itself and be less hyperactive. This lowers anxiety, fear, and stress. The result is a sense of greater well-being and improved quality of life. Less distress and better coping.

12

PROFESSIONAL MIND THERAPY APPROACHES

Mental health is a continuum, and people may fall anywhere on the spectrum.

- Amy Morin -

Mind therapy techniques are usually most helpful when planned and used with the guidance of a professional, e.g. audiologist or psychologist. If you're in formal therapy, your care provider will give you counselling and specific treatment approaches for your individual hyper ears needs.

A team approach can be very useful for people with hyper ears. This could include an audiologist and psychologist. This way the audiologist can focus on sound therapy and general management or coping techniques, with more distressed people referred to a psychologist as needed for counselling therapy.

Cognitive Behaviour Therapy

For decades, cognitive behaviour therapy (CBT) has been studied, used, and recommended for people with hyper ears distress. Some sound therapy approaches like Neuromonics and Progressive Tinnitus Management use CBT style counselling.

CBT and CBT style coping tools are sometimes called different names, e.g. cognitive behavioural therapy, cognitive therapy, behaviour or behavioural therapy.

Counselling or behavioural therapy helps emotional distress, e.g. anxiety, sadness, depression, negative feelings, difficulty sleeping. CBT lowers distress and improves well-being and quality of life. People on waitlists cope worse than people taught how to use CBT techniques.

The distress cause isn't important. Mental techniques are similar for chronic pain or chronic hyper ears. Four main CBT technique categories used alone or in combination are cognitive, distraction, relaxation, and guided imagery. This book has specific chapters on each of these technique categories.

cCBT Self-Help Programs
Because mental illness is so widespread worldwide, there are licensed cCBT programs in different languages, usually developed by psychologists. People can do programs online. The more distressed a person is, the more likely they'll need one-on-one support from a counselling therapist. cCBT can help tide a person over if there's a waitlist for therapy.

In the world of psychology, the approach is to get people access to the help they need, then study and fine-tune programs. Science shows if people with mild to moderate distress work all the way through a cCBT program, practicing and using techniques daily, they could get as much benefit as if they'd seen an actual therapist. Online CBT courses include Pathway to Coping, Cognitive Behavioural Therapy Online, Life Skills Online, CBT Training Online,

MoodGym Training Program, Online CBT for Anxiety, Beating The Blues.

For example, MoodGym is about $40 Australian for 12 months of access. The Australian National University developed it. MoodGym is currently available in English and German. It includes CBT based online apps and interactive tools, including a self-help book that helps people learn and practice techniques to manage and prevent anxiety and depression. Independent science shows MoodGym lowers depression and anxiety in adults. Experts say MoodGym is a good option for people who can't access CBT locally or who are on a waitlist for therapy.

In the UK, Living Life to the Fullest has online CBT based courses, books, and other resources. The Canadian Mental Health Association distributes it in Canada.

In Scotland, the National Health Service offers an 8 week CBT based program called Beating The Blues that's free with a referral from a family doctor. Beating The Blues is also available in the US.

The University of New Brunswick in Canada offers an online CBT based course called Pathway to Coping. Its goal is to improve mental health by helping people learn to cope with less stress, frustration, anxiety, and hopelessness. People with better coping skills have better mental health than people who don't. It's about $250 for 2 years of access to complete the course.

I know from personal experience that mild or moderate depression can spiral into the depths of despair when there is no support or info given on coping tools and resources. Stopping depression or anxiety from getting worse, even if that means using self-help cCBT, is easier than trying to recover from severe mental health issues left untreated for whatever reason, including sitting on a waitlist or not being able to find or afford local therapy.

Weise et al. (2016) state, "Implementing [c]CBT for tinnitus into regular health care will be an important next step to increase access to treatment for patients with tinnitus." I agree. Except it should be implemented for tinnitus and decreased sound tolerance to increase treatment access for everyone with hyper ears.

Elbert et al. (2014) say it's time to start using eHealth as part of care provider daily practice. Distressed people need good quality computerized self-help programs now. Not years from now. Then more evaluation can be done on real world benefits for people with hyper ears, and cCBT programs and smart games can be improved as needed.

But there are still issues to work out. Which program or smart game features give the most benefit? Are programs and smart games being developed with open-captioned multimedia and text based content for people in hyper ears, hearing loss, and Deaf communities? It needs to be designed to teach self-help tools with or without sound turned on. Are these smart games and programs being developed for hyper ears in people of different ages: children, teens, young adults, and adults?

Should cCBT programs be available to public or only to target populations of distressed people? Youth prefer a more general delivery without stigma. Research shows cCBT helps everyone have more positive mental well-being, even people without any anxiety or depression to start with. A universal, open approach could certainly be useful.

What is the best way for care providers to use cCBT for tinnitus-decreased sound tolerance healthcare? Who, when, and how? Science on guided self-help found people who used a CBT style self-help workbook with weekly care provider guidance by telephone had 32% less tinnitus distress compared to people on a waitlist. This approach was estimated to be 3 to 5 times more cost-effective than CBT group therapy. As an alternative to psychological therapy, Progressive Tinnitus Management uses a self-help workbook with CBT based techniques, and weekly audiologist guidance can easily be done by telephone.

It's still rare to find psychologists, audiologists, or tinnitus-hyperacusis therapists offering guided self-help as a lower cost therapy option, at least in North America. Care providers should consider this cost-effective approach to provide the most accessible services possible for people with hyper ears. Especially people who are stuck on a waitlist, who don't live near a hearing or hyper ears clinic, or who find it easier and more comfortable to do self-help at home with telehealth guidance.

Emotional Freedom Technique (EFT)
EFT, tapping, or psychological acupressure helps anxiety and post traumatic stress disorder (PTSD). It's believed tapping helps restore body energy balance and relieves symptoms from negative experiences or emotions. EFT coaching sessions help people identify issues and goals to accept yourself despite the problem. They teach the EFT tapping sequence on the body. Science on military veterans with PTSD showed significant improvement within one month of EFT coaching sessions. More science is recommended on how EFT results compare to CBT or other cognitive therapy.

Hypnotherapy
Experts say only certain types of hypnosis help tinnitus, but those types of hypnotherapy can help people as much as using anti-anxiety drugs or doing Tinnitus Retraining Therapy. Hypnotherapy dates back to the 1700s. It uses mental concentration, with guidance and suggestions from the therapist, to help the subconscious mind change patterns of thoughts or behaviours. People being hypnotized are completely aware of their surroundings and can "wake up" any time they want.

People use hypnotherapy for pain relief, coping better with stress, and having a more positive mental outlook. It works better for some people than others. Experts believe it's most effective when used with other mental techniques.

Some hypnotists use regression therapy to take people back to before their tinnitus. They look for any trigger and deal with thoughts related to that. Sub-routine hypnotherapy looks at why the brain hyperactivity causing tinnitus is happening. CARPETS is a desensitization hypnotherapy approach said to help tinnitus loudness and distress. Hypnotherapists teach the person self-hypnosis to help with ongoing relaxation and calm.

Different hypnotherapy products for tinnitus are on sale, including Dr. K. Hogan's Tinnitus Reduction Program (CD/DVD program). He wrote the book *Tinnitus: Turning the Volume Down*. Self-hypnosis CDs/MP3 downloads are available, e.g. Turn Down Tinnitus. There are also self-hypnosis apps, e.g. Anxiety Free.

Relaxation Therapy
This therapy helps people with hyper ears cope better with anxiety or stress. It focuses on teaching relaxation techniques including progressive muscle relaxation, deep breathing, guided imagery, and mindfulness practice. Science shows relaxation therapy can be helpful for people with hyper ears.

After Relaxation Therapy, people had less tinnitus severity and less distress, anxiety, and depression, but results didn't last unless the person learned cognitive techniques too. Therapists recommend The Relaxation and Stress Reduction Workbook to help people learn step by step relaxation techniques. There's a version for kids.

Self-Regulation Therapy (SRT)
SRT was developed to relieve uncomfortable or painful emotional and/or physical symptoms including symptoms caused by traumatic events. It's offered by some counselling specialists. Treatment balances or regulates the nervous system by reducing excess activation. Excess activation comes from accumulated fight-or-flight response energy that the person didn't release when the stressful event happened.

Humans bottle up their reactions to upsetting, frightening, or traumatic experiences instead of experiencing and letting out these natural physical reactions, e.g. try to hold back or hide tears, trembling or physical symptoms when stressed. When left unreleased, energy from these reactions is stored in the nervous system causing different symptoms like tinnitus, hyperacusis, anxiety, depression, fatigue, and pain.

SRT is reported to balance the nervous system and give people a sense of control and well-being. Sometimes people notice temporary heat, tingling, trembling, or an increase in pain or other symptoms after a session releases excess energy. This settles as the nervous system starts balancing energy better. Some therapists offer modified SRT for stress management.

Sudden onset tinnitus-hyperacusis can be a stressful event or related to a traumatic event, e.g. head injury, acoustic trauma. It's unknown if SRT is more helpful for sudden onset tinnitus-hyperacusis than for other types, e.g. gradually developing.

MINDFULNESS BASED THERAPIES

Mindfulness based therapies are showing promising results for tinnitus. They should also help for hyperacusis, although there is not much science on that. Unlike CBT, these therapies focus on the thought process instead of working on changing thought content. Mindfulness is about being aware without judgement—in the moment—of your physical body and your thinking.

Acceptance and Commitment Therapy (ACT)
This is a mindfulness based therapy that teaches people skills to let go of painful thoughts and memories. It helps people become mindful, and helps people accept their distress or painful feelings, find what they value, and use that knowledge to work towards a better quality of life.

Depending on amount of distress, ACT can range from a few 20 to 30 minute sessions, several one hour sessions, or long-term therapy. Science on ACT for treating tinnitus in people with normal hearing found better tinnitus acceptance, and significant improvement in tinnitus distress, anxiety, and sleep compared to people on a waitlist. The What's Up? app includes CBT and ACT style exercises.

Mindfulness Based Stress Reduction (MBSR)
Dr. Jon Kabat-Zinn developed MBSR in the 1970s for managing chronic pain and other conditions like anxiety, depression, stress, and PTSD. It uses mindfulness meditation, and has positive effects on brain and immune function. Bookstores have different MSBR books and workbooks.

Mindfulness Based Tinnitus Stress Reduction (MBTSR)
In 2009, Dr. J. Gans developed MBTSR to help people with tinnitus distress that doesn't respond to traditional therapies. It teaches people to bring conscious attention to their present awareness. It helps people stop dwelling on the past or thinking negative thoughts of the future. Experts report MBTSR lowers tinnitus annoyance and severity, and reduces anxiety, fear, depression, and sleep problems.

There is an 8 week online MBTSR course. It costs about $845, although it goes on sale sometimes. People do the course from home when it's convenient. The program includes deep breathing, yoga, relaxation, and meditation. The course uses Jon Kabat-Zinn's book *Full Catastrophe Living*.

Mindfulness Based CBT
This is used for managing chronic pain and depression. It's based on Jon Kabat-Zinn's MBSR program. Mindfulness based CBT teaches meditation techniques in an 8 week course, usually in a group format. People with tinnitus taking this approach had less tinnitus severity and less distress, anxiety, and depression with benefit lasting up to 6 months after the course ended. Professionals in some countries offer

similar programs called Mindfulness Behavioural Cognitive Therapy. There are books and workbooks on mindfulness based CBT for chronic pain that could be useful for people with chronic hyper ears.

Mindfulness Meditation Self-Help Apps

There are lots of apps offering mindfulness based meditation. These include Insight Timer, Headspace, Pause, Sanvello (also includes CBT), Depression CBT Self-Help Guide, and The Mindfulness App. The 10% Happier app includes meditations by some of the top mindfulness teachers in the world, e.g. Joseph Goldstein, Sharon Salzberg, and George Mumford.

PROFESSIONAL MIND THERAPY SUMMARY

Guided Self-Help

- Books and Workbooks: How to Manage Your Tinnitus workbook (CBT based), Full Catastrophe Living (mindfulness based), The Relaxation and Stress Reduction Workbook, Tinnitus: Turning the Volume Down (hypnotherapy based), and other books or workbooks on CBT, mindfulness based stress reduction, mindfulness based CBT, hypnotherapy, relaxation, and stress reduction.
- Computerized CBT programs, e.g. Beating the Blues, CBT Training Online, Cognitive Behavioural Therapy Online, Life Skills Online, Living Life to the Fullest, MoodGym Training Program, Online CBT for Anxiety, Pathway to Coping.
- Emotional Freedom Technique (coaching sessions).
- Hypnotherapy: e.g. Tinnitus Reduction Program (CD/ DVD program), Turn Down Tinnitus (CD/MP3 download), Anxiety Free (self-hypnosis app).
- Mindfulness Based CBT programs.
- Mindfulness Based Stress Reduction.

- Mindfulness Based Tinnitus Stress Reduction (MBTSR) program.

Therapy (face-to-face or telehealth)

- Cognitive Behaviour Therapy based counselling (e.g. Progressive Tinnitus Management, Neuromonics).
- Habituation based counselling (e.g. Levo, Widex Zen Therapy).
- Cognitive Behaviour Therapy.
- Computerized CBT programs.
- Mindfulness Based CBT programs.
- Mindfulness Based Therapies: e.g. Acceptance and Commitment Therapy, Mindfulness Based CBT, Mindfulness Behavioural Cognitive Therapy.
- Hypnotherapy, e.g. CARPETS, regression, sub-routine approaches.
- Relaxation Therapy.
- Self Regulation Therapy.

13

COGNITIVE TECHNIQUES

My therapy has come from paying attention to my life.

- Oprah Winfrey -

Emotions or feelings show in our background thoughts, inner voice, or self-talk. Self-talk is often full of negative thoughts, especially when people are dealing with chronic conditions. Negative self-talk, including "what if" thinking, can be full of fear about how we'll cope in the future.

For example, it's snowing. One person thinks, "I can hardly wait to go for a walk in the snow." Their emotional reaction is positive. Another person thinks, "I'm scared to drive home. What if I get in an accident?" Their emotional reaction to the same snowstorm is negative. It's our thoughts that lead to whether we have a negative or positive emotional reaction.

In the same way, having hyper ears doesn't cause the emotion. The emotional reaction comes from how the person thinks about their hyper ears. The focus of cognitive techniques is not to change people into a sunshiny person full of positive thinking. The goal is to change from unhelpful negative thinking to realistic neutral thinking. Fight thoughts with different thoughts. This includes thoughts caused by misophonia dislike and fear triggers.

Experts explain this using a traffic light analogy. Red means the thought is unhelpful; it makes you upset, e.g. "Today is going to be awful." Green means the thought is helpful; it doesn't make you upset, e.g. "Good thing I have coping tools I can use." These are examples of green thoughts:

- What type of cookies should I eat tomorrow?
- This lemon froyo is really good.
- Where should I go for a walk?
- The red orange fall leaves look beautiful.
- I'd like to do that as a hobby.
- What supplies do I need for my next project? Or recipe?
- I got the spice just right on my Pad Thai.
- I love riding my horse in Zelda.
- That bird is different. I wonder what it is? I'd like to know.
- Googling, surfing, surfing, surfing. Rufous-Sided Towhee. Huh.

Over treatment, a person's self-talk changes from red to green thoughts. This process is like weeding a garden. Unhelpful negative thoughts are plucked out like weeds. Cognitive techniques are easiest to learn with professional guidance.

Sometimes people avoid activities because they have negative thoughts about what might happen. People predict they'll have a problem, e.g. my hyper ears will be worse if I go to the shopping centre. Some people with hyper ears distress become isolated from avoiding social and work activities they fear will make things worse. In cognitive therapy, the counselling professional helps encourage people to try activities.

A person may be worried about going out to see a movie at a movie theatre because they think it will be too loud. They could try seeing a movie that doesn't have a lot of loud gunfire or special effects, and see if the volume is still too loud. They could see a movie but wear social hearing protection (more info in Hearing Protection chapter) and see if it would be comfortable enough at least now and then. They could choose to watch a special movie at home set to a comfortable volume. The counselling specialist helps guide people through this process while problem solving any concerns that come up.

Jan's View

I've had counselling from psychologists and psychiatrists in the past. Sometimes it was helpful. It really depended on the specific care provider. Some were useless, and it was a waste of time to see them. One told me, "Exercise is over-rated." Seriously? Says who?

I've gone to cognitive behaviour therapy tinnitus management workshops. They were helpful for everyone there to learn techniques, share ideas, and support each other. The first workshop I went to made me cry. I realized I've never talked about my tinnitus to anybody face-to-face. I think I had a lot of buried grief brought out at the workshop hearing everyone's stories.

CBT Books & Workbooks
Different cognitive behaviour therapy (CBT) style self-help books and workbooks are sold in bookstores. Check best-of lists, reviews, or ratings.

Mind Therapy Self-Help Apps

Apps come and go, so some disappear from app stores and new ones arrive from different developers. Choosing one or more comes down to which app has exercises and techniques that help you, and that you're going to use consistently.

There are tinnitus specific mind therapy apps, but not developed by tinnitus-decreased sound tolerance scientists yet. For example, Relax Melodies app has a tinnitus module you can pay for in an app upgrade. It calls tinnitus a discomfort and affliction. In over 30 years, I've thought many things about my tinnitus, but never that it was a discomfort. I've never heard anybody distressed by tinnitus say it was "uncomfortable."

Calling tinnitus an affliction—causing pain, suffering, wretchedness, torment—goes against tinnitus therapy approaches and cognitive behaviour therapy. I don't like the negative words. I won't pay to check out this module.

Many apps have CBT style cognitive exercises. I included these because they're in several top app lists, have good reviews, and have high online user ratings for helpfulness: 7 Cups Of Tea, Depression CBT Self-Help Guide, Happify (game based), Lantern, Mindshift (for teens to adults), MoodKit, SAM, Sanvello, The Worry Box, What's Up (includes Acceptance and Commitment Therapy exercises), Worry Watch– Anxiety Journal.

I've been using the free trial version of the Sanvello app, developed by psychologists. It includes cognitive behaviour therapy (CBT) based Guided Paths: 7 education lessons on CBT and how to use it. It's a basic intro to CBT. It has a section on Thoughts: cognitive style mental exercises to help thought patterns be less negative.

I figured I already knew cognitive techniques from past counselling, books, courses, and workshops. I only checked the app out for this book; not because I needed any new coping tools. But knowing how to do something and doing it are two different things.

Jan's View

The Sanvello Thoughts Reframe technique takes less than 5 minutes. I used it at bedtime to reframe my top daily anxiety, and after a few days I noticed it helped my mind stop spinning with the same worries over and over. I can shut down negative thoughts easier during the day. I found out my thought traps are Mind Reading, Fortune Telling, and Labeling & Judging. It helps to know what bad mental habits you're falling into, and how to get into better mental habits.

Happify is an interesting app that focuses on positive thinking, but it uses games and activities. These include clicking only on positive words floating on and off screen or hidden object games. It has an assessment questionnaire. After you fill it out, it lists your top strengths. Mine were love of learning, bravery, and curiosity. I think that's true. It's a good reminder that I have positive qualities when I'm feeling sad and defeated. It made me feel better than a different app questionnaire that told me to get professional help.

An advantage of apps is being able to set reminders. At first I set up daily reminders, so I didn't forget to use the app while getting into my new daily routine. It's easy to start using the techniques without the app once you know how. If I'm having a high anxiety day, I go back to the app for a refresher, and keep using it until my anxiety lowers. Apps are my thought security blanket.

When choosing apps, think of how many categories of CBT it offers. For example, Sanvello has cognitive, relaxation, and guided imagery techniques; Having multiple features in one app lowers the number of apps you'll have on your phone or device.

Sanvello has relaxation sound tracks with different sound types, e.g. coloured noise, nature. I like the White Noise app better for relaxation sound quality than Sanvello. Personal preference. I have 4 apps on my phone for my sound therapy and mind therapy exercises.

Another consideration is what your care provider recommends. If you're getting professional CBT, your psychologist might recommend an app to help you stick with a new routine of mental habits during therapy or after it ends. My family doctor recommends apps, and wants feedback on which help me cope better.

14

DISTRACTION TECHNIQUES

When there are thoughts, it is distraction: when there are no thoughts, it is meditation.

- Ramana Maharshi -

While cognitive mind therapy uses strategies to help a person think differently about their tinnitus-hyperacusis, distraction mind therapy uses strategies to help a person switch their thoughts away from hyper ears by thinking about something else. For example, learning the lyrics to a song. It's hard for people to focus on more than one thing at a time. Distraction divides your attention. Taking your focus off your hyper ears includes misophonia dislike or phonophobia fear reactions.

There's an expression that what you focus on increases. It's certainly true the more people focus on their hyper ears, the more distressing it can be. Some authors describe a mental condition called "flow state". Flow state is the opposite of focusing. Flow state is like being on automatic pilot. For example, imagine you're driving home from the store.

It's a trip you've taken many times. You reach your driveway and realize you can't remember the drive. You were in flow state. Your body functioned automatically, and your background thoughts were free to roam.

In contrast, imagine you're driving home from the store in the middle of a fierce storm. All your thoughts are completely focused on each part of the trip. Each turn of the steering wheel. Each touch on the gas or brakes. You arrive home exhausted from the stress of worrying over the drive.

When you worry over hyper ears like a dog with a bone, then flow state is lost. When people regularly focus on their hyper ears, it leads to more stress, anxiety, and depression. It's important to do everything possible to spend less time checking on tinnitus and less time thinking about your hyper ears. Easier said than done. This can be a hard habit to break.

Counselling specialists can teach people specific distraction techniques that help them shift their focus away from their hyper ears. It's best if people try different techniques to find the ones that work best for them.

By using distraction techniques, the goal over time is to think less and less about the hyper ears until you reach the end of the day and realize you haven't had any particular thoughts about it. Or think less and less about misophonia triggers when they happen. Outside of therapy, distraction strategies can be used for self-help.

Alphabet Distraction
If you need to force yourself to think something different, the alphabet distraction works. First choose a category. It can be something general or something specific to you. Name something in that category from A-Z, using every letter of the alphabet in order. The harder the category, the more distracting it will be.

You can use whatever categories you want. It doesn't have to be the same every time. You can pick easy categories or hard categories. If you can't come up with a name, just move on to the next letter. Don't worry if you make a mistake. This is just thought control. With practice you'll get better at thinking of a name for each letter. For example:

- Fruit: apple, banana, cantaloupe, date, e = don't know, fig, grape...z = don't know.
- Vegetables: a = don't know, broccoli, celery, d = don't know...yam, zucchini.
- Shows or Movies: try naming titles, characters, actors.
- Music: try names of songs, bands, lead singers, instruments.
- Gender neutral names. Traditional girls or boys names.
- Capital cities: I don't do this category because I'm really bad at it.
- Countries: Australia, Brazil, Canada...US, Venezuela, Waikiki, X = don't know, Yemen, New Zealand. I'm not very good at countries either so I make do.
- Living Things: You get the idea. Make it harder by picking a particular type. Cats or dogs. Birds. Do you like fishing? Pick names of fish.
- Plants: Can you name flowers? Plants in general? Trees? Botanical or common names?
- Sports: Types of sports. Team names. If you're into sports, try naming pro athletes in your favourite sport e.g. golf, hockey, football.
- Whatever category you like.

The category doesn't matter. The key is forcing your mind to think about something neutral instead of your hyper ears. With regular practice, people often find that in the middle of doing the alphabet distraction, their thoughts stray to other things like plans for the day, shopping lists, what to cook for dinner. By regularly practicing thinking about something different, it becomes easier to stop your thoughts from always settling on hyper ears. The alphabet distraction helps break that mental habit.

Another way to make it harder, or more attention grabbing, is to learn a sign language alphabet. Sign each letter of the alphabet as you go through the alphabet distraction. The signed alphabet can help with more than communication breakdowns.

Jan's View

I learned the alphabet distraction at an Arthritis Society of Canada 8 week self-help chronic pain management course. I thought it sounded stupid. But I tried it. Going for walks or climbing stairs, I would alphabet away. Forcing myself not to think thoughts like how much it hurt, what if the pain got worse, what if...

The more I used the alphabet distraction, the better it worked. One day while climbing stairs, I realized I wasn't paying attention to my pain even though I wasn't doing the alphabet distraction at the time. My thoughts were on what I was doing later that day. I was automatically thinking other things.

I tried the alphabet distraction for my constant negative tinnitus thoughts. It helped. I still use it when needed. This was before scientists proved chronic pain tools also help people with chronic tinnitus-hyperacusis, especially mind therapy techniques. It's interesting because many people with hyper ears have chronic pain.

---

10 Second Rule

If you're thinking about your hyper ears, you've got 10 seconds. Then it's like dropping a cookie, chip, or carrot stick on the floor. After 10 seconds it's trash. Gone. The 10 Second Rule stops you from focusing on your hyper ears. Helps lower hyperactivity. This rule gives you time to think, what are you up to now, hyper ears? FU T. Or whatever. Then you must think about something else.

Is is time to take the dogs for a walk? I need to make chocolate chip cookies. What is the answer to 10 across? According to Shakespeare, love is 5 letters ending in d. Any good book giveaways on Goodreads? Time to pet the cat. I wonder if the hummingbird will visit my garden today. A = Avatar, B = don't know, C = Carrie, D = Deadpool, E = Elf, F = Failure to Launch...

Crafts

Experts say crafts like crochet or knitting can be very helpful for depression. I was given a book on crochet for depression published by a woman named Betty. I thought it was a strange idea in a strange little book, with no consistent formatting or instructions. But when I tried crocheting, it helped me cope better.

I think it's the multiple senses including the 6th sense of thinking. There's the colour and feel of the yarn running past my fingers, thinking how to do stitches, counting stitches and rows, seeing a project grow, feeling more productive than a lump on the couch doing nothing with my days. Knitting gives the same effect.

Betty wrote even if you unravel the whole thing at the end, the process of crocheting helps with mental well-being. Unfortunately, Betty stole the patterns from other books, and her book is not for sale any more.

Jan's View

I do cross-stitch. Stitching coloured floss on canvases to make a picture. I like counted cross-stitch instead of pre-stamped. I follow a grid, and count squares to make sure I'm stitching the pattern properly.

I rarely think of my hyper ears when I'm doing this hobby. When I'm finished, it helps me feel productive since I have something to hang on my wall. They're not perfect. I make mistakes all the time. But nobody else knows if my finished canvas doesn't match the pattern.

Projects don't have to be perfect; it's the thought distraction activity that counts.

Games

People use different games for distraction. Card and board games are fun. So are gaming systems whether you're racing cars or battling a dragon. It's easier than ever to load game apps on a computer, tablet, or phone. This wasn't available when my hyper ears started.

Some games are better than others. People can pick what's interesting or enjoyable. Many have a soundtrack or sound effects if that's comfortable for listening. Mind therapy plus sound therapy combo.

Jan's View

Game apps help me. For cards, I have trouble shuffling because of pain and stiff fingers. Apps shuffle for me, so I can play cards again. I rarely notice my hyper ears when I'm playing any game, whether it's solitaire, Yahtzee, word puzzles, number puzzles, or Stardew Valley.

One portable gaming system I use is a handheld Nintendo DS. The screen is bigger, so it's easier to see what's going on in games than on my phone. DS are small, lightweight, and more portable than a tablet. There are loads of different DS games. I don't like fighting games generally, so my choices are puzzle or fantasy. Sherlock Holmes. The Hobbit. Professor Layton. Zen games.

Recently, I became addicted to Animal Crossing on DS. I've never thought about my hyper ears while playing. Most of my senses come into play, from choosing and making decisions, touching my DS, watching the screen. For hearing, it has a soundtrack of music and sound effects I turn on or off depending on my mood.

It's a world building game where I'm in total control of my town of animals. I've put in the Eiffel Tower, and a white flower garden in homage to Gertrude Jekyll. I collect fossils, ore, art, and fish to display in my museum. Or sell to pay for my clothing, furniture, and town projects.

If I don't like somebody in my town, I shun them for 2 weeks and they move away. If only getting rid of hyper ears was so easy.

Hobbies

The most common distraction technique is doing activities or hobbies. Sitting around doing nothing pleasant only leaves a person with time on their hands to think about their hyper ears. The more you can keep yourself occupied with activities or hobbies you enjoy, the better the distraction. Try to identify when your tinnitus is more noticeable or you're paying attention to your hyper ears. During those times, keep busy with pleasant, meaningful activities, especially where you need to use your mind.

If you don't have activities or hobbies, find things to do that interest you and distract you. For example, bird watching can be an interesting distraction, whether you have a birdfeeder in your garden or just look for different birds on a walk around your neighbourhood. Some people enjoy learning to identify the birds they see. But even just counting how many birds you see on a walk can be an easy neutral method of distracting your thoughts.

Other examples include exercise, cooking, reading, shopping, cross-word puzzles, photography, gardening, fishing, golfing, woodworking, doing volunteer work. Activities or hobbies will be as different as the interests of different people with hyper ears.

My hyper ears change from day-to-day. So a distraction that works one day, might not work as well at a different day or time. I pick distraction activities depending on how much my hyper ears are grabbing my attention. I use sound therapy at the same time if possible. Combining mind therapy and sound therapy works better than either alone.

I spend a lot of time reading. If my tinnitus is still at the front of my mind while reading, I pick something harder to read. Something I have to concentrate on. Or something that draws me into the world within the book. Away from my hyper ears temporarily.

Crossword puzzles or Sudoku are the same. If they're too simple, they're not always enough to distract me. I try to pick something harder.

I enjoy baking desserts. When I'm picking a recipe, gathering my ingredients, and preparing everything, I don't think about my hyper ears. My mind is too busy making sure I don't forget something or add the wrong amount. That I'm following the recipe. Imagining the hot melty chocolate chip cookies or lop-sided cake soon coming out of the oven.

Learning a new language is a big distraction. With language apps, you can pick any language you want. I chose Swedish on Duolingo. When I'm busy with hej ursäkta, my hyper ears is the last thing on my mind. I want to learn American Sign Language because it's used in Canada. I want to learn to sign for many reasons. Including I know it would help me forget about my hyper ears for a while.

Notice how my hobbies and activities don't mean running around exhausting myself. I choose what I do. I choose when to do them, and for how long. Sometimes it's only 10 minutes at a time. Every bit helps.

Laughter

Norman Cousins wrote a book called *Anatomy of an Illness as Perceived by the Patient,* which describes how he took charge of a disease through humour and treatment. It's hard to think of concerns or problems while you're laughing. Laughing is good for a person's health and sense of well-being.

Certified Laughter Leaders offer formal therapy using the power of laughter to lift spirits, heal, and bring better physical health. It includes breathing exercises. You can add laughter into your life by using what makes you laugh. Choose funny TV shows or comedy movies to watch. Find reading material that's funny.

Making yourself smile and laugh even when you don't feel happy are techniques for battling anxiety, depression, and stress. Grin at yourself in the mirror each morning as you get ready for the day. Practice making yourself laugh. Experts call this fake it until you make it.

As Zen master Thich Nhat Hanh once said, "Life is both dreadful and wonderful... Smiling means that we are ourselves, that we have sovereignty over ourselves, that we are not drowned in forgetfulness. How can I smile when I am filled with so much sorrow? It is natural—you need to smile to your sorrow because you are more than your sorrow." Whether you're happy or just putting on a show to manage feeling sad, smiles and laughter are an effective and inexpensive technique of distraction mind therapy.

Jan's View

In 2017, I was very depressed and decided to guinea pig myself with an experiment I called Fight Sad with Sad. I thought you fight fire with fire, sound with sound, thoughts with thoughts. Why not fight sad with sad? Get the tears out in one big cryfest.

Given my tower of teary tissues, I thought my experiment needed to last a few days. This experiment wasn't based on science. The idea popped into my head. I thought it seemed good. What could go wrong?

I read the saddest books I have. Guaranteed tear jerkers. The Memory of Running by Ron McLarty. A brother struggling to cope with his sister's mental illness. Watership Down. I bawl at the end.

I listened to my saddest songs of heartbreak and death. Songs I can't sing along to for my tears and sobbing. Nothing Compares 2 U. Glenn Gould on piano playing Bach's Brandenburg Concertos. What Hurts The Most. Shouldn't Be This Way. Chopin's Tristesse. If You're Reading This.

I watched my saddest shows, guaranteed to make me cry. Forest Gump. My Sister's Keeper. 13 Reasons Why. Moulin Rouge.

Let's just say, this was the worst experiment ever. My major depressive disorder got much worse. I switched to fighting sad with comedy. It took ages to get back to my sadness level before this experiment started. Don't try it. Never.

This was a good reminder not to guinea pig myself unless I'm trying something hyper ears scientists and care providers recommend.

Sign Language Music Videos

More and more bands are releasing music videos in sign language. Bands are taking interpreters on the road for live shows, sometimes with multiple interpreters around the stage so everyone can see the signing. It's hard to pay attention to tinnitus when you're singing signing along to a favourite song and it's deep, bass beat. People sense lower frequencics by vibration. Feeling the sensation more than hearing low notes. Deaf people are better at this.

For music, the interpreters adapt their signing to match the lyrics and tempo of the songs, whether it's rap or techno pop. The signing is very exciting to watch. Von Buren (2017) says, "Sign language is a full body language, from the facial expressions to the movements of the hands and arms, making it the perfect language to portray emotional messages such as song lyrics."

I think it's a good way to learn sign language, after learning the alphabet. Find a song you like with a signed and captioned music video. Learn to sign it. Imagine a concert with the whole audience singing signing. Imagine the words and phrases people would learn. Then be able to use in daily life.

Strange Distraction
This is how it works. Sit down. Lift your right foot an inch above the ground. Start rotating it clockwise. Now use your right index finger to trace a figure eight in the air in front of you. Once you can do these actions at the same time, you'll have spent time not thinking of your hyper ears.

15

RELAXATION TECHNIQUES

It is requisite for the relaxation of the mind that we make use, from time to time, of playful deeds and jokes.

- Thomas Aquinas -

Relaxation tools are any method or activity that helps you feel calmer, less tense, less stressed out. Stress can make any chronic condition worse. It isn't always clear whether hyper ears makes people feel stressed and then distress goes up, or whether stress makes hyper ears worse and then distress goes up. Like the riddle of the chicken or the egg, it's hard to tell if the hyper ears or the stress came first. The only thing that matters is they often increase together.

People can use relaxation techniques to lower stress, be more relaxed, and better able to cope. Sometimes very distressed people have felt tense for so long they've forgotten what relaxation or calm feels like. Learning relaxation techniques can help people know what it should feel like. Then they can better recognize when they're feeling tense, and when they need to use relaxation techniques.

Counselling specialists can teach people specific relaxation techniques helpful in specific situations, e.g. sleep, stressful events, misophonia triggers. People try different techniques to find the ones that work best for them.

The more you practice relaxation, the better the relaxation tool works. Many people only try something once or twice, or quit long before finding out how well a particular technique could work for them.

Counselling experts say relaxation techniques are not as helpful if used on their own. They work best when combined with other mind therapy techniques like cognitive, distraction, or guided imagery.

Binaural Beats
These are a way of changing brainwaves to switch a person into a relaxed state. People with normal hearing, hearing loss, or in the Deaf community can use binaural beats. Always check with your doctor before trying binaural beats to make sure it's safe for you. People with certain mental health conditions or medical conditions including epilepsy, heart disease, or a pacemaker should never use binaural beats.

Physicist Heinrich Wilhelm Dove discovered binaural beats in 1839. He found when signals of 2 different frequencies are presented separately, one to each ear, our brain tries to make sense of the difference. It makes you hear a 3rd tone: a binaural beat at a frequency that's the difference between the 2 pure tones. For example, if a frequency of 120 Hz is presented to your left ear, and a frequency of 110 Hz is presented to your right ear, your brain hears a binaural beat at 10 Hz.

This changes your brain waves to the binaural beat frequency, changing your level of consciousness or wakefulness. It's called brain entrainment or whole brain synchronization. Instead of the left and right sides of the brain working separately, like usual, both sides synchronize or work together. Experts say this helps increase blood flow in the brain and balances our nervous system.

Psychologists and hypnotherapists are using binaural beats for therapy. Other brain entrainment beats include isochronic tones (rapid pulses of sound) and monaural beats (described below).

There are 4 types of binaural beat frequencies or frequencies of brain activity when people are awake. These different brainwave states give different results:

- **Gamma Waves** (30–70 Hz) put people into a highly alert state with super concentration on tasks. Too much gamma wave activity can cause stress and anxiety. These binaural beats are not recommended for people with hyper ears.
- **Beta Waves** (12–27 Hz) make people alert, but too much can cause anxiety, stress, bad sleep, and release of fight-or-flight chemicals. Definitely not recommended for people with hyper ears.
- **Alpha Waves** (8-12 Hz) put people into a relaxed state of mind. People feel less stressed, less anxious, and calmer. This might be helpful for people with hyper ears, depending on what they are doing at the time.
- **Theta Waves** (3-8 Hz) are the brain activity needed for meditation. Theta waves quickly put people into a state of deep meditation and deep relaxation, calming the mind, and reducing anxiety and stress. Science shows 30 minutes a day of Theta meditation significantly improves people's general health and well-being.

Children aged 0 to 12 naturally have alpha and theta brainwaves so experts think they should be safe for children to listen to for relaxation, but there's not a lot of science yet on this. Gamma and beta wave binaural beats should not be used by children; scientists don't know if it could negatively change their normal brainwave activity over time.

Binaural beats work best when using stereo headphones in a room with no other sounds or distractions. Guttman (2003), at The Monroe Institute, studied binaural beats. He found they helped with relaxation for Deaf people. The relaxation effect was best when the headphones were not placed over the ears. The best location, for comfort and ease of use, was one inch above and slightly behind each ear. Another comfortable location suggested was over the carotid arteries in the neck. In the experiment, they felt for the pulsing of the arteries and placed the headphones over the pulsing. This location helped put the person into a relaxed, meditative state.

The problem with pure tone binaural beats is they don't sound very nice. Most people use binaural beats with added natural sound effects or music. Binaural beat meditations are available in apps, CDs, MP3s, or computer downloads. Be very careful which binaural beats you try because sound quality can be bad. Many people complain the binaural beats on most YouTube videos don't work. Experts say that's because the sound isn't properly engineered.

Start slowly if you use binaural beats. They can make people feel very weird after listening, especially the first few times they try it. Some people report flying through space, seeing vivid colours or images, and even meeting unearthly beings, although this is more common when using pure tone binaural beats. If it feels strange, stop.

I-DOSER Software Binaural Dose store has a variety of binaural beat MP3s for download at under $10 to $20; their website idoseraudio.com includes online chat with a Dose Advisor. There is also an iOS and Android I-DOSER app.

Binauralblog.com features articles on mindfulness tech, including binaural beats and different relaxation exercises.

Alban (2018) recommends free downloads Zen 12 (12 minute binaural beats meditation) and OmHarmonics (10 minute binaural beats meditation). Binaural Beats Freak (2018) says companies Binaural Beats Meditation (BBM) and Enora have good reputations and recommends Deep Meditation-BBM with layered vocals and eastern inspired music, Stress Release–Enora with layered music, sounds and effects, Anxiety Release–BBM with flute and keyboard music (recommended to use before stressful events), and Zen Focus–BBM with running water, piano, and nature sound effects. Use caution. Make sure binaural beats are medically safe for you before trying.

Cannabidiol (CBD)

This is a compound in cannabis that doesn't make a person high like the psychoactive cannabis compound THC. In a 2011 study, the National Institute of Health concluded controlled use of CBD is safe and non-toxic in humans.

People have used CBD to cope better with inflammation, pain, anxiety, depression, seizures, and other medical conditions. Side effects include dry mouth, increased Parkinson's tremor at high doses, low blood pressure, light-headedness, and/or drowsiness. CBD can change how your liver processes prescription drugs. If you're on prescription drugs, always check with your doctor before taking CBD.

Cannabis comes in different strains with different proportions of CBD versus THC. Some strains are CBD-dominant, CBD only, or CBD pure for symptom relief without the high. Specific strains are often prescribed or sold for specific medical conditions.

Options include prescription medical cannabis, recreational CBD pure cannabis, CBD e-cigarette vape juice, CBD oil, hemp CBD oil, etc.

Medicinal and recreational cannabis is legal in some countries, or parts of some countries.

Comfort, Emotional Support, Service Animals

Many people feel more relaxed when they're with their pet. It's comforting. My cats have always been my comfort animals. An allergy doctor once told me I had to get rid of my cat because of a severe allergy. I refused. So he told me when my cat died, I could never get another cat. When that sad day came, I really wasn't going to get a cat again. But my anxiety and depression got worse. Within a year, I had to get another comfort cat.

Emotional support animals are used by people who can't be separated from their pet, because it puts their emotional well-being at risk. These animals help ease anxiety or depression. They're used in Animal Assisted Therapy. Dogs and cats are most common, but other types of animals are also used for emotional support including birds, lizards, and monkeys.

Service animals are specially trained and medically certified for people with anxiety, depression, PTSD, or other conditions. Hearing dogs are trained for people with severe hearing loss or Deafness, and can also help people cope better with tinnitus. Service animals can serve in places other animals aren't allowed to go. Refusing to allow a service animal entry is discrimination against people with physical or emotional disabilities.

Air travel has become a big issue for people using emotional support and service animals. Different airlines have different rules and require-ments. Some don't allow animals at all, and some make the animal travel in air cargo. If allowed, documents needed usually include rabies and health certificates, as well as documentation from a medical or mental health professional certifying the need for the animal, e.g. the pet calms the owner and reduces risk of emotional problems while travelling.

Deep Breathing

When people feel stressed or anxious, they don't breathe as deeply as they should. One of the easiest and most helpful relaxation tools is deep or belly breathing. With deep breathing, you slowly breathe out as deeply as possible and then slowly breathe in as fully as possible. Deep breathing is done sitting or lying in a comfortable position for a few minutes at a time, e.g. 5 to 10 minutes. Other people can't tell if you are using deep breathing.

It's easy to practice during the day, e.g. in a lineup at a store, while sitting at a stoplight in a car, during a TV commercial. With practice, it's an effective relaxation technique to use before falling asleep or when you're feeling stressed or tense. The more you practice, the better it relaxes you. This is one example of how to do deep breathing.

Breathe out. Close mouth.

1. Breathe in through your nose slowly for a count of six: one, two, three, four, five, six, or until lungs feel stretched full of air like a full balloon.
2. Blow air out your mouth slowly for a count of six: one, two, three, four, five, six, or until lungs feel completely empty with no air left inside, like an empty balloon.
3. 1 round of deep breathing = 5 complete breaths in and out.

If you're short on time, even a few proper deep breaths in and out can help with relaxation. You can do more than one round at a time if you want. Use a time limit, e.g. deep breathing for 5 or 10 minutes or however long you want. When could you use deep breathing? Three times a day? At a stoplight? When you feel stressed or tense? Are your shoulders so tight they're almost up to your earlobes? Deep breathing.

Deep Breathing Apps

There are many self-help apps that include relaxing breathing exercises to use during the day or before sleep. Depending on the app, you can adjust the length of the inhale/exhale under settings.

Breathe2Relax uses a visual aid to teach deep breathing techniques; it was developed for military veterans with PTSD and is highly rated. I like it because it's easy to use, and quick to open if having an anxiety or panic attack.

Sanvello includes a deep breathing exercise, and Essence is another popular app that has a visual aid to help with timing breaths in and out. It uses a 4/7/8 technique: inhale through your nose for four seconds, hold your breath for seven seconds, then exhale through your mouth for eight seconds.

Hearing aid manufacturers offering free apps with deep breathing exercises include the Beltone Tinnitus Calmer app, Resound Tinnitus ReliefTM app, and Widex Zen Tinnitus Management app.

Left Nostril Breathing
Ancient yoga masters discovered people don't breathe evenly through their nostrils. We always breathe slightly more through one nostril than the other, and this changes constantly over the course of our day. Stronger right nostril breathing is linked to a logical or alert state of mind, and stronger left nostril breathing is linked to a relaxed or drowsy state of mind and less anxiety.

Right for relax = close off the right nostril. If a person is anxious or stressed, they can gently press down and close off their right nostril so they're breathing more through the left nostril.Everyone is individual, so a few people are more relaxed closing off the left nostril.

Meditation
When practiced regularly, meditation can calm the mind and bring feelings of relaxation and well-being. People do meditation in a quiet,

peaceful place. If possible, people with hyper ears benefit from using relaxation sound while meditating, e.g. water sounds, nature sounds, and gentle instrumental music.

There are many types of meditation. People can start meditating with a meditation teacher or class, but many people learn to meditate on their own. People spend 5 to 10 minutes on a meditation. It doesn't matter if you can't clear your thoughts. Recognizing there's a swirl of thoughts going on can help.

Regular practice means daily or several times a week. If possible, choose a regular time of day to practice. Some people find meditating at bedtime helps with relaxation.

Meditation Self-Help Apps
There are many self-help guided meditation apps available. Stop, Breathe, and Think includes info on how to meditate, which is helpful for people who've never meditated before. Smiling Mind also gives an intro to meditation and has programs for kids and different age groups.

Apps often include relaxing background sounds or music. Meditations can be long or short. For example, Aura has daily personalized 3 minute meditations, and instructions are open captioned so it's accessible. Free Beltone Tinnitus Calmer app and Resound Tinnitus ReliefTM app include short guided meditations.

People interested in more science or neuroscience based meditation might rather use apps like Meditation for Fidgety Skeptics or Headspace. Other popular apps for guided meditations include Ananda–Personalized Meditations, Calm, Buddify, and Insight Timer.

If you can't hear meditation audio instructions, there are free meditation scripts online to read, e.g. exploremeditation.com has Theta Frequency Guided Meditation and Relaxation Meditation scripts.

Monaural Beats

This is a type of brain entrainment that can also improve relaxation when using alpha and theta wave frequencies. Instead of 2 different frequencies sent to each ear to create the binaural beat frequency, with monaural beats the actual beat frequency is sent to one or both ears. People with single-sided or asymmetrical HL can use monaural beats.

The monaural beat pulses on and off in a specific pattern. People can listen to monaural beats with headphones or through a speaker for ambient room noise. This can be more comfortable for people who don't like using headphones when trying to relax.

There is little data on the effect of monaural beats since most scientists have studied binaural beats. Chaieb et al. (2017) found a significant improvement in anxiety for people listening to monaural beats compared to controls. Monaural beats are believed to be better, having a stronger effect on brain waves than binaural beats.

Different websites have monaural beat MP3s for brainwave entrainment. These include surginglife.com (monaural beats plus music), unexplainable. com (monaural beats plus white noise), pineal-wave.bandcamp.com (pure monaural beats). I don't know how good the sound quality or relaxation effect is for these MP3s.

Always check with your doctor before trying monaural beats to make sure it's safe for you, especially if you have mental health conditions or medical conditions like epilepsy, heart disease, or a pacemaker.

Monaural Beats Video Games

A new video game using monaural beats is coming out on Steam, iOS, and Xbox One. It's called SmashET. It uses simple game play and 5 different monaural beats options to help lower anxiety and improve relaxation, concentration, and sleep. Many people like playing a relaxing game with mental health benefits instead of something formally targeting their mental health. Other companies are also offering monaural and binaural beat video games.

Multimedia

There are lots of different relaxation apps, CDs, MP3s, music, shows, and videos in different formats. They're under categories like healthy lifestyle, chronic pain, sleep, tinnitus, or relaxation in libraries or stores.

News Breaks

When I first heard about news breaks as a relaxation method, I thought it sounded stupid. If I took a break from watching or reading the news, how would I know about current affairs? But most news is negative, upsetting, depressing, or maddening. Injuries, illness, crime, murder, war, discrimination, politics. People with hyper ears need to avoid negative, upsetting, depressing, maddening things. Is that putting your head in the sand like an ostrich? Maybe. But if it helps with coping better...

Jan's View

The first time, I tried a total TV news and newspaper break for 1 day. It worked. I felt more relaxed. I tried it longer. It still worked. I realized if anything major happened, I would hear it on the radio or see a headline somewhere on social media. If I think it will upset me, I don't check the full story.

I've used news breaks for weeks at a time. Sometimes I decide to avoid certain news sources or shows. Sometimes I only check the national or local news banner until it repeats and then I turn it off. Sometimes I stick to community news. I've never missed anything important. And I've avoided a lot of negativity.

Recently, I've made an effort to focus on funny, strange, or interesting news to read about. It gives me things to think about that aren't upsetting.

Progressive Muscle Relaxation (PMR)

This technique helps relax the body and calm the mind. It takes 10 to 15 minutes to do and people can relax muscles any time of day. Many people find it helpful to do before bedtime. PMR is a body scan technique used to tense and relax different muscle groups one at a time in a specific order. Some instructions start with the head and work down the body to the toes. Others start with the toes and work up to the head. The more regularly you practice PMR, the better it works.

This is one example:

1. Inhale and flex toes for 5 to 10 seconds. Flex muscles but not enough to hurt. Exhale and completely release the muscle tension. Relax for 10 to 20 seconds.
2. Keep working your way comfortably through muscle groups: feet, calves, knees, thighs, butt, stomach, chest, arch back, fingers, hands, arms, shoulders flexed towards ears, then face muscles including eyebrows raised, tightly closed eyes, wide open mouth to flex.
3. For each muscle group, slowly inhale while tensing for 5 to 10 seconds then slowly exhale while relaxing for 10 to 20 seconds. Some muscle groups might feel similar when you tense and relax them. Feet might seem similar to toes. That's okay.

After you're finished, take a few moments to see what it feels like to be more relaxed. The goal is to feel that way more often, so you're coping better with less tension.

Relaxation Apps

There are lots of apps with relaxation techniques, including deep breathing and PMR exercises. Apps come and go, so some disappear and new ones arrive from different developers. These apps are currently in several top app lists, have good reviews and high online user ratings for helpfulness:

- Ananda Personalized Meditations.
- Aura.
- Beltone Tinnitus Calmer.
- Breathe2Relax (highly recommended).
- Buddify.
- Calm.
- Essence.
- Headspace.
- I-DOSER (binaural beats).
- Insight Timer.
- Meditation for Fidgety Skeptics.
- Mindshift (teens to adults).
- Sanvello
- Smiling Mind.
- Stop Breathe Think.
- Stop Panic and Anxiety Self-Help.
- Self-Help for Anxiety Management.
- Widex Zen Tinnitus app (includes progressive muscle relaxation).

It's helpful to have an app guide you through relaxation techniques. Once you learn them, you don't have to use the app every time. For example, I use the PMR exercise on Sanvello. I like having a consistent way to do it every time so I can train my brain and body to relax.

Other Relaxation Techniques
People don't find the same things relaxing, so specific techniques vary from person to person. The following examples are just a few ideas of what works for some people. Have a warm shower or bath. Go for a

walk, or do some gentle exercises that make you feel good when you are finished.

Hug or cuddle somebody. Pet a dog or a cat. Have a nice cup of tea or a cool drink. Take 5 or 10 minutes and just sit or lie down in a pleasant place with no interruptions. Think about what makes you feel relaxed or at ease and try to make a point of setting aside time to relax during your daily life.

16

GUIDED IMAGERY TECHNIQUES

Visualization is daydreaming with a purpose.

- Bo Bennett -

Guided imagery or visualization is a mind therapy technique used for chronic pain. With guided imagery, a person shifts their attention to specific mental images or pictures instead of their tinnitus or hyper ears distress. It helps with relaxation and people say it creates a calm inner oasis. It's important to practice regularly for this technique to be most effective.

Some people can do guided imagery more easily than other people. Counselling specialists can help a person get good at developing imaginative mental images or scenes that involve all the senses, e.g. sight, touch, smell, taste, hearing. Experts say imagination techniques are not as helpful if used on their own. Guided imagery works best when combined with other mind therapy techniques.

Multimedia

Options for home practice include books and audio or audio-visual devices like MP3s, CDs, or DVDs. They're under the categories of relaxation, meditation, guided imagery, or creative visualization. Tools describe different imagery or visualization techniques and walk a person through them step by step.

Pleasant Imagery

Anyone with hyper ears can use this by imagining a scene enjoyable for them. With practice, people can use their imagination to picture different scenes to help take their mind off their hyper ears. For example, a person could imagine petting their cat. They could imagine how the cat looks, the softness of the fur, the warmth, smell, or sound of purring.

Some people use their imagination to picture pleasant memories. For example, people can remember a special vacation, an enjoyable family gathering, or favourite place in detail. Sometimes people use favourite pictures, paintings, or photographs of people or places they love to help them create positive mental images.

Other people use their imagination by choosing a pleasant daydream. For example, what would your dream vacation be like, or how would you play each hole of your favourite golf course?

Jan's View

While struggling with severe health issues, my partner imagined where we could go camping: Barkerville, British Columbia to pan for gold; Drumheller, Alberta to see dinosaur bones. It helped switch thoughts away from pain, and on to something positive in the future.

While travelling with a tour group in Wales in 2017, the cat people would chat about how much we missed our cats. "I made a recording on my phone of my cat purring," I announced somewhat proudly. "I listen when I miss him."

I didn't tell them I don't just listen. I use imagery along with the video. Imagining I'm holding his soft warm vibrating body in my arms. Pressing kisses against his ginger fur. Picturing how I make him purr louder when I give him a squeeze as if he's part bagpipe. Imagining his slightly stinky cat breath smell. My uncontrollable sneezes from his fur.

This guided imagery mind therapy tool is personal. Nobody ever recommended it. I came up with it in 2017, based on what I know about mind therapy techniques. Another new coping tool that works well for me at home and away from home.

A good guided imagery example is from a person who loved hiking with his family, but noticed his tinnitus because it was so quiet outdoors. He was always thinking negative thoughts when hiking, e.g. What if my tinnitus bothers me so much I can't hike with my family anymore? The relaxation techniques he had learned didn't help, so he focused on distraction techniques. Pleasant conversation with hiking companions; identifying birds or animals from their sounds or tracks; counting or identifying plants, birds, or animals along the hike; rock hunting along the trail if interested; alphabet distraction wish list of places to hike.

Another idea was to focus on his senses. Trying to imagine describing the hike to someone. What landmarks did he see? What specific colours and shades would describe things around him like the ground, plants, sky, people, animals? What sensations was he feeling like crunch of trail underfoot, warmth of sun on skin? What can he smell along the hike like crushed foliage, dirt? What is his favourite part of the hike? The idea is to focus and be mindful in the moment. He could use this later as a pleasant guided imagery visualization.

Tinnitus Imagery

Imagine a scene that involves all the senses including sound effects similar to your tinnitus. For example, if your tinnitus sounds like a buzz, you might imagine bumblebees in a garden full of flowers.

Another technique is to imagine tinnitus as something specific and then change it. When you change your tinnitus image, the tinnitus may change. Different people might think of images like an ear on fire, a hornet, or a chainsaw. One person might imagine pouring water on the ear to put out the fire. Another person might imagine squashing the hornet with a rolled-up magazine. Another might imagine the chainsaw turning into a soft power drill. Or imagine smashing the chainsaw to pieces with a sledgehammer.

One person had tinnitus that sounded like a train whistle. She would imagine a mountain scene with a railroad track running through it with a train whistling away. She found with practice this helped make her tinnitus thoughts more neutral, along with using other relaxation and distraction techniques.

Guided Imagery Self-Help Apps

Guided imagery techniques are included on apps like Headspace, Smiling Mind, Calm, Stop Breathe Think, Beltone Tinnitus Calmer, and Widex Zen Tinnitus Management.

PART IV

BODY THERAPY TOOLS

17

DENTISTRY

Health is the soul that animates all the enjoyments of life, which fade and are tasteless without it.

- Lucius Annaeus Seneca -

Oral health is very important for the hearing system. Bacteria in the mouth from bad oral health can get in the bloodstream, cause inflammation, and stop blood from flowing to the inner ears. Blood circulation problems cause high blood pressure or other heart disease that's linked to sensorineural hearing loss. Brushing teeth and flossing regularly are important as well as following your dentist and dental hygienist's recommendations. For procedures like cavities or root canals, find a dental office where the staff will accommodate your tinnitus-hyperacusis needs.

Dental Equipment & Hearing Protection
Noise levels of ultrasonic tools used to clean teeth are usually less than

85 dB (but often incorrectly reported at up to 98 to 107 dB loudness depending on the source). This can be uncomfortably loud; ultrasonic tools are linked to hyper ears flare-ups in some people. If asked, most dental offices will clean teeth using manual tools instead of ultrasonic devices.

Other dental tools can be loud, including high speed suction at 72 to 75 dB, and drills at 88 to 102 dB depending on the manufacturer. This can make tinnitus worse temporarily and be painful for people with hyperacusis. Some people are able to tolerate 5 minutes on-5 minutes off or other timing intervals.

Dr. Nagler's Tinnitus Corner (2015) shared advice from Dr. Jack Vernon (2001): "Earplugs will block some of the air-conducted sound that goes through the ear canal. But the majority of the sound from a dental drill is conducted to the inner ear by the bones in the face and head. You could ask your dentist to drill in short spurts, 5 seconds on and 10 seconds off. (To our knowledge, no dentist has refused to do this for patient when the patient asked.) The exacerbation of tinnitus by loud sound is a time-intensity function. Although you cannot control the sound intensity of the high-speed drill, you can control the length of time that you are exposed to it."

Amalgam (Mercury) Dental Fillings

These are silver coloured metal fillings that have a high percentage of mercury. Science suggests mercury vapour from these fillings can damage the hearing system over years. Some people with tinnitus report lower tinnitus severity after having their amalgam fillings replaced with fillings that don't contain mercury.

There can be complications or side effects from having mercury fillings removed. Dentists experienced in this procedure can discuss risks, safety precautions, and how to detoxify your body after removal.

Jan's View

Many years ago, I had all the mercury fillings taken out of my teeth. I had to take special pills for the detox. Luckily the dentist told me I might be more sensitive to the detox than average since I have hyper ears and chronic pain. They suggested I go 50% slower than recommended on their handouts. I'm glad they did; even the 1/2 dose knocked me off my feet for a few days. I don't think having the mercury fillings removed made any difference to my hearing or hyper ears, but I think it was good prevention of future hearing health problems. I make sure new fillings are never mercury.

Neuromuscular Dentistry

Dental treatment for problems with the jaw joint or Temporo-Mandibular joint (TMJ) can help people with hyper ears. If you have symptoms like face, neck, or jaw pain, headaches, or clicking jaw noises, a dentist could check for TMJ disorders.

Neuromuscular dentistry focuses on correcting jaw misalignments or jaw dysfunction from TMJ problems or TMD (TemporoMandibular Dysfunction). It helps improve TMJ position and function, typically by using special appliances that guide the jaw and attached muscles into a relaxed position.

With current tech, clinics can do computerized scans to custom fit appliances like nightguards. People wear mouth nightguards (occlusal guards/splints, bite splints) to line up the upper and lower teeth into the proper position. Some nightguards help stop teeth grinding or clenching. Many people with tinnitus and jaw problems report improvement after TMJ treatment.

Jan's View

I've been treated for TMJ dysfunction for years. I've been through tech changes in nightguards from the old hard plastic taken from teeth molds to the new custom scanned thermoplastic material that softens with heat when worn. The latest ones are comfortable and fit better.

18

DIET & SUPPLEMENTS

Let food be thy medicine and medicine be thy food. - Hippocrates

-

Experts sometimes tell people with tinnitus to avoid certain food (e.g. sugar, salt, chocolate) and avoid drinks with alcohol. But something that affects one person's tinnitus can have no effect on somebody else. Many people won't change their diet if the change will increase distress at the loss of something nice like enjoying a chocolate bar or glass of wine.

Research doesn't show a significant effect from caffeine, but some people with tinnitus would disagree. Caffeine makes their tinnitus worse. Caffeine is in coffee, tea, and chocolate, but read labels carefully because it can also be in energy drinks and some types of mints.

Science using animal models found a daily dose of caffeine hurts recovery after noise damage. Even if caffeine doesn't make tinnitus worse, people exposed to acoustic trauma or chronic noise over time might want to consider cutting or reducing caffeine for better hearing health.

If you need to lower or cut your caffeine intake, do it gradually to avoid withdrawal headaches. Don't go overnight from 12 cups of coffee daily to zero cups of coffee. Instead, you could cut a cup of coffee a day over a few weeks until your caffeine intake is down to a reasonable amount (e.g. 1 to 3 cups a day) or no caffeine at all if you're very sensitive. If you're able to enjoy reasonable amounts of caffeine, don't have it within 6 hours of bedtime, otherwise it can make it hard to fall and stay asleep.

Some people cut out certain food or drinks to see if their tinnitus improves. After about a week, people try the food or drink again to see if it affects their tinnitus. The problem is tinnitus goes up and down so much for no particular reason, it's hard to tell if improvement is from the diet change or a normal tinnitus change. People need to repeat the process a couple of times to see if the food or drink is really affecting the tinnitus. If it turns out a food or drink does affect their tinnitus, people can make the decision whether they want to change their diet all or some of the time.

People who eat a banana a day have less hearing loss because bananas are a good source of potassium for hearing health.

People who eat a healthy diet have less hearing loss than people who eat an unhealthy diet. Scientists studied women using 3 different diet systems: Alternate Mediterranean Diet, Dietary Approaches to Stop Hypertension (DASH), and Alternative Healthy Eating Index. Women using the Mediterranean and DASH diets were 30% less likely to have moderate or severe hearing loss. These diets are high in fiber (vegetables, fruits, whole grains, nuts, legumes) with low sugar and salt. The Mediterranean diet includes more fish and olive oil. The same results likely apply to men.

DIETARY SUPPLEMENTS

People often try dietary supplements for tinnitus. Coelho et al. (2016) found 70% of people reported no tinnitus benefit after taking dietary supplements. Out of the people surveyed; 19% reported improvement, and 6% reported side effects including bleeding, diarrhea, and headaches. Experts don't recommend dietary supplements to treat tinnitus, even though some might help a limited number of individuals. Don't take mega-doses of any supplement. Supplements don't replace a healthy diet. Get medical clearance before taking any.

Antioxidants help protect cells in our bodies from damage, maintain health, and prevent disease. Some science suggests antioxidants protect hearing from noise damage.

Food sources of antioxidants include green leafy vegetables like spinach and kale, or orange and red coloured fruits and vegetables like carrots, sweet potatoes, mangos, and tomatoes. Some meats, fish, breads, grains, nuts, dairy products, and oils contain antioxidants. A diet that includes recommended daily amounts of antioxidants is likely helpful for overall health including hearing health.

Companies might advertise antioxidant supplements as a "hearing protection" pill. While these products might protect the hearing by strengthening the ears' natural defenses, anyone exposed to hazardous noise should always use proper hearing protection.

Iron Deficiency Anemia (IDA) is when red blood cells don't have the hemoglobin they need to carry enough oxygen through the body. Anemic adults are twice as likely to have sensorineural and mixed hearing loss. This is likely because anemic people don't have the high blood oxygen levels needed for the inner ears to stay healthy. That means quick diagnosis and treatment for IDA is very important for people's hearing health.

IDA can happen at any age and in people of any ethnicity. Symptoms include weight loss, fatigue, headache, and dizziness. IDA is most common in pregnant women and women who menstruate. Chemotherapy, kidney disease, sickle cell anemia, and genetics can cause IDA.

Scientists don't recommend iron supplements as hearing loss treatment. More science is needed on how iron might protect our hearing.

People should be able to get enough iron from a healthy diet, with help from a dietician if needed. Iron rich food includes meat, fish and poultry, dried beans, peas and lentils, some fruits and vegetables, and iron fortified grain products like flour, pasta, or breakfast cereal. Dietician websites usually have full lists of food sources of iron.

Lipoflavonoids are a vitamin product that includes a lemon extract (citrus bioflavonoid) plant base, vitamin C, and other B vitamins. Some people say lipoflavonoids will help ear conditions like imbalance, Meniere's, or tinnitus. Evidence-based science shows lipoflavonoids do not give any more benefit than a placebo, despite positive reports from people using lipoflavonoids as a dietary supplement.

Magnesium deficiency is linked with tinnitus-hyperacusis and increased risk of noise-induced hearing loss. Magnesium increases blood circulation, and some people call it the calming or anti-stress mineral. Food sources of magnesium include nuts, whole grains, legumes, and green leafy vegetables. People could consider taking a regular daily vitamin and mineral supplement with magnesium to maintain healthy levels in your system. If taking a magnesium supplement, check with your doctor or pharmacist to make sure it's in a form that's absorbable by the body.

Vitamin B12 Some people who get noise-induced hearing loss and tinnitus from chronic noise exposure might be low in B vitamins. Your doctor can check this. Some people low in B12 get weekly B12 injections from their doctor to help reduce tinnitus severity. If you're taking a regular daily vitamin and mineral supplement, consider one with good amounts of B complex vitamins with more B12 compared to other B complex vitamins in the supplement.

Zinc levels may be low in some people with tinnitus. The highest concentration of zinc in our bodies is in the inner ears. Studies have shown that people with low zinc levels had a decrease in tinnitus after taking zinc supplements. People may want to consider taking a regular daily vitamin and mineral supplement that contains zinc to maintain healthy levels in their bodies. Some experts say if you try a zinc lozenge and it doesn't have much taste, you could be low in zinc. If it tastes bad, your zinc levels are probably fine.

The Tonaki Tinnitus Protocol claims to cure tinnitus in 21 days if people drink their special smoothie recipes. The ingredients are said to fix missing hearing nerve "fat" or myelin sheath. The ingredients are found in food most people already eat. Marketing includes bashing the healthcare industry and "testimonials" using pictures from purchased stock photos online. Website operation-wellness.com calls this product a scam. In my opinion, it looks like cure ale. Any benefit is likely no more than the placebo effect.

ADAPTOGENS

Adaptogens are a plant or herbal tonic that help the body fight chronic stress. They come in pills or powders people add to recipes. Naturopathic doctors decide what adaptogens might help individuals. Adaptogens don't replace a healthy diet. Get medical clearance before taking.

Ashwagandha is used in Ayurvedic medicine first developed in India. It's supposed to help men and women with memory, exhaustion, and bad sleep. Ashwagandha is an anti-oxidant and anti-inflammatory that can help fight the effects of chronic stress on our bodies.

Ginseng: Maca or Peruvian is a broccoli-like adaptogen with a nutty flavour. It's said to help anxiety and depression in post-menopausal women.

Ginseng: Asian or Siberian (eleuthero) are said to improve physical and mental energy.

Holy Basil (tulsi) has been used in South Asian folk medicine. It's supposed to help fight chronic stress inflammatory effects.

Lemon Balm is similar to mint and often used in tea. If you plant it in your garden, it will spread everywhere including flower beds and lawns; it's really hard to get rid of after that happens.

Licorice is another anti-inflammatory used in Ayurvedic medicine. It's supposed to make effects of other herbs stronger, so it's often used in combination formulas.

Rhodiola (golden or arctic root) is a traditional medicine in China, Serbia, Scandinavia, and the Ukraine. It's usually used in teas or extracts and is said to help lower physical and mental fatigue or exhaustion from stress.

HERBAL SUPPLEMENTS

These are some common herbal supplements people take for tinnitus or hyperacusis. Get medical clearance before taking.

Black Cohosh is an herbal remedy most often used to treat menopausal symptoms and arthritis. People with tinnitus sometimes use it. Research hasn't found any benefit.

Gingko Biloba is the most popular herbal treatment for tinnitus and is said to be helpful for hearing and concentration. If tinnitus is from blood circulation problems, gingko is more likely to help.

Europeans use gingko biloba along with other treatment approaches. Large scale research studies have found no benefit in general but some people do report less tinnitus after taking gingko biloba. Available studies used different dosages or had study method flaws, making it hard to prove any benefit. Gingko biloba can interact with prescription medications, and can have side effects including indigestion, depression, and potential cardiovascular or heart related effects.

St. John's Wort is an herb used for tinnitus treatment. It's used to treat mild to moderate depression. Science hasn't found tinnitus benefit in general, but it might help some people. St. John's Wort can have side effects or interact with prescription medications.

Valerian is a sedating herb used for thousands of years for anxiety and insomnia. It's believed safe and not addictive or habit-forming.

TINNITUS SUPPLEMENTS

Different manufacturers sell tinnitus supplements with different dietary and herbal ingredients. Benefit depends on ingredient quality so manufacturer reputation is important. Even if these products don't change tinnitus-hyperacusis, they can help improve hearing health. Avoid cure sales. Don't take supplements without clearance from your medical doctor.

Tinnitus 911 is a supplement with a combination of plants, vitamins, and minerals. There is no independent scientific evidence to support this product helps or cures tinnitus as claimed. Their website used to use scare tactics, saying if you didn't use the product you would get dementia; saying if you didn't buy right away, they might run out completely or not have any to ship. The website home page used to have a testimonial from a man named Charlie Gains giving a rave review. In the footer tiny fine print, it stated "Any likeness to a real Charlie Gains living or dead is entirely coincidental."

This is all allegedly, because they've revamped to a slicker website as of 2017. There are loads of online reviews saying this product is a scam. In my opinion, this is cure ale. For a well researched review by scientist Joe Cannon, see supplementclarity.com.

Arches Tinnitus Formula
Manufacturer—Arches Natural Products.
Company in Operation—1998 to date.
Ingredients—antioxidants, zinc, gingko biloba.
Cost— $40 per bottle or discount for multiple
$129 for 3 month supply starter kit (4 bottles).
Tinnitus Stress Formula—$40 per bottle (high potency vitamin B complex).
Tinnitus B12 Formula—$30 per bottle (high potency B12).
Antioxidant Formula—$40 per bottle.
Tinnitus Combo Kit—$170 3 month supply of Arches Tinnitus, Stress, and B12 Formulas.

Mr. B. Keates developed the original Tinnitus Formula about 25 years ago based mainly on European science. He founded the company with Mr. B. Curtis. Key ingredients include antioxidants, zinc, and gingko biloba.

Arches doesn't claim their product cures tinnitus. They offer a 3 month supply, which suggests they know that's often the length of time to see improvement. Their website tinnitusformula.com has science-based info on tinnitus supplement ingredients. Arches has a tinnitus news-letter called Quiet Times and an "Ask Barry" section.

Arches is doing clinical trials to determine tinnitus benefit for people using their Arches Tinnitus Formula. Care providers can contact Arches to be added to the clinical trial if you're interested in participating.

19

EXERCISE

Along with physical benefits, exercise can distract attention from tinnitus, reduce stress and anxiety, improve mood, and help with relaxation.

Exercise doesn't mean major athletics or aerobics. Gentle activities like walking, swimming, or stretching are helpful. Many people with hyper ears find gentle exercises help with flexibility, strength, cardiovascular fitness, and overall wellness.

Sometimes people notice tinnitus temporarily goes up after exercise. This is common after people safely elevate their heart rate with a cardiovascular workout. Exercise benefit outweighs any temporary change. Check with your doctor if you have any concerns, or before starting any new exercise routine.

Biking is a quiet environmentally friendly exercise. People with bad balance sometimes use three wheeled bicycles, three wheeled electric bicycles, or three wheeled electric scooters people sit on to ride. They're easy to use, especially if you have chronic pain or fatigue.

Gardening is good exercise that uses the major muscle groups, e.g. legs, arms, stomach, back, shoulders, neck. It helps flexibility and makes joints stronger. Many people enjoy puttering around in the garden deadheading even if they can't do heavier garden work.

Laughter is good exercise. Experts say 1 minute of laughing gets your heart rate up as much as 10 minutes on a rowing machine.

Qigong, quigong, or quijong means energy cultivation. It's a daily routine of body movements, breathing, and meditation used since before recorded history over 5,000 years ago. Qigong is based in Chinese medicine, philosophy, and martial arts. The exercises build up healing energy called qi or chi. This lowers stress, helps mental illness including depression, gives people more energy, better health, and a better sense of well-being.

Science on quigong for tinnitus found people who completed 5 weeks of quigong training reported significant improvement in tinnitus severity with effects lasting at least 3 months after the training ended.

Swinging Not that type of swinging! I mean using a swing set or porch swing and swinging gently, but only if your doctor or ear specialist says it's safe for you. Swinging can help exercise the balance system since the brain needs to match up sensory info from open eyes and inner ear balance systems. If swinging ever makes you lightheaded or dizzy, safely slow and stop.

If on a swing set, hold on tight. Start very slow and gentle. Feel the air against your face and your body movement. Your feet against the ground propelling you. The outdoor colours and smells.

I like to get going fast and pretend I'm flying. It's the fastest I can go in real life, and it makes me feel better. I only swing at the playground if I have kids with me using the swings, or when there are no children. Otherwise it looks weird to have a lone adult swinging at the playground. If you're going to use a public swing set—and you're not a child or teen—do it at an appropriate time.

Tai Chi or Tai chi chuan is a Chinese system of gentle physical exercise and stretching developed about 2000 years ago. It uses a series of movements that flow into each other without pausing. The gentle flowing poses are sometimes called meditation in motion. Experts say Tai chi improves relaxation, balance and agility, reduces stress, and helps wellbeing. This helps some people by reducing stress and increasing feelings of relaxation.

Yoga is an ancient Indian exercise practice. It's a method to gain control over the body and mind. Yoga includes physical techniques or postures, breathing techniques, and mental techniques, e.g. meditation. There are different types of yoga classes depending on fitness level. Experts recommend yoga for people with hyper ears. Yoga can lower stress and increase feelings of relaxation. Some poses will make tinnitus louder or sound different.

Jan's View

My T jumps around in loudness and pitch when I do yoga. If I make myself into a pretzel, balancing on one leg, with my head hanging upside down turned a certain angle, my T goes away. It's nice while it lasts, but not practical in daily life.

Fitness Activity Trackers are wearable tech usually worn on the wrist. They log fitness activities or health, e.g. count footsteps, heart rate, body temperature. They help some people stay motivated to follow fitness programs. Trackers can wirelessly connect to Bluetooth enabled devices. Science suggests they might help with weight loss when tracking diet, but it's unclear if using fitness activity trackers changes how much people exercise.

20

PHYSIOTHERAPY

It does not matter how slowly you go as long as you do not stop.

- Confucius -

Pain management is an effective treatment tool for hyper ears. Many people with tinnitus-hyperacusis have chronic pain, including headaches and arthritis. Any effective treatment for pain can improve well-being and coping abilities in general. Physiotherapists are often care providers for people with hyper ears.

Somatic Tinnitus
Somatic tinnitus is from neck or jaw problems can cause pain and tinnitus called somatic tinnitus. People with somatic tinnitus can change how their tinnitus sounds with head or neck movements like clenched jaws, tongue stuck out, and/or turning or flexing their necks. It's estimated 36 to 43% of people with tinnitus have somatic tinnitus. That seems low to me.

A 2016 systematic review of studies on physiotherapy for neck and TMJ treatment found significant benefit for making tinnitus less severe. Treatments included manipulations, triggerpoint treatment, neck or jaw exercises, splints, and bite adjustments. Although results looked positive, more research was recommended with larger sample sizes, current high tech treatments, better criteria for including subjects, and better consistent tinnitus treatment outcome measures. No universal treatment outcome measure for tinnitus science is bad for physiotherapy science too!

Targeted Bimodal Auditory-Somatosensory Stimulation
Scientists at the Kresge Hearing Research Institute at University of Michigan, US, are studying a new treatment for somatic tinnitus called Bimodal Stimulation. It works by changing brain activity causing tinnitus. The treatment uses a combo of 2 senses: hearing and touch.

People listen to sound matched to their tinnitus pitch and loudness precisely timed with mild electrical impulses, usually on the neck or cheek. The electrical impulses come from electrodes with small pads attached to the skin.

A clinical trial on 20 subjects used the sound plus electricity device for 30 minutes a day for 4 weeks. Results were compared to the same subjects only listening to the sound for 30 minutes a day for 4 weeks. None of the subjects reported any improvement when only listening to sound, but they likely knew they weren't getting active treatment.

With active treatment, 50% of subjects had significantly less tinnitus distress, reporting softer tinnitus and tinnitus that sounded less annoying. By the 4th week of treatment, subjects' tinnitus loudness was softer by an average of 12 dB. Two subjects reported their tinnitus went away completely—very unusual for any other current tinnitus therapy. All the subjects' tinnitus went back to usual about a week after treatment ended.

The scientists are studying which people might get the most benefit, if the treatment will work on non-somatic tinnitus, and the best length of treatment. It's not clear if longer treatment will help benefit last longer after treatment ends. The University of Michigan has patented the device. No word yet on what it will be called or cost when it becomes available clinically or for at home use.

21

PRESCRIPTION DRUGS

I believe in prescription drugs. I believe in feeling better.

- Denis Leary -

There are currently no approved prescription drugs for tinnitus-hyperacusis. Researchers are working on drugs to cure hearing loss and tinnitus or hyperacusis from different causes.

Many drugs prescribed for anxiety and depression have tinnitus or hyperacusis as a side effect. Discuss any concerns with your doctor. Follow your family doctor or ear specialist's recommendations for any drug treatments, including over-the-counter medications.

Sedley et al. (2015) looked at how tinnitus is mapped in the brain. In an interview with Knox (2015), co-author Gander said, *"We found essentially that almost all the hearing parts of the brain are involved plus a number of other areas of the brain related to processing emotion and memory and attention...Maybe the reason tinnitus is so treatment-resistant is because it's involved with so many parts of the brain."*

In a 2015 Tinnitus Today interview, Dr. P.J. Jastreboff who developed the neurophysiological model of tinnitus said, *"I believe it will be impossible to find a medication to cure tinnitus (meaning removing the tinnitus perception) because the neurophysiological mechanisms involved in tinnitus perception are too intertwined with the normal function of the auditory system (e.g., it is possible to evoke tinnitus just by spending a few minutes in a very quiet environment). I remain skeptical about medications for the cure of tinnitus."*

Acamprosate is a drug used to treat alcohol addiction. Since a Brazilian study in 2005, people have reported acamprosate could improve or cure tinnitus. The problem is the sample size for the Brazilian study was 25 people. These results have never been repeated or verified by any other research studies. Acamprosate has serious side effects including depression and suicide. It's also ototoxic, causing hearing loss, tinnitus, dizziness, and auditory hallucinations. Experts do not recommend acamprosate for tinnitus.

Ototoxic Drugs cause ear or balance system damage, e.g. hearing loss, tinnitus, imbalance, or vertigo. These include cisplatin or platinum-based chemotherapy for head and neck cancers. Ototoxic "mycin" antibiotics include streptomycin, tobramycin, gentamicin, neomycin, and vancomycin. Furosemide or Lasix is an ototoxic drug used to treat fluid build-up from heart, liver, or kidney disease.

Quinine and salicylates, like in aspirin, are ototoxic. Salicylates are in many over-the-counter medications and prescription drugs. Some people taking regular daily low dose aspirin report tinnitus or worse tinnitus that gets better when they stopped taking aspirin.

Ototoxicity depends on different factors including how large a dose, how long a person takes the drug, genetics, and family history of drug related ear problems. Doctors try not to prescribe ototoxic drugs for the elderly or people with hearing loss. When needed, doctors prescribe the lowest dose possible, closely monitor the dose by testing drug levels in the blood, and hearing is tested before and during treatment. This includes standard audiometry and extended high frequency audiometry.

If ototoxicity is detected, drug treatment is stopped unless the condition is life-threatening and there are no safer alternatives. Sometimes hearing loss and imbalance recover, at least partly.

22

BODY THERAPY APPROACHES

*To keep the body in good health is a duty... otherwise we shall
not be able to keep our mind strong and clear.*

- Buddha -

Over the centuries, people around the world have tried different
tinnitus body therapies. Egyptians poked reeds into the ears. Assyrians
chanted spells. Romans filled ears with earthworms boiled in goose
grease. The Welsh used hot bread fresh out of the oven, torn in half and
held over the ears. There are better tool options now. And options that
won't do any more than greasy boiled earthworms or hot bread.

There are body therapy options for physical health, hearing health, and
specifically for tinnitus-hyperacusis. Relaxation approaches are helpful
for misophonia (and phonophobia). When people are in as good health
as possible, it's easier to cope. Avoid fads and trends. Eat healthy.
Drink lots of water. Don't smoke. Make lifestyle choices that make you
feel good.

Since people with hyper ears are higher risk for chronic pain, and dental or jaw problems, professional care providers often include dentists and physiotherapists. Some tinnitus body therapies or treatments are not science-based. Make sure anybody you're seeing for body therapy is certified and/or licensed.

Acoustic Stimulation (PAXX)
This tinnitus treatment is said to lower hearing system hyperactivity and help people habituate to tinnitus. It uses a PAXX device with earbuds. Sound is customized for each person's tinnitus and hearing loss. People use the device daily for 3 months, then every other day for 3 to 12 months, and then as needed. It costs about $700 and is sold in over 20 countries. Trial periods may be shorter than the 3 months some people need to know if the device helps or not.

Acoustic Trauma Emergency Drugs
Scientists are working on emergency intra-tympanic drug delivery for the military. The needle delivery is similar to Epi-pens for allergic reactions. After acoustic trauma, military personnel could jab the needle through their eardrums to deliver a saline solution drug as soon as possible after the exposure. These drugs help maintain inner ear health and reverse any inner ear noise damage.

Acupuncture
This is an ancient Chinese healing system where a licensed acupuncturist uses fine needles inserted into the body at specific therapy points. Science is mixed on whether acupuncture helps lower tinnitus severity, but it can improve relaxation and that can improve coping.

Jan's View

I've used acupuncture for a serious stress-related health problem. Acupuncture didn't change my tinnitus or hyperacusis. But it helped me become deeply relaxed; this carried over into my daily life, so I was less stressed out and coped better.

Acupressure

This is a healing system like acupuncture that can improve relaxation. It uses gentle pressure on specific pressure points on the body instead of needles. Different books or courses on acupressure show therapy points for the ear or tinnitus.

Aromatherapy

This ancient approach is used to heal and balance people's body systems. In ancient times, people burned aromatic plants to smoke illness out, and different ancient civilizations used aromatic plants and extracts. Now aromatherapy uses essential oils, either alone or in combination. Effect of aromatherapy for anxiety or pain is still uncertain based on science.

People sometimes use essential oil atomizers (e.g. diffusers, electric diffusers, nebulizers) to spread a fine mist of oils into the air. Aromatherapy might help with general well-being.

If you have pets, always check with your vet before using essential oils since some are toxic, and the scent can be very irritating to cats, dogs, birds, and other pets who have much better senses of smell than humans.

For babies and children, experts recommend getting professional advice on safe essential oils, and instructions on how to dilute and use them including never in ears, never by mouth, and never in bath water.

Autogenic Training (AT)

German psychiatrist J.H. Schultz developed AT in 1932. AT is a stress management and relaxation technique. With meditation you focus on your breathing, and with progressive muscle relaxation you focus on relaxing your muscles. With AT you focus on different areas of the body.

Experts say with regular practice, AT calms the body's overactive fight-or-flight stress response. People using AT report a better quality of life and better mental health. AT helps psychosomatic or mind-body disorders, e.g. anxiety and depression. World-class athletes and NASA astronauts use AT for peak performance training.

AT is usually used with guided imagery and other mental techniques, so it's hard to find science on benefit of AT alone. AT is a very structured process. It can take months of regular daily practice, 3 times a day, to see the full health benefits. Autogenic training teaches your body to respond to your mental commands when you're feeling stressed. It's a form of self-hypnosis.

When doing AT, the person sits or lies down comfortably. They do a series of 6 mental exercises to create specific sensations in different parts of the body. The sensations are associated with being physically relaxed, e.g. heaviness in arms and legs, warmth in arms and legs, calm regular heartbeat, calm regular breathing, warm stomach, cool forehead. With practice, people can use mental commands to calm their body into an AT state of relaxation. This helps lower stress.

People with heart conditions, severe mental or emotional disorders, and children under 5 should not use AT. Sometimes doing self-help AT can make anxiety worse. Autogenic therapists like psychologists give professional guidance for training exercises. It's possible to find AT mobile apps or AT MP3s from reputable developers. Use caution and check with your doctor first before trying AT.

Biofeedback
With biofeedback, people train their mind to control various body

functions including blood pressure, muscle tension, heart rate, etc. It's very useful for treating stress-related conditions. The results are similar to Autogenic Training, except no devices to monitor body functions are needed with AT.

Since tinnitus-hyperacusis are aggravated by stress, biofeedback could be helpful for some people. By gaining control over their body, people often feel more in control of their life in general. Even with practice, some people are better at using biofeedback techniques than others. Some experts say biofeedback is not helpful when used alone, but helps in combination with other coping strategies.

Brain Surface Implants
This is an invasive experimental treatment. Experts don't recommend invasive treatments for tinnitus, because there are so many non-invasive effective treatments like sound therapy, mind therapy, and body therapy approaches. With Brain Surface Implants, neurosurgeons place electrodes on the brain's surface. Scientists don't know the best spot to place the electrodes yet to reduce tinnitus. There are serious brain surgery risks.

Chiropractic
Manual adjustment techniques, usually along the spine, treat back pain, neck pain, headaches, and migraines. Some people say chiropractic helps their tinnitus. In people with tinnitus and musculoskeletal pain, chiropractic could help general coping since pain relief gives better well-being overall.

Cochlea Destruction
In rare cases, doctors use surgery to destroy the cochlea, e.g. past treatment for single-sided, very severe Meniere's. In one case, a musician with single-sided sudden hearing loss also had hyperacusis and diplacusis or impaired pitch perception. Doctors destroyed his cochlea on that side. It helped the hyperausis and diplacusis, but he was off balance for the rest of his life.

Cranio-Sacral Therapy
Gentle skull manipulations treat conditions like headaches, migraines, jaw pain, and repeated ear or sinus infections in children. It may be available through osteopaths or chiropractors. This approach might help with pain relief and general health for people with tinnitus and head pain.

Cure for Deafness
In 2018, scientists at Harvard Medical School confirmed a sensor protein TMC1 (transmembrane channel-like 1) is key for converting sound waves reaching the inner ear hair cells into electrical signals. This important discovery greatly adds to what is known about inner ear biology. Dr. P. Barr-Gillespie, a professor of otolaryngology and director of the Hearing Restoration Project at Oregon Health & Science University, stated, "it's going to be a really important piece in moving forward to understanding various causes of deafness." This type of research will help scientists work towards finding cures for Deafness and hearing loss that might also help tinnitus and decreased sound tolerance.

Deep Brain Stimulation (DBS)
This is an invasive experimental treatment not recommended by experts. DBS is used for people with Parkinson's, tremors, or other medical conditions. Scientists stimulate the brain with electromagnetic energy from surgically implanted electrodes. Most data is from people who were getting DBS treatment for something else, but also had tinnitus. Some people had less tinnitus during and after DBS. Some didn't. Scientists don't know yet which part of the brain is best to stimulate for tinnitus.

Desyncra for Tinnitus uses neuromodulation (described later in this chapter). It's available in different countries, and the cost is several thousand dollars. Trial periods may be shorter than the 3 months some people need to know if the device helps or not.

Eardrum or Intra-Tympanic Drug Delivery
Drugs delivered through the eardrum can now be used for some inner ear disorders. Doctors inject drugs like steroids through the eardrum for conditions including Meniere's disease or sudden sensorineural hearing loss. I hate shots and needles, but I would get this if it helped.

That's why after sudden hearing loss, the faster people get to emergency services for treatment, the more likely the hearing loss will recover. Early evidence shows related sudden onset tinnitus might get better, but there's no evidence these steroid injections help tinnitus alone with no other condition.

e-Cigarettes Or Vaping
Non-organic vape juice used in e-cigarettes almost always has Propylene Glycol (PG) in it. PG is an ototoxic alcohol-based solvent that can cause hearing damage including tinnitus, hyperacusis, and hearing loss. It's not an allergy or sensitivity; ototoxic chemicals damage the hearing system. There are other unhealthy chemicals in vape juice including antifreeze and cancer causing ingredients. There are no warnings about PG risk to hearing health on package labelling.

Manufacturers list VG/PG Ratio for vape juice flavours. VG/PG Ratio is how much vegetable glycerin versus PG is in the e-juice. Organic or 100% VG e-juice shouldn't contain PG or only in tiny amounts. Max VG may or may not have PG depending on the manufacturer. VG is thicker with a sweet flavour, shorter shelf life, and possible equipment maintenance issues from build-up on coils, wicks, or other components.

When governments and experts discuss e-cigarette safety, they don't consider PG hearing health damage to vapers of all ages. PG should be banned in vape juice given the high risk of hyper ears and hearing loss.

Don't use vape juice with PG. It's not worth the risk. It might not do anything obvious to some people. But there's no way to know ahead of time if you're going to be the one with a permanently damaged hearing system. Stick to organic vape juice or 100% VG vape juice if you use e-cigarettes.

New science shows significant risk of lung disease from vaping. E-cigarettes are likely not safe to use.

Jan's View

I started vaping in November 2016 for anxiety. I'd heard vaping could be calming, so I thought I'd give it a try. I got myself set up with mint vape juice. Vaped a little, 2 or 3 puffs, once or twice a day. Some days none. It helped my anxiety.

I started feeling caterpillars crawling in my ears. I kept touching my ears expecting to feel fat fuzzy wriggling bodies stopping up the holes. How could that be from vaping?

Then I was googling around and found lots of reports on vaping and the ears: vaping causes tinnitus, makes tinnitus worse, makes tinnitus better, causes hyperacusis, makes hyperacusis worse, causes hearing loss, makes hearing loss worse; makes anxiety worse, makes anxiety better. I kept doing a little vaping.

In December 2016 I hit a very stressful patch and started vaping at least 10 times a day. Minimum 3 puffs a time. Up 80% more than before. My tinnitus got so bad it was screeching like when it started in 1986. My hyperacusis was the worst ever all day every day. I couldn't hear sometimes because people kept talking too fast and too soft. Vaping appeared to have an extremely negative effect on my hearing health. This caused a severe emotional reaction including anxiety and depression.

I couldn't believe after so many years of effort learning to cope better with my hyper ears, everything was worse, and it was my own fault. I went into major flare-up toolbox action: constant sound therapy 24/7; mind therapy techniques. By early 2018, over 18 months after first vaping, my tinnitus and hyperacusis settled down. But they were still worse than before. My hearing hasn't come back.

Eye Movement Desensitization & Reprocessing (EMDR)
The UK Norfolk and Norwich Teaching Hospital is studying EMDR to treat tinnitus. Experts use this psychological treatment for phantom limb pain, when people feel pain in a missing or amputated limb.

Feldenkrais Method
This uses gentle therapy touch and group training in a series of movements to improve posture, breathing, and well-being. It's used for chronic neck, shoulder, and back pain, as well as imbalance in elderly people. Some people say these movements can re-program the brain and reset neuromuscular pathways. Based on an Australian systematic review of available science, it's unclear if Feldenkrais helps any specific health conditions.

Food Allergies
Food can cause different reactions including tinnitus, headaches, stomach problems, and respiratory problems. Allergic reactions can happen immediately (e.g. hives, anaphylactic shock) or can cause a more chronic reaction (e.g. headaches, arthritis, asthma, fatigue, depression). People can also have food intolerances when they react negatively to a certain food, e.g. stomach problems from lactose intolerance, migraines from red wine. If you suspect you have food allergies or intolerances, you should see an allergy specialist. Treatment for food allergies can improve overall health and can reduce tinnitus in some cases.

Gene Therapy

Scientists around the world, including the UK, US, and Switzerland, are using genes for growing inner ear hair cells to treat sensorineural hearing loss. The scientists use intra-tympanic drug delivery to inject the gene treatment through the eardrum into the cochlea. Trials on rodents showed hearing improved by 20%. Since ethical scientists don't damage existing hearing, they are doing early human trials on volunteers with little to no hearing. Treating hearing loss with this gene therapy might cure tinnitus. If and when this therapy becomes clinically available, people predict high cost. For example, new gene therapies to treat blindness or leukemia cost over $500,000 per person.

Heat-Not-Burn Tobacco
This is the latest trend supposed to take over the e-cigarette market. It's produced by big tobacco companies. Users heat leaf tobacco until it's an aerosol they can inhale. In a 2017 news article, Dr. M. Stanbrook, a respirology specialist at Toronto Western Hospital, Canada, said "This is really nothing more than a marketing effort on behalf of the tobacco industry to keep people using tobacco products to expand the smoking population and getting people to stay on these products that might otherwise quit." Heat-not-burn tobacco still has harmful toxic and cancer causing ingredients and is not recommended.

Homeopathy
Dr. Edward Bach developed homeopathy in the 1700s. It's a form of naturopathic treatment that uses gentle flower or plant-based remedies to promote self-healing. Science hasn't found an explanation for Bach remedy effectiveness, but it's accepted there's a physical basis for its benefits. This approach might help with health and general well-being. There is no scientific evidence showing homeopathy helps specific health conditions.

Inner Ear Membrane Reinforcement Surgery
The Silverstein Institute in Sarasota, Florida, is studying hyperacusis treatment options including surgery to reinforce the inner ear round and oval window membranes with body tissues from the patient. There

are different theories on how this surgery works to help lower hyperacusis. Experts think the surgery might be helpful for people with
hyperacusis that hasn't responded to other treatments or therapies. This
needs more research.

Inversion Therapy
Inversion or upside down therapy uses the force of gravity to stretch
the body and increase oxygen and blood flow to the upper extremities
including the brain and hearing system. People often use an inversion
table that they adjust for their height, lie on, and tilt. They can be partly
inverted with their feet higher than their head or completely inverted
tilted upside down.

You don't need to be totally upside down for inversion therapy as long
as you're lying with your body on a slant with your feet higher than
your head. Some people use a slant board. This is a sturdy board with
one end placed on the ground and the other end placed safely and
securely on an elevated surface, e.g. first step of a staircase, leaning on
a bed.

People often notice louder tinnitus when inverted or tilted. The therapy
stimulates the inner ear balance system including upper regions that
don't get much stimulation from everyday positions like standing or
sitting.

Inversion therapy for 5 to 15 minutes a day is said to help lower
back pain, headaches, stress, and depression as well as give better
circulation, mental alertness, and balance. People who use inversion
therapy often say it gives them better physical and mental well-
being.

When people first try inversion therapy, they often feel like they're
right upside down even when their head is tilted only slightly below
the horizontal position. With regular inversion therapy, people have a
more accurate sensation of their head and body position. Inversion

therapy is not recommended for people with medical conditions like heart disease or eye disease.

Always get clearance from your medical doctor or ear specialist before trying inversion therapy. Follow manufacturer recommendations if you're using an inversion table. If you're trying inversion therapy, start out with a very gradual tilt and only increase the tilt slowly. Any comfortable tilt that places your feet higher than your head is reasonable for ongoing therapy.

Jan's View

I like using an outdoor lounge chair. I can lie down, and tilt it partly back so my feet are higher than my head. If nothing else, it's relaxing. I've also used an inversion table, and it helps my balance. If you forget to adjust the table for your height and it's set too tall, the table thunks upside down and you can't get back up again. You're stuck like a bat settling in for the night with all the blood rushing to your head. Squeaking for help. Not that anything like that ever happened to me.

Low Level Laser Therapy (LLLT)

LLLT uses light in the visible to near visible range of the spectrum (red and near infrared). It's been used for many years in Europe to treat inner ear problems like vertigo, imbalance, and inner ear related tinnitus. The laser beams are cool and reportedly comfortable. They're aimed into the ear canal. The idea is the light or laser irradiation stimulates cells leading to regeneration and healing.

Many people with tinnitus report lower tinnitus pitch and/or loudness after treatment. But some people report worse tinnitus after treatment at least temporarily. While some scientists suggest LLLT can improve hearing, other studies haven't confirmed this. Four double-blind placebo controlled studies have found no difference in reported tinnitus improvement between laser therapy and placebo.

One issue is that available studies have used different treatment protocols, e.g. power output, laser strength, positioning, light dosages, length of session, treatment frequency. There have been study method flaws. This makes it hard to prove benefit. More consistent research could show if laser or light therapy treatments help tinnitus, and which treatment protocols are best. LLLT should be viewed cautiously until more consistent scientific data is available. If you're considering LLLT, get clearance from your medical doctor or ear specialist first.

Magnetic Field Therapy
Some people suggest placing rare earth magnets in the ear canal to treat tinnitus. Research studies find no benefit.

Massage
This is most commonly used for short or long-term pain relief. Less pain means coping better. Massage can help lower stress, and improve relaxation. Sometimes massage can change how tinnitus sounds.

Middle Ear Bone Disconnection Surgery
In this hyperacusis surgery, doctors disconnect the chain of middle ear bones in one ear. Surgery is considered if people have severe distress from a rare single-sided hyperacusis caused by sudden severe single-sided hearing loss. The effect is like using an extreme noise reduction earplug. Patients report the surgery gives relief.

Migraine Treatment
People who get migraines are more likely to have tinnitus-hyperacusis. Tinnitus often gets louder and hyperacusis much worse during a migraine. Medical treatment can lower the frequency and severity of migraines. Fewer migraines can help with better hyper ears coping and well-being overall. Sometimes what feels like a migraine is a severe

tension headache from too much stress or distress; relaxation tools can help with coping either way.

Naturopathy

Naturopathic medicine is a professional therapy including diet, exercise, and supplements. Therapy focuses on our natural healing abilities. There is no scientific evidence to show that naturopathy is effective for hyper ears, although it might help certain individuals.

Neural Therapy

Neural Therapy was developed in Germany about 30 years ago. It's a naturopathic healing approach mainly used for pain. For tinnitus-hyperacusis, naturopathic doctors inject a safe pain killer into trigger points around the ears. This is supposed to reset hearing system brain activity. Injections don't work for everyone. There is very little scientific evidence on neural therapy for hyper ears.

Neurofeedback

This is also called neurobiofeedback, brain biofeedback, EEG biofeedback, or brain training. People with tinnitus-hyperacusis have hyperactivity or abnormal brainwaves. Neurofeedback trains people to use their mind to control their brain activity. Some tinnitus clinics internationally offer it.

Providers test the person's brain activity with a QEEG (Quantitative Electro-EncephaloGram) using electrodes on the scalp. For neuro-biofeedback treatment, the electrodes are used again so the person can watch their ongoing brain activity. Training teaches the person how to lower tinnitus related brain hyperactivity. This process takes about 2 to 3 months of weekly 1 hour appointments. It's unclear yet if neurofeedback could be used for hyperacusis.

Neuromodulation

Acoustic coordinated reset (CR) neuromodulation was developed in Germany. It's used for tonal tinnitus between 200 Hz to 10 kHz.

Therapy is supposed to change or reset how neurons in the brain are firing, to help lower hearing system hyperactivity causing tinnitus.

Treatment takes 36 weeks, with therapy tones adjusted at appointments for greatest benefit. It usually takes a few weeks to notice treatment results. For people with hyperacusis and tinnitus, the hyperacusis is treated first. Clinics internationally are using neuromodulation.

This therapy can't be used if people have too much hearing loss to hear the tones. It can't be used for people with Meniere's disease, hearing disorders with active symptoms, pulsatile tinnitus, tinnitus from TMJ problems, psychiatric problems, or other specific conditions.

People report lower tinnitus severity and annoyance after neuromodulation, but there's little scientific evidence-based research. Brain imaging studies have been inconclusive, and so far haven't proven neuromodulation works as claimed.

Webber et al. (2017) did a systematic review of available science, and found poor methods, inconsistent analysis, and low level of evidence. Studies used different treatment outcome measures so data couldn't be pooled or easily compared to other proven treatments. Webber et al. pointed out that the same authors did the articles and studies on the same patients with a total sample size of 329. Webber et al. concluded, "The available evidence is insufficient for clinical implementation of acoustic CR neuromodulation."

Neuromodulator listening soundscape is available at myNoise.net.

Optical Cochlear Implants
Cochlear Implants are electronic devices surgically implanted inside the cochlea that give a sensation of sound. They are mainly used by people with profound hearing loss or Deafness. Currently cochlear implants use electrical signals to stimulate hearing.

Scientists are developing optical cochlear implants. This science uses optogenetic therapy to implant proteins containing vision or optic fibers into the hearing system. Laser light is used to stimulate hearing instead of acoustic stimulation.

In 2018, German scientists at the Institute for Auditory Neuroscience at the University Medical Center Göttingen used this method on adult Mongolian gerbils that have a similar hearing system to humans. After training, the gerbil's responses to optical stimulation were close to normal hearing, and there were no negative side effects. More research is needed before optical cochlear implants become available for human trials.

Osteopathy
This is a system of manipulative therapy. Manipulation techniques are used to treat the whole body, not just the spine. This therapy approach might help with lower pain and better health in general for people with hyper ears and body pain.

Outer Ear Transplants
People who don't have outer ears or who lose an ear in an accident can now get outer ear transplants. Doctors use a person's own cartilage (e.g. from the ribs) to reconstruct an ear and grow it under the person's skin, e.g. the forearm. After it grows, doctors attach the ear to the person's head. New blood vessels form in the cartilage. With time the person gets back feeling in their outer ear, and the new ear collects and conducts sound down the ear canal. It's unclear if this type of transplant will help any related tinnitus.

Paired Vagus Nerve Stimulation (VNS)
The vagus nerve runs through the neck, connecting the brain to other parts of the body. With VNS, an electrode is implanted to electrically stimulate the vagus nerve. VNS is used to treat epilepsy and depression, and being studied for tinnitus. Most VNS for tinnitus science is

being done by private companies hoping to develop and sell VNS devices. VNS is typically an invasive experimental treatment.

The Serenity System® In 2011, scientists at The University of Texas at Dallas, US, found VNS stimulation paired with sound got rid of tinnitus in rats. Paired VNS uses VNS to make the brain release neuro-chemicals. It's paired with sound therapy signals that happen at the same time as the VNS electrical stimulation. Paired VNS is believed to rewire damaged hearing system pathways and lower brain hyper-activity.

Dr. W. Rosellini founded a company called MicroTransponder that is a neuroscience-based medical device company. They produced The Serenity System®: a wireless device for Paired VNS T therapy where the electrodes needed for VNS are attached to the neck in a short outpatient procedure. The sound therapy is loaded on a laptop, the person listens to it using headphones. Paired VNS therapy is done over 12 weeks for 2 1/2 hours daily. Time can be divided into 2 separate sessions per day.

Physicians and audiologists provide Paired VNS. Audiologists do a tinnitus evaluation so sound therapy is customized based on the person's hearing ability and tinnitus match. For VNS, as described at microtransponder.com, the physician places the device in the upper chest wall and a spiral lead is wrapped around the vagus nerve. A few days later, the physician programs the device.

There are double-blind placebo controlled studies at 4 sites on people aged 22 to 65 with chronic unilateral or bilateral tinnitus. Everyone had already tried at least one tinnitus therapy approach unsuccessfully, with an average of 4 previous failed tinnitus treatments. With Paired VNS, 56% of people had significantly less tinnitus distress, and everybody improved at least one category on the Tinnitus Handicap Inventory, e.g. changed from severe to moderate or moderate to slight distress. Safety and risks were the same as VNS for epilepsy or depression.

There is a small risk of vocal cord paralysis that typically gets better over time if it happens.

Paired VNS can't be used by people with severe hearing loss, Meniere's disease, ear tumours, or middle ear problems. It can't be used by people who may be pregnant or plan to be pregnant, may need an MRI during the therapy period, are using drugs that might impact the vagus, or have a significant history of cardiovascular disease.

As of 2018, this therapy is still in clinical trials being done in Europe (Deutsch, English). For current info on where clinical trials are happening in the world, check microtransponder.com.

3D Printed Middle Ear Bones
Scientists are studying 3D printing to make replacement middle ear bones. This could be a very helpful treatment, or even cure, for people with hearing loss and tinnitus or hyperacusis from middle ear bone problems, including causes like otosclerosis or fractures.

Pulsed Electromagnetic Field Stimulation (PEMF)
In the former Soviet Union, cosmonauts used PEMF to reduce bone loss while in space. Countries like Switzerland, Germany, and Austria later added PEMF in their healthcare systems to treat specific conditions. It is now commonly used worldwide.

PEMF uses non-invasive magnetic brain stimulation technology. Science suggests PEMF changes brain activity to reduce tinnitus symptoms. PEMF is also used for diabetic neuropathy, healing (cells, vascular, tissue, bone), depression, and pain management. Treatment lowers fatigue and improves sleep. It is often used for people not helped by medication or other treatment approaches.

Pai (2018) reports most of the science is by commercial device manufacturers. In one study, subjects with chronic pain used a PEMF device for two to five weeks, for twenty-five to thirty minutes daily. The treatment eliminated depression in 32% of subjects. Subjects reported 61% less pain and 75% improvement in quality of life. Pai states PEMF is safe to use, and can be combined with other approaches for different health conditions.

When compared to other brain stimulation approaches like Deep Brain Stimulation or Repetitive Transcranial Magnetic Stimulation (rTMS described below), PEMF is easier to use, lower cost, and treats the body as well as the brain.

Cleanhearing Sono (cleanhearing.com) is a patented PEMF home treatment system for tinnitus and related conditions, e.g. headache, depression, and TMJ disorder. Austrian engineer Gerald Neuworth developed the device to help his own tinnitus.

People use the stand-alone portable Sono device and headphones, twice a day, for thirty minute sessions. Treatment takes three to four months. If they want, Sono users can download a free sound enrichment app that notches sounds or personal music based on the person's tinnitus pitch match. The Sono device should be on sale in 2020.

Quantum Entanglement Clips
Some manufacturers are making wearable "quantum entanglement" clips. Manufacturers say these clips improve balance problems, strength, and joint function. They can't explain how it works, and have no science to back their claims. Independent scientists call the product snake oil.

In 2018, CBC News Marketplace tested clips with help from the Canadian University of Toronto's Institute of Biomaterials and Biomedical Engineering. There was no difference in balance or grip strength when people used the quantum clips, placebo clips, or no clips. Quantum entanglement clips won't help balance problems, no matter what the advertising claims. Don't waste your money.

Reflexology

This is a therapy where massage or pressure on reflex points in the feet or hands stimulates and balances energy flow through the body. Scientific reviews found no benefit for any specific health conditions. People report reflexology helps lower stress and makes them feel more relaxed.

I've used a self-help reflexology book for chronic pain points. It lowers my muscle tension and related pain. Because it makes my muscles relax, it helps me fall asleep easier.

Regrowing Inner Ear Hair Cells

In 2017, American scientists at Massachusetts Institute of Technology, Brigham and Women's Hospital, and Massachusetts Eye and Ear, were using a drug cocktail to regrow intestinal structural support cells when they noticed the cells are very similar to the inner ear ones. They tried the drug cocktail on mice, and it worked to regrow damaged hair cells that processed sound. The scientists believe these drugs—injected through the eardrums—will regrow inner ear hair cells.

Testing and government approval of new drug therapies can take many years. Some scientists from this study have formed a company called Frequency Therapeutics, and they hope to test the new drug therapy on human subjects around 2018 or 2019. If it works, this could be a cure for sensorineural hearing loss from common causes of inner ear damage like genetics, age, and diseases. Experts believe this could cure some cases of tinnitus and hyperacusis.

Reiki

This Japanese technique of stress reduction and relaxation promotes healing for different health conditions. The practitioner places their hands on or near the body for an injury or problem area. Treatments are said to give feelings of relaxation, peace, and well-being. A series of treatment may be needed for chronic conditions. Providers may recom-

mend regular treatment to maintain well-being. This approach might
help with stress relief and relaxation.

Reltus Ear Massaging Device

This product is advertised for tinnitus treatment. Scientists compared
effects of sound therapy through headphones versus the Reltus
vibrating device. Residual inhibition of tinnitus happened for both the
auditory and vibration testing. But the Reltus made a sound that
caused the residual inhibition with no effect from the massaging
itself.

SAD Light Therapy

Seasonal Affective Disorder (SAD) is depression from shorter, darker
fall and winter days. The farther people live away from the equator, the
higher the risk of SAD, especially in Earth's northern hemisphere.
Experts believe SAD is from too little exposure to bright light. People
with other types of depression can get SAD.

Lifestyle changes like spending more time outside, exercise, and
healthy diet are helpful. Treatments include CBT, antidepressant
medications, acupuncture, and light therapy or phototherapy.

SAD lights are 25 times brighter than regular household lights.
Medical experts recommend people use the SAD light at least 30
minutes a day, morning and evening for more severe cases. Side effects
include irritability, insomnia, headaches, and eyestrain.

Jan's View

I've used a SAD light for about 5 years from October to
February. The light therapy helps prevent SAD that triggers my
major depressive disorder. I like using the light while I'm eating
breakfast or doing a crossword. My eyes are sensitive so I don't
look at the light. I sit close by and make sure it's shining on me.

The bright light is also great for crafts or hobbies with small parts like model ship building.

Saunas

These are small rooms used for high heat sessions. Heat can be dry or wet if steam is added. Sweating in a sauna helps flush toxins from the body, helps the immune system, lowers muscle pain, makes people feel relaxed, and science shows regular sauna use could help prevent dementia. Saunas won't directly change tinnitus-decreased sound tolerance, but they can help with overall relaxation and well-being. Some fitness centres and recreation centres open to the public have saunas.

Sensorineural Therapy

Scientists used to think acoustic trauma damaged hearing nerve cells, inner ear hair cells, and structural supports. Damage to structural supports inside the inner ears isn't treatable.

But Stanford University School of Medicine animal model studies using modern imaging tech haven't found structural support damage after acoustic trauma. They've only found damage to the hearing nerve cells and inner ear hair cells. Scientists could treat or reverse this damage after developing better hearing loss treatments and cures. This research is part of the Stanford Initiative to Cure Hearing Loss.

Sensorineural therapy is a very important area of research internationally for people in the military with acoustic trauma.

Shiatsu Therapy

Shiatsu therapy is based on Oriental traditional medicine. The treatment approach and philosophy is similar to acupuncture. Instead of needles, providers apply pressure to specific body areas to balance energy flow and heal. Scientific reviews show no benefit for specific health conditions. Shiatsu could help by improving relaxation and general well-being.

Repetitive Transcranial Magnetic Stimulation (rTMS)
Research is mixed on whether rTMS is routinely helpful for conditions
like tinnitus. TINNET and tinnitus clinical practice guidelines don't
recommend it. It's still clinically available in some countries, e.g.
Canada. rTMS is a non-invasive technique that uses an electromagnetic
coil to stimulate electrical currents in the brain.

The device is placed against the scalp over tinnitus related brain areas.
It makes a very loud sound, so people need to wear earplugs during
treatment. Some say rTMS is painless; some say it feels like getting hit
in the head. Facial muscle twitching can happen with active or placebo
rTMS treatments. Some people think they can guess whether they're
actually getting rTMS or not, but scientists have found people do no
better than chance at guessing whether they had real or placebo
treatment.

When rTMS research was pooled together and systematically reviewed
in 2011, there was very little evidence to support rTMS was any better
at helping tinnitus distress than a placebo. More research was recommended to see if rTMS was really helpful for tinnitus. The authors
pointed out that while rTMS might be safe for short term treatment,
there is no data on safety of long-term treatment with rTMS.

Another systematic review of rTMS in 2016 found some tinnitus
benefit with rTMS. But there was high variability between the studies
reviewed for method and outcome measures. The Tinnitus Functional
Index is often used as a treatment outcome measure, so results can't be
compared to many other proven treatments. More research with large
sample sizes and long-term follow-up was recommended. Scientists
need to study best coil placement for tinnitus best stimulation
frequency and intensity, as well as how often patients should get treatment for the best benefit.

Folmer et al. (2015) say rTMS isn't a replacement for other currently
available treatment options or therapies. They suggested rTMS be

combined with current therapies, or be considered for people who
haven't had any benefit from other available treatment options.

Stem Cell Therapy
Scientists are looking at using stem cells to treat hearing disorders
including tinnitus. Research is still being done using animal models to
find the best way to harvest embryo stem cells, program the stem cells,
and transplant the stem cells back into damaged auditory areas. The
biggest challenge is transplanted cells usually die.

In 2015, Japanese scientists found a way to inject the stem cells into rat
hearing nerves so the stem cells didn't die after being transplanted.
Stem cells spread through the hearing nerve from the cochlea to the
brain, repairing the hearing pathway and restoring some hearing.

Experts think it will be about 10 years before stem cell therapy
becomes clinically available for hearing disorders or tinnitus. Some
companies are already selling over-the-counter stem cell tinnitus treatment in gel capsules. There's no reason to think taking a capsule
absorbed in your stomach, instead of direct hearing system injection,
will even work. There is no science on safety or benefit in humans.

TinniTool Laser
This device is available to rent or buy for home laser ear treatment.
Advertising says this laser can help tinnitus, hearing loss, Meniere's,
and middle ear problems. Again, four double-blind placebo controlled
studies have found no difference in tinnitus improvement between laser
therapy and placebo.

Tinted Light
Scientists at the University of Leicester, UK, are studying the effect of
tinted light on tinnitus. About 40% of people report that looking at
certain tints or colours of light improved their tinnitus while looking at
the light. More than 1 tint helped some people. In ongoing clinical
trials, the scientists will compare tinnitus in 3 light conditions: white

light, dark or low level light, and self-selected tinted light. This is interesting research. Tinted light has been studied for Seasonal Affective Disorder, e.g. blue light. Pink tinted glasses are sometimes recommended to help prevent migraines.

Tobacco

People who smoke tobacco—including children—have a higher risk of hearing loss. Risk increases the more cigarettes are smoked per day. Smoking while pregnant can cause hearing loss in the baby. The good news is a large 2018 Japanese study, on people aged 20 to 64, found quitting smoking drops hearing loss risk to the same as non-smokers within a short time after quitting.

Transcranial Direct Current Stimulation (tDCS)

This is a non-invasive treatment using electrodes on the scalp, said to target brain hyperactivity causing tinnitus. Low level electromagnetic pulses are sent through the skull into the brain to stimulate neural activity. People notice a tingling sensation on their skin.

A 2012 systematic review by scientists in Belgium, Korea, and New Zealand found 40% of people reported softer tinnitus after tDCS, with loudness dropping on average by 13%. Effects haven't lasted very long after the treatment. Recent double-blind placebo controlled studies found no difference between active treatment and placebo.

A 2016 Finnish study looked at whether treatment at home could be useful. Subjects did 20 minutes of treatment or sham treatment for 10 days in a row, using a headcap with electrodes. For two people, tDCS made their tinnitus louder, and one person got slight skin burns from using the electrodes wrong. Everyone else in the treatment group showed significantly less tinnitus distress.

The sham treatment group also showed significantly less tinnitus distress. The authors suggest being able to do treatment at home was a key factor. They recommended adding data logging to the tDCS device to confirm people followed study rules during treatment sessions, e.g. length of treatment, proper electrode placement. More research was recommended to see if there are subgroups or categories of people with tinnitus who might benefit more from tDCS than others. Because studies using at home treatment are safe and easy to use with similar results to studies done in hospitals, the authors suggested at home tDCS could be a useful way to do long-term treatment research.

BODY THERAPY TOOLBOX SUMMARY

Body therapy starts with a healthy lifestyle. Many tools help more with wellness, relaxation, or stress relief than directly changing tinnitus-decreased sound tolerance. But this can still lead to better coping and improved quality of life. Other tools target the brain although science is still in experimental or early clinical stages for many treatments. Being able to do treatment at home significantly lowers tinnitus distress, even when treatment doesn't change tinnitus at all.

Available treatments depend on what country you live in, and what local clinics are offering. For example, a tinnitus clinic in Montreal Canada has audiologists, psychologists, and physiotherapists on staff. As well as sound therapy and mind therapy approaches, tinnitus services include QEEG brain activity testing, acoustic stimulation, neurofeedback, and rTMS. Treatment is at hourly rates or in packages that cost about $6,500 depending on what's included.

I believe more team approach clinics will start to offer body therapy options as well as sound and/or mind therapy. Clinics will usually come up with fancy names to use in marketing even though other clinics might offer the same thing by a different name. Look past the name at what the treatment actually is. Consider the science. Consider the source. In the end is the cost worth the potential benefit of coping better?

Self-Help

- Healthy diet: bananas, antioxidants, iron rich, magnesium rich, avoid food allergies or intolerances.
- Dietary supplements or formulas: antioxidants, B12, magnesium, potassium, zinc.
- Herbal supplements or formulas: adaptogens, gingko biloba, St. John's wort, valerian.
- Quit smoking or using tobacco; avoid heat-not-burn tobacco.
- E-cigarettes: only use vape juice with no PG (propylene glycol); risk of permanent lung damage.
- Exercise: walking, stretching, biking, gardening, laughing, qigong, swimming, swinging, Tai chi, yoga.
- Specialty treatments: Pulsed Electromagnetic Field (e.g. Cleanhearing Sono), inversion therapy, SAD light therapy, sauna.
- Pain management: headaches, migraines, physical pain.

Therapy (face-to-face or at home)

- Tinnitus-decreased sound tolerance management clinic: may include acoustic coordinated reset neuromodulation (e.g. Desyncra), acoustic stimulation (e.g. PAXX), neurobiofeedback, bimodal stimulation for somatic tinnitus (when clinically available), Repetitive Transcranial Magnetic Stimulation (rTMS)
- Dentist: includes dental healthcare, hearing protection at appointments, on-off drilling, no ultrasonic cleaning, safe mercury filling removal and detoxification.
- Neuromuscular dentistry (TMJ/TMJ dysfunction): includes splints, nightguards.
- Physiotherapist: includes treatment for physical pain, somatic tinnitus.
- Psychologist: includes autogenic training, biofeedback, Eye

Movement Desensitization and Reprocessing, CBT for Seasonal Affective Disorder.

- Physician: includes Paired VNS (e.g. The Serenity® System).
- Neurosurgeon: includes brain surface implants (invasive), deep brain stimulation (invasive), Transcranial Direct Current Stimulation (tDCS).
- Specialty therapies: acupressure, acupuncture, aromatherapy, chiropractic, cranio-sacral therapy, Feldenkrais, naturopathic medicine (e.g. dietary and herbal supplements, homeopathy), Low Level Laser Therapy, massage, osteopathy, reflexology, reiki, shiatsu, tinted light.

PART V

SLEEP TOOLS

23

SLEEP BASICS

Sleep is the golden chain that ties health and our bodies together.

- Thomas Dekker -

Signs of bad sleep include problems falling asleep, waking up in the middle of the night and finding it hard to get back to sleep, waking too early, feeling tired when waking up in the morning, early morning headaches, and depression. Anyone who has a sleepless night wakes up feeling tired and not rested, but it's much worse with insomnia when sleep problems happen regularly over time.

Chronic bad sleep causes higher stress and anxiety making it harder to cope. Causing a cycle of more bad sleep. Easily leading to insomnia for people with hyper ears. Over 50% of people with chronic tinnitus have sleep problems, with worse insomnia than people in general. I would expect the same for people distressed by hyperacusis. The worse the hyper ears distress, the worse the sleep. People have difficulty coping with their personal, social, and work commitments when they're always tired.

Jan's View

I've had insomnia for decades. Sometimes I have trouble falling asleep. Usually I wake up during the night many times. Often I wake up and can't get back to sleep, so I putter around until I feel tired again. But there are now some really helpful sleep tools that I know can help anyone struggling with insomnia.

There are 2 types of sleep: REM (Rapid Eye Movement) and non-REM (NREM). When sleeping, we go through cycles of NREM and REM sleep. With REM sleep, the eyes move quickly in different directions. People usually dream while in REM sleep. During REM, there is temporary paralysis of the body, e.g. arms and legs, so people don't act out their dreams. REM sleep behaviour disorder is when people move and kick during REM sleep because the muscle paralysis doesn't happen properly.

NREM sleep is healing restful sleep. As people age, they tend to get less NREM sleep falling from about 2 hours in people under 30 to only about 30 minutes in older adults. NREM sleep has several stages that each last about 5 to 15 minutes. In stage 1, the first 5 to 10 minutes of falling asleep, the eyes are closed and it's easy to wake up. In stage 2, the body falls into a light sleep, then deep sleep in stage 3 where it's harder to wake up, and people feel disoriented if woken up suddenly.

During the deep sleep NREM stage, the body repairs and heals tissues, bone, and muscle, and also strengthens the immune system. People with emotional distress from hyper ears need NREM sleep to help lower the chronic immune system stress from fight-or-flight reactions. NREM helps people feel more rested after sleep.

The first REM sleep usually happens about 90 minutes after falling asleep and lasts about 10 minutes. The body should cycle NREM-REM over and over several times during sleep, with REM sleep lasting up to an hour by the final cycle.

During REM sleep, our brains process memories and learning as well as help balance our emotions. REM sleep should make up about 20 to 25% of an adult's sleep cycle, and over 50% of a baby's. Not enough REM sleep is linked to worse coping skills, migraines, and obesity.

A healthy adult needs 7 to 9 hours of sleep a night. Children need more. Short sleep (<6 hours), interrupted sleep, and poor quality sleep mean less NREM and REM sleep cycles. People cope better and have better physical, mental, and emotional health when they get enough REM sleep; it's very important for people with hyper ears who have bad sleep night after night.

There are lots of options people can try to sleep better and get enough NREM and REM sleep. Your daily routine can affect your sleep. Some activities help people sleep better. Some don't. The environment you sleep in also makes a big difference; background noise, temperature, and lighting can all disturb sleep. The more you use relaxation techniques and have a set bedtime routine, the easier it is to fall asleep and get back to sleep after waking up when you want to sleep longer. This includes people with hyper ears and shift workers who can be disturbed by noise outside their bedroom while trying to sleep.

Trying one tool or option isn't going to help bad sleep as much as tool combos, used regularly at the same time or in the same day, e.g. as a bedtime routine. People can use many of the mind therapy tool options to help relaxation and sleep, including Tinnitus-Decreased Sound Tolerance Management, Progressive Tinnitus Management, Tinnitus or Hyperacusis Activities Treatment, Tinnitus or Hyperacusis Retraining Therapy, Cognitive Behaviour Therapy (CBT), Mindfulness based

CBT, Mindfulness based therapies, Hypnotherapy, and Relaxation
Therapy.

REGULAR ROUTINES

These are some general guidelines for daily routines that help everyone
sleep better. Get in the habit of following them as much as possible for
better sleep. These are mostly free and easy to do.

- Get up at the same time every day. This is the most important
  rule for getting good sleep. It's the best way to set your
  internal clock to properly synchronize your 24 hour sleep-
  wake cycle.
- Take a warm bath—not hot—before going to bed. When the
  body cools off after, it signals the brain it's sleep time.
- Sleep in a cool room. Cooler body temperatures help with
  deep sleep. Experts recommend room temperatures of 16 to
  19 degrees Celsius (60 to 67 degrees Fahrenheit).
  Temperatures above 24 degrees C (75 degrees F), especially
  if humid, cause bad sleep. I turned off the furnace without
  telling anybody to see if a cooler bedroom would help my
  insomnia. There was much whining and complaining about
  the chill when the temp reached 65 degrees F. I told them I
  would turn the furnace back on. I didn't tell them I set it to
  67 degrees F. Nobody complained. So 67 degrees it is for
  sleep.
- Sleep in a dark space. Any light, even from an alarm clock,
  phone screen, or soft moonlight, makes it hard to sleep.
- Save your bedroom for pleasure, relaxation, and sleep. Other
  activities like work projects, studying, budgeting, eating, or
  arguing should happen somewhere else.
- Don't use hearing protection for sleep. Tinnitus seems louder
  while wearing hearing protection, which is not helpful when
  trying to sleep. Over time, using hearing protection daily or

regularly for sleep makes tinnitus and hyperacusis worse. The Hearing Protection chapter has more info on overprotection.

- Leave cell phones in another room unless you're using them for sleep sound. Phones should be set to Do Not Disturb.
- Avoid naps, if possible. Napping messes up your internal clock and makes you sleep less and sleep more poorly.
- Avoid caffeine at least 6 hours before bedtime.
- Quit smoking. Smokers are 4 times more likely to wake up feeling tired than non-smokers.
- Avoid drinking moderate to high amounts of alcohol since it makes sleep quality worse by reducing REM sleep.
- Do mild to moderate exercise in the late afternoon or early evening, e.g. walk, gentle stretching. People who exercise sleep better than people who don't exercise regularly.
- Unwind long before bedtime. Slow down and do relaxing activities.
- Keep regular routines before bedtime. This helps make you sleepy. For example, read a book for 15 minutes while lying in bed right before falling asleep or trying to fall asleep.
- Give yourself 20 to 40 minutes to fall asleep. If you haven't fallen asleep, then get up and do something relaxing or slightly boring for 30 to 60 minutes until you feel tired.
- Don't check the time if you wake up. Clock-watching makes people more awake and less sleepy.
- Don't let pets like dogs or cats sleep on the bed, if possible.

These are guidelines, not rules. There are always exceptions, depending on the individual. I've had horrible nightmares forever. My cat is my comfort animal. He sleeps on my bed. Close to calm me when I have a terrifying dream. He doesn't disturb my sleep. Except when he wakes me up while attacking my twitching feet during a dream.

You know yourself best. The experts have good advice. But there are times you have to adjust things for your individual needs.

SLEEP AIDS

Sleep aids help people sleep better by creating a comfortable, dark environment. They help people feel more calm and relaxed, so it's easier to fall asleep and stay asleep. These are the most commonly used options people use to sleep better.

Blackout or Darkening Window Coverings
These block light from coming through windows and help make the bedroom much darker for sleep. This helps everyone, including shift workers needing to sleep when it's light outside.

Blackout window coverings come in different patterns and styles, including drapes, curtains, blinds, roman shades. They should cover the whole window with no cracks to let light through, especially at the sides or edges. These products are often thermal insulated because of the thickness needed to be room darkening.

I like room darkening window coverings. I've used thermal insulating drapes with a heavy backing, and they cut the light making it easier to sleep. They also help block drafts around the window.

Calming Exercise
This helps with relaxation before bedtime. This includes gentle stretching and yoga calming or sleep poses. Science shows cognitive behaviour therapy works better than yoga alone for relaxation. Calming exercises alone won't help enough for people with more severe sleep problems.

Cannabidiol (CBD)
This cannabis compound with medical benefits doesn't make people feel stoned or high. CBD-dominant or CBD pure strains have very little psychoactive THC content.
Science shows cannabis helps people fall asleep faster and increase

length of sleep without making the person feel groggy the next day. It's still unclear how cannabis does this. If people use cannabis nightly and then stop, they get worse insomnia and more vivid dreams.

Medicinal and recreational cannabis is legal in some countries, or parts of some countries. Options include prescription medical cannabis, recreational CBD, CBD e-cigarette vape juice, CBD oil, hemp CBD oil. Sativa-dominant strains are often recommended. Always check with your doctor before taking CBD.

Comfort Bedding

There are lots of companies offering sheets, pillows, and mattresses advertised as extra comfortable to help people sleep better. Regular pillows, sheets, and mattresses are fine too, as long as they're comfortable.

For sheets, some people prefer the softness of bamboo material to other fabrics. For pillows, if you have neck pain, any comfortable pillow that lowers pain will help you sleep and cope better. There are many brands and styles, including foam, bamboo, and water base.

Jan's View

I've tried so many types of neck pillows over the years, with some helping more than others. I found a Mediflow waterbase neck pillow you fill with water that had rave reviews online, and advertised as science-based. It cost about $70 for 2 pillows, and they were easy to fill up with water to a comfortable firmness.

The sloshing from inside the pillow when getting settled was strange, making me feel like I was on a sinking ship. But I didn't hear it during the night. From the first night, I wasn't always waking up and plumping my pillow to get comfortable. It helped my neck pain.

Then a month or two later, my waterbase pillow sprung a leak. A big leak, soaking the bedding and mattress. Nobody online had mentioned that problem. I solved the mystery when I caught the cat attacking the pillow. Double hammering it with both paws and claws like he was playing Beethoven's 9th Symphony: da da da DAH. The cat didn't like the sloshing.

Something to keep in mind if you have a cat and get a waterbase pillow. When putting together a coping toolbox, things don't always turn out as expected.

Dental Nightguards or Splints

Talk to your dentist or neuromuscular dentist to see if this is an option for you. These are helpful if you grind your teeth or clench your jaw during sleeping.

Eyebrow Acupressure

This technique is sometimes used to help people fall into a deep sleep. After getting comfortable in bed and ready to fall asleep, gently massage between your eyebrows.

Herbal Teas

Drinking caffeine-free herbal tea at bedtime can be relaxing and calming. Teas sold for sleep time usually include herbal ingredients like chamomile or valerian. I hate the smell and taste of chamomile, so I can't use most sleep or bedtime teas. Personal preference.

Lavender

Studies show lavender scent helps adults with insomnia fall asleep easier and sleep deeper. Stores sell different lavender products including scented room sprays, scented products used in daily warm bath before bed, or scented candles. Don't use scent if you're allergic and never leave a candle unattended.

People sometimes use essential oil atomizers (diffusers, electric diffusers, nebulizers) to spread a fine mist of oils into the air. This approach might help with general well-being. Some essential oils are toxic, or the scent can be very irritating to cats, dogs, birds, and other pets. People can also put a drop of pure lavender oil on a cotton ball and tuck it inside a pillow case for lavender scent while sleeping.

Jan's View

I grow English lavender in my garden. It's got the best scent over other varieties, which sometimes have no smell. If you're buying lavender to grow, sniff it before buying. Find a variety that smells nice.

If you pick the lavender when it's blooming, you can dry and use in potpourri. Some people put it inside small sachets to tuck in a pillowcase.

I use lavender scented detergent for my bedding. It's individual. If you hate the smell of lavender, don't use it. Pick a smell or scent that makes you feel relaxed.

Monaural/Binaural Beats-Delta Waves

Monaural or binaural beats can be used to help people fall asleep. This technique can be used by adults as long as it's safe medically e.g. no epilepsy, heart disease or pacemaker.

For sleep, the best brain entrainment frequency is delta waves. Delta waves (0.5-3 Hz) are the brain activity needed for stage 3 NREM sleep. These beats are slow and low pitched, sending the person into a deep, dreamless sleep. This pattern of brain activity during sleep gives the most relaxation and healing benefit. With proper delta wave sleep, people typically wake up feeling well rested.

The challenge with binaural beats is they work best through stereo headphones. This is not a comfortable way to sleep. Binaural beat generators for sleep usually have added natural sound effects or music. These are available in apps, CDs, MP3s, computer downloads, and YouTube videos, although sound quality may not be great depending on how sound was engineered. Apps include iAwake, with a 40 minute Deep Delta module. Relax Melodies and Sleep Pillow apps also have binaural beats modules that can be used at bedtime for getting to sleep.

Monaural beats can also be used for Delta wave sleep, and no headphones are required. There are different sources of sleep monaural beats online. For example, surginglife.com has a 1 hour Peaceful Sleep Induction Music CD or mp3, along with a 4 minute sample. Transcendingvibrations.com has an Induce Sleep (Pure Monaural Beats) on mp3 or unlimited streaming. Monaural beats video games, e.g. SmashET, uses monaural beats to help people relax for sleep.

Always use caution and get medical clearance from your doctor before trying beats for sleep.

Sleep Mask
If the bedroom isn't dark enough for good sleep, sleep masks that block light can be a low cost, helpful option for people in general and shift workers. Sleep masks should be lightweight and comfortable, with a strap to keep the mask in place without putting pressure on the eyes, face, or head. Many people recommend face masks with a small air vent for the best sleep comfort and contoured eye pockets, so the mask isn't touching eyelids or lashes during REM sleep.

Jan's View

In 2018, I got $10 Bucky brand sleep masks for my family. The product had rave reviews online. The sleep mask makes everything dark although the strap needs to be tight to stop slipping or falling off my head while sleeping. Everyone thought the fit was comfortable, the masks made everything dark, and the small vent helped keep things cool. There are lots of other brands and styles of sleep masks.

Sleep Side

Closing off the right nostril is linked to a relaxed and drowsy state of mind. When people lie on their right side, it shifts breathing towards a sleepy state. Many people fall asleep faster and more deeply if they go to sleep lying on their right side. We're unique, so there are people who get sleepy on their left side.

Once you're ready to fall asleep, turn gently onto your sleep side and get comfy. If you're not sure which your sleep side is, try your right side for 10 minutes versus left side for 10 minutes. It should be easy to tell which side makes you more relaxed and drowsy.

If you wake up before you want to, and aren't on your sleep side, turn on your sleep side again to get back to sleep. Don't toss and turn. Figure out your sleep side and use it. The more you do this, the easier it will be to fall back asleep if you wake up in the night. It's a way of training your body and brain that right side means sleep.

Jan's View

I thought this sounded silly until I tried it. I tested both sides and I relax best when sleeping on my right side. Combined with other parts of my bedtime routine, this helped me fall asleep faster. When I wake up in the middle of the night, I'm almost always on my left side. I turn back on my right side, and it helps me fall back asleep faster.

I've been using the sleep side technique every night for years

now. The longer I've used it, the faster I fall asleep. It's free,
safe, and easy to do.

Weighted Gravity Blanket

These blankets were first used as therapy for people with autism. The
deep even pressure of heavy weighted blankets can help lower fight-or-
flight stress hormones and increase relaxation hormones that help
people feel calm and sleep better. Weighted gravity blankets stop
people from moving around as much while sleeping, including fewer
movements from restless leg syndrome. They're now used to help
people cope better with anxiety and insomnia.

Different sizes and weights are available for children, teens, and adults.
Therapists usually recommend a blanket that's 10% of the person's
body weight. Manufacturer websites usually have recommended
weight charts based on age and weight or height. Weighted blankets are
meant to be used by one person or two people snuggled close together.
They're not like a regular double, queen, or king-size blanket, so they
don't come in those sizes. They'd be way too heavy if they did.

More and more companies are selling weighted gravity blankets with
different options, e.g. washable covers, choices of colours or patterns.
Hypoallergenic glass, plastic beads, or sand pellets are usually used for
weight. The more the pellets are stitched in place or in small pockets,
the better for people with hyper ears who could be bothered by the
sound of pellets shifting. Check reviews online for detailed pros/cons
of weighted blankets from different manufacturers.

Jan's View

In 2018, I tried a weighted blanket for the first time. Along with
my insomnia, I have restless legs syndrome where my legs
twitch uncontrollably, worse when lying down. I have REM

sleep behaviour disorder. During REM sleep, I kick and punch; I have long conversations.

I ordered a 60 inch by 80 inch 20 pound weight of blanket made with glass beads and a removable washable cover. I don't like plastic near me, especially for hours at a time. So the glass beads were a plus.

This blanket was heavier than 10% of my body weight, but I wanted it to be more on the heavy side because of my twitching and moving during sleep. My weighted blanket cost about $250. When the box arrived, it was heavy. Too heavy for me to lift. Unfolding it to spread over the bedsheet and under the comforter was difficult; I had to get help.

I tried it out right away even though it was only the afternoon. There was no problem with noise from beads shifting around inside my blanket. I've seen rave reviews of how weighted blankets instantly put people to sleep. It didn't make me feel sleepy. It felt nice. Other people thought my blanket was too heavy, and worried I'd stop breathing.

Night 1 to 5, I slept without waking. It had been a long time since I slept that many nights in a row. I was less twitchy while trying to fall asleep because the weight of the blanket kept me in place. I'm told my REM sleep behaviour disorder was better than without the blanket. Was I sleeping better?

Each morning I had pushed the weighted blanket off me in the night. The more I used it, the more uncomfortably heavy it felt. I realized ordering a blanket heavier than 10% of my body weight was a big mistake. Plus I want to be independent. I don't want to have to ask for help to get a blanket on or off the bed. I sent it back.

When my partner saw me packaging it up to return, they looked very worried. "Why are you sending it back?"

"Too big. Too heavy. Exchanging for a smaller lighter one."

They were happy I was replacing it. It told me the change in my sleep wasn't my imagination. They noticed I was sleeping better too and thought I should keep using a weighted blanket.

I ordered a 15 pound blanket that was still about $250. While I waited for it to arrive, I was back to twitching and restless legs syndrome. I couldn't fall asleep. I kept waking up in the night, waking up early, and sleeping worse.

The smaller, lighter weighted blanket is more comfortable. I took the fuzzy cover off, because it was too hot. Then I noticed something gritty on the bed sheets. There was a small hole in my weighted blanket, and pellets were spilling out. I used duct tape to fix it. I blame the cat for ripping my blanket. Or the dog's toenails. If the material was a thicker better quality or I kept the cover on all the time, I don't think it would have ripped.

My insomnia hasn't gone away and never will, given my REM sleep problems, but I'm a fan. Even though the weighted gravity blanket was expensive, it's helping me sleep better without sleeping pills. Definitely in my toolbox.

REST AND REFUEL BREAKS

Better sleep isn't always enough for energy management while awake. Chronic stress from hyper ears can drain physical and mental energy. People with hyper ears are often more tired or fatigued than people in general, similar to people with chronic pain or fatigue that need rest and refuel breaks.

If fatigue is a problem, you might need to look at how you're using up your energy in a day. Break your activities down into smaller chunks of time, separated by rest breaks, to keep your energy up.

Experts don't recommend napping because it can make sleep worse. Rest and refuel breaks help refill our mental and physical energy gas tank. They can be as simple as taking 10 or 15 minutes during your day to do deep breathing, progressive muscle relaxation, meditation, mindful meditation, or guided imagery, with relaxation sound playing if possible.

If you're exhausted, a napper, or wish you could nap, this could be a tool to consider. It doesn't have to be done lying down or in a bedroom. Any comfy spot you can close your eyes in peace to use relaxation or sleep relaxation music could work. Another option is using no percussion music from a relax or sleep app. The more you use the same music tracks, the better it works.

Jan's View

It's hard not to nap when you're struggling with fatigue like many people with hyper ears insomnia. During the day, I often feel exhausted. A few years ago, I was napping 2 hours a day when my doctor ordered me not to. I had to wean off naps slowly over several weeks. Using alarms and slowly reducing the nap time.

But I still nap occasionally. Sometimes I'm so exhausted I just have to crash with no time limit. Other times, I set a timer for 15 or 30 minutes so my nap doesn't mess up my sleep later, or use this time for a rest and refuel break without napping.

I use relax or sleep music apps picking tracks that run from 15 to 60 minutes. I set a timer on my phone if needed. I set myself up like for sleep in a dark, comfortable room. I still have some mind spin while resting, but that's pretty normal. Sometimes I zone out into a meditative state, but I don't rest past the music turning off or past my timer.

Does it mess up my sleep period at night? I don't think so, but this is guinea pigging. What I know, is that these rest and refuel breaks leave me feeling a bit more refreshed and more alert. My mood is a bit better. Sometimes even a 5 or 10 minute rest and refuel break picks me up enough to cope better in the hours after.

SLEEP DISORDER TREATMENT

In some cases, people with hyper ears have trouble sleeping because of a sleep disorder. Doctors can refer people to a sleep specialist or sleep clinic for evaluation and treatment. The person with hyper ears might have the sleep disorder, but a partner with a sleep disorder can disturb sleep too.

The most common sleep disorders include snoring and sleep apnea. When the airways become partly blocked while sleeping, it causes snoring. Sleep apnea is when a person stops breathing briefly but repeatedly while sleeping.

Over-the-counter snoring aids are available, e.g. strips that go on the nose, or nightguards. Air purifiers can improve bedroom air quality to help breathing, reduce mild snoring, and give a more restful sleep.

Medical treatment for snoring or sleep apnea includes surgery, airway machines, or dental appliances. The surgery is very painful and has a limited success rate. People can use airway machines that force air into the nose at night while a person is sleeping. Only 50% of people keep using these machines regularly.

Dental appliances are similar to appliances used to stop teeth grinding while sleeping. They're worn in the mouth while sleeping to hold the jaw in a position that helps keep airways as open as possible. These appliances are effective for stopping snoring and can help mild to moderate sleep apnea. A sleep specialist or sleep clinic can evaluate if you have a sleep disorder and what treatment is best for your individual needs.

SLEEP TOOLBOX SUMMARY

Tools for sleep focus on calming the mind and relaxing the body. Watch out for new safe science-based sleep or insomnia tools; there's a big consumer market for them. Too many people sleep badly.

Using a coping tool routine is one of the biggest factors for fighting insomnia.

The more you stick to a bedtime routine, the more you train your brain to settle into sleep mode. Don't quit if you still have bad sleep or insomnia. The more consistently you use a sleep routine, the better it will work. Cutting the number of sleepless nights.

Jan's View

My sleep routine has changed over time with new products and new tech. The key is I use the same routine every night as much as possible. I always have sleep sound therapy turned on to play the whole time I'm sleeping. I use my sleep-mood tracker app.

Before sleep, I watch comedy shows on TV with my sleep sound on in the background. Then I read for a while. Because I do this every night, reading makes me feel sleepy.

If I have anxiety or mindspin, I do cognitive techniques. For relaxation techniques, I lie on my back and do belly breathing and progressive muscle relaxation. I've been doing this for months, training my brain, so I'm often almost asleep by the time I finish the progressive muscle relaxation. I turn on my sleep side and drop off to sleep fairly quickly. If not, sometimes I need to go back to reading until I feel sleepy or repeat the relaxation techniques.

If I wake up during the night, I turn on my sleep side. If I need to I repeat belly breathing, progressive muscle relaxation, eyebrow acupressure. If I can't fall back asleep within about 60 minutes, I get up and do something until I'm sleepy enough to try going back to bed again. Sometimes a hot drink with no caffeine helps.

I'm not saying you should follow my routine. But find a routine that works for you and use it.

Be patient. Coping better with sleep and insomnia takes time. Bedtime sleep routines end up being a tool combo, whether you're using cognitive techniques, relaxation techniques, and/or sleep sound therapy.

- Take time for daytime rest and refuel breaks to help with energy management.
- Don't use hearing protection for sleep.
- Follow guidelines for better sleep routine.
- Use sleep aids as needed.
- Dietary or herbal supplements help some people get through patches of bad sleep, if ok'd by doctor .
- Use cognitive and relaxation techniques to help your mind and body prepare for sleep.
- Use constant comfortable relaxation sleep sound therapy.
- Distraction sound that shuts off automatically after falling asleep can help some people, e.g. TV, music.
- If necessary, on a temporary basis, use a non-addictive over-the-counter sleeping pill or talk to your doctor about prescription drugs to help with sleep.
- If sleep problems continue, you (and your sleep partner if you have one) should get referred to a sleep clinic to evaluate and treat any sleep disorder.

There are so many options to help people sleep better. More details on sleeping pills or supplements, techniques, and sleep sound therapy are described in other chapters in this section.These are only some of the possibilities:

Self-Help

- Regular sleep routine: e.g. no caffeine within 6 hours before bedtime, unwind with relaxing activities, calming exercises, gentle stretching or yoga, warm bath before bed, cool dark bedroom, cognitive and relaxation techniques at bedtime, sleep sound therapy, regular wake up time .
- Sleep aids: blackout or room darkening window coverings, cannabidiol (CBD), comfort bedding, dental nightguards/ splints, eyebrow acupressure, herbal teas, lavender scent, sleep mask, sleep side, weighted blanket .
- Dietary and herbal supplements: lipoflavonoids, L-theanine, melatonin, tryptophan, chamomile, valerian, kava (medical supervision required).
- Sleep sound therapy: air appliances, water appliances, bedside sound generator (e.g. Marsona, Sound Oasis), audio/media devices, YouTube darkscreen sleep sound (e.g. Weightless by Marconi Union), sound pillow, pillow speaker, Smart pillow, SleepPhones®, sleepbuds.
- Over-the-counter sleeping pills.

Guided Self-Help

- Insomnia or cognitive behaviour therapy for insomnia (CBTi) books and workbooks.
- Sleep and sleep sound apps: include Breathe2Relax, Essence, Calm, Headspace, iAwake, myNoise, Pacifica, Sleep Pillow, Sleep Time, Tinnitus Sound Therapy Pro, Tinnitus Therapy Lite, White Noise, Widex Zen Therapy.

- Binaural beats for sleep: apps with no percussion music plus binaural beats include iAwake, Relax Melodies, Sleep Pillow.
- Monaural beats for sleep: include Peaceful Sleep Induction music, Induce Sleep (Pure Monaural Beats), monaural beats video games, e.g. SmashET.

Therapy

- Cognitive Behaviour Therapy for Insomnia (CBTi): face-to-face, telehealth, online, computerized.
- Sleep sound therapy and/or counselling therapy: e.g. Levo Tinnitus System, Progressive Tinnitus Management, Tinnitus or Hyperacusis Activities Treatment, Tinnitus—Decreased Sound Tolerance Management, Tinnitus or Hyperacusis Retraining Therapy.
- Prescription sleeping pills (no benzodiazepams).
- Sleep disorder treatment.
- Specialized therapies described in Mind Therapy Tools chapter: include hypnotherapy, mindfulness based CBT or mindfulness based therapies, Relaxation Therapy.

24

SLEEPING PILLS & SUPPLEMENTS

I love sleep. My life has the tendency to fall apart when I'm awake.

- Ernest Hemingway -

Over-The-Counter and prescription sleeping pills can help people fall asleep or help them stay asleep. They have side effects, with some lasting longer in the body depending on the pill and the individual. Some are more addictive or habit-forming than others. Never mix sleeping pills with alcohol.

Sleeping pill side effects can include feeling foggy or drowsy the next day—especially in women—forgetfulness or trouble concentrating, dizziness or imbalance, depression, headaches, constipation, muscle aches, blurred vision, dry mouth, nausea, and rebound insomnia. Rebound insomnia is when a person stops taking sleeping pills and sleep is worse than before they used sleeping pills.

Some sleeping pills have the side effect of causing tinnitus-hyperacusis or making them worse. Check with your pharmacist or doctor. Very detailed side effect information is available online. If you have tinnitus-hyperacusis, you're likely at higher risk of hearing related side effects than people in general.

People with hyper ears need lower doses than other people. Experts recommend starting with the smallest dose and working with your doctor to increase the dose to one that helps sleep with as few side effects possible. If taking sleeping pills over time, people's bodies can get used to them. If they need a higher dose to sleep, side effects can be worse. That's one reason why people shouldn't take sleeping pills for months on end.

Discuss any sleep problems and options available with your doctor. Work with your doctor to find the best choice for you. Sleep drugs can help improve coping while people find and use other tools and techniques to cope better with bad sleep. Use of prescription drugs should only be phased out gradually under medical guidance.

Over-The-Counter (OTC)
The main ingredient in OTC sleeping pills is sedating antihistamine, usually either Diphenhydramine or Doxylamine. These are short term help for bad sleep, only used for a night or two or at most up to 2 weeks. People can feel groggy the next day. Experts suggest only taking them if you have at least 8 hours before doing activities that require you to be alert and concentrate, e.g. driving, operating equipment. If used regularly over time, OTC sleeping pills can cause forgetfulness and headaches.

Prescription (Rx)
Compared to OTC sleeping pills, Rx sleeping pills are strong sedatives that have more side effects, are more addictive, and there is a higher risk of rebound insomnia where people can't sleep without them. If coming off Rx sleeping pills, people need to taper off gradually under

their doctor's guidance. Slowly lowering the dose until they're not taking them anymore. If a person suddenly stops taking Rx sleeping pills, they can have terrible withdrawal symptoms including anxiety, nausea, sweating, shaking, and rebound insomnia.

Rx sleeping pills can cause allergic reactions, memory problems, new or worse depression, and suicidal thoughts. People can also sleep walk, sleep drive, and sleep eat with no memory of it the next day. If any of these happen, talk to your doctor as soon as possible.

Benzodiazepines are controlled substances approved to treat anxiety and insomnia. They are addictive physically and mentally, and are linked with dementia. Benzodiazepines help people sleep, but there is less deep sleep and REM sleep. Some people feel groggier the day after taking benzodiazepines than they do the day after a bad sleep.

Experts say after 3 or 4 weeks of taking benzodiazepines every night, they work as well as placebo sugar pills. When a person stops taking benzodiazepines, insomnia will come back unless they start using other coping tools and regular routines including relaxation techniques to sleep better without drugs. These aren't going to be that helpful if the insomnia cause is a sleep disorder that needs evaluation and treatment.

In his 2015 ATA interview, Dr. P.J. Jastreboff warns that if people are taking medications like benzodiazepines (more than 1.5 mg per day), habituation doesn't happen because the drugs stop brain activity from getting less hyperactive. Discuss any concerns with the prescribing doctor, educating them on this fact if necessary.

Non-benzodiazepines are newer medications that work like benzodi-azepines to treat insomnia. They're controlled substances, but have fewer side effects and less risk of addiction then benzodiazepines.

Melatonin Mimics are the newest type of sleep medication. They work like melatonin to help people fall asleep. They don't help people stay asleep. The risk of addiction is low, but there are side effects like dizziness or depression.

Antidepressants Since antidepressants have a sedating effect, some doctors prescribe them for sleep problems even though they aren't approved to treat insomnia. Side effects include worse depression and suicidal thoughts, especially in children or teens.

Jan's View

In 2012, I was prescribed Celebrex, Tramadol, Elavil, Ativan, Cymbalta, Lyrica, and cyclobenzaprine. These drugs are a combination of major pain killers, anti-inflammatories, anti-anxiety, anti-depression, and sleep aids. It isn't surprising I turned into a zombie.

My neurologist says 90% of people are not helped by Rx medication for depression and chronic pain. People with hyper ears taking these meds are left with side effects like imbalance, grogginess, and worse depression. Mental anguish from pills is added on top of hyper ears distress. The problem is a depressed person doesn't always realize the pill is making things worse.

When starting or changing Rx meds, if you aren't less depressed with the Rx med, talk to your doctor. If somebody you know doesn't seem less depressed after starting or changing Rx meds, talk to them about it.

If you're worried the person is thinking of hurting themselves, ask. It's better to ask than not. Listen. Sometimes having somebody to listen—another person, helpline, professional—is what the person with hyper ears needs most.

Doctors should ask about depression on follow-up appointments. Be honest. It's not helpful to take something that only gives you side effects without any benefit.

DIETARY AND HERBAL SUPPLEMENTS

There isn't much science on supplements for sleep, and supplements aren't regulated to make sure they're safe over time or work as claimed by the manufacturer. Dietary supplements with the most research backing include lipoflavonoids, L-theanine, melatonin, and tryptophan. Herbal supplements with the most research backing include chamomile and valerian. Supplements might include a single ingredient or be combined dietary and herbal ingredients.

Natural doesn't mean safe. Supplements can have side effects or interact with other medications, medical conditions, or medical treatments including surgery. Discuss sleep problems with your doctor, and get medical clearance before trying any sleep supplements. Make sure doctors and specialists caring for you know about your dietary or herbal supplements.

Lipoflavonoids are a vitamin supplement with lemon extract, B vitamins, and vitamin C. A small number of people report better sleep and less tinnitus distress when taking lipoflavonoids.

L-theanine is an amino acid in green tea that could help with deep sleep. Since you'd have to drink huge amounts of green tea to notice any results, people usually use an L-theanine supplement.

Melatonin is a hormone that helps reset the body's inner clock. Experts recommend low doses of melatonin (e.g. 1 to 3 milligrams). Take melatonin a few hours before bedtime instead of right before bed. Experts recommend melatonin for sleep problems from jet lag or shift work. Some companies are coming out with melatonin insomnia products like sprays.

When I weaned off prescription sleeping pills, I used melatonin, and it was helpful. People shouldn't take melatonin month after month. It's for shorter bouts of insomnia, unless recommended by your doctor.

Tryptophan or L-tryptophan is an amino acid used to increase serotonin levels in the brain. Serotonin tells your body it's time to fall asleep. Jerry Seinfeld knows this is the amino acid that makes people feel sleepy after turkey dinners.

Chamomile is a gentle sedating herb used in herbal sleep supplements.

Valerian is a sedating herb used for thousands of years for insomnia and anxiety. Valerian is believed safe and not addictive.

Kava is an herbal sleep supplement for stress-related insomnia. It isn't commonly used. People taking kava must be under medical supervision, because kava can cause liver damage. I have seen Kava listed as an ingredient in over-the-counter sleep aids like teas. Big problem if consumers don't know the risk.

25

COGNITIVE BEHAVIOUR THERAPY FOR INSOMNIA

Insomnia is a vertiginous lucidity that can convert paradise itself into a place of torture.

- Emil Cioran -

Science proves cognitive behaviour therapy (CBT) helps people cope better with hyper ears. CBTi is cognitive behaviour therapy that helps people cope better with insomnia. Scientists are still studying which CBTi program components are most helpful for people with hyper ears. CBTi is offered by psychologists or counselling specialists in individual or group sessions. Cognitive, distraction, relaxation, and guided imagery techniques can help.

CBTi style self-help books are available in bookstores. This includes books on how to sleep better and insomnia workbooks. Check reviews or recommendations.

Any of the mind therapy apps mentioned in the Mind Therapy Tools chapters can be used for CBTi. Many of them have specific modules with guidance and exercises for better sleep. These apps aren't specifically for hyper ears, but they help most people sleep better no matter why the person has a sleep problem.

Check out different CBT style mind therapy apps to see which cognitive techniques help you the most for falling asleep and staying asleep.

Cognitive Techniques help people examine how their thoughts affect their sleep. Mindspin or negative self-talk at bedtime can make it hard to fall asleep, and harder to fall back asleep if people wake up before they want to. The goal of cognitive techniques is to help reduce or stop negative thoughts that interfere with sleeping. CBT style apps can be very helpful for this.

Jan's View

When I started using self-help apps for sleep, I was surprised how helpful the cognitive techniques were. This included guidance on reframing negative thoughts into realistic statements. Right before sleep, I like using the reframe thoughts guide on my Sanvello app.

I use the app prompts to pick whatever negative thoughts are spinning in my mind or my biggest worry. Usually I'm catastrophizing, predicting the future, taking blame, or overgeneralizing. I decide what I'd say to somebody else in the same position and say it to myself. "I can only do my best. It probably won't work out that badly. I can always improve things in the future."

After practicing this technique at bedtime, I noticed during the day I could use the realistic reframing immediately when I had negative thoughts. It helped lower my constant mindspin and worry. Some apps describe this as putting your worries away, as if shutting them into a box, so they're not stopping sleep.

Distraction Techniques are the least helpful for insomnia. Examples include counting sheep or counting backwards from 100 by 3s. Thinking about something so boring it puts you to sleep.

Jan's View

Counting sheep has never worked for me, but I accidentally found a way to bore myself asleep. I was researching parts used to build a stereo system for writing the Hearing Sound System chapter. Source component, woofers, mid-range, tweeters, power amplifiers, integrated speakers, dynamic microphones. I'm not an audiophile. I'm not interested in this topic, other than how it relates to hearing.

I couldn't fall asleep that night, so I thought about stereo systems, and what I would include in the chapter. I was trying to remember as much detail as possible. Before I knew it, I fell asleep. Much faster than usual. Every time I try it, it helps me fall asleep.

If you try a distraction technique, pick something boring. It's easy to find books at the library or info online. For me, no offense intended, it could be a furnace filter replacement manual, tax code, global economics, or philosophy. Pick what bores you. You could try reading it in bed before falling asleep. Or try to remember what you read while trying to fall asleep. The boredom might just put you to sleep.

Relaxation & Guided Imagery Techniques While distraction techniques can help some people with sleep problems, relaxation and guided imagery techniques are most helpful. CBTi relaxation tools are any method or activity that helps you feel calm and deeply relaxed so you can fall asleep and stay asleep. Psychologists or counselling specialists can teach people specific techniques for sleep. The more you practice and use the technique regularly at bedtime every night, the better the relaxation tool works.

Sleep Apps

There are lots of sleep apps on iOS and Android, for people of all ages. Some free, free with upgrades, by subscription, or at a set price. As always, things to consider when choosing apps include reputable developer, high user ratings, and being included in best-of lists. Popular apps include Calm, Happify, Happy Not Perfect, Headspace, iAwake, Sleep Pillow, Sleep Time. The Widex Zen Tinnitus Management app includes sleep exercises and info on sleep routines.

Accessibility problems for the Deaf and hearing loss communities are the same as for other mobile apps. Depending on the app content section, apps might have visual indicators, text-base, or open captioning. Some sleep apps are accessible, some are partly accessible, and some aren't accessible, depending on each person's hearing. People need to check individual sleep apps until app developers take accessibility for the hearing loss and Deaf communities into consideration.

There are several types of relaxation content used in sleep apps:

- Deep or belly breathing exercises.
- Progressive muscle relaxation (PMR).
- Meditation, mindful meditation, guided imagery.
- Sleep-mood trackers (also on some fitness apps).
- Sleep stories (slow, soothing, unexciting).
- Sleep sound.

Jan's View

There was no internet, mobile phones, or sleep apps back when I was taking CBT courses. Nothing to guide me or keep me motivated to use them even though deep breathing and progressive muscle relaxation (PMR) at bedtime had helped me fall asleep faster and sleep better in the past. I had put them under the category of flare-up tools and forgotten them.

In early 2018, I checked out sleep apps. I didn't expect much. To be honest, I was only trying them as research for this book. They reminded me to do relaxation techniques at bedtime. It was easy doing the techniques a consistent way every night guided by an app. It only took 6 minutes for deep breathing and PMR. A quick tool combo.

Once I knew the routine, I didn't need the app anymore. The more I use the techniques nightly, the faster it works. No judgement, but I'm not interested in the meditations and guided imagery app components, even though they help many people with sleep. Just my personal preference.

Many experts recommend mood trackers for people with anxiety or depression. I tried sleep-mood trackers to track my sleep versus mood. I didn't realize how strong the link was before I used this app feature. When I try new sleep tools, like my weighted blanket, this feature helps track benefit. It's rewarding to see when I sleep more than 1 or 2 nights in a row.

The sleep stories are unexciting tales, read very slowly and soothingly, usually by famous people. Some people enjoy these and find them relaxing. They're not for me. I'd rather listen to an audio book or read an ebook. No horror and nothing exciting that revs up the heart rate or gets the mind racing.

26

SLEEP SOUND THERAPY

Take care of the sense and the sounds will take care of themselves.

- Lewis Carroll -

Sound isn't always available in our environment, so sleep sound helps people create their own soundscapes. This is useful in any quiet rooms, especially bedrooms, where the person with hyper ears spends time. The hours spent sleeping are an easy and effective way to add to total duration of daily sound therapy.

For hyper ears, there are 2 big reasons experts recommend using sleep sound for people who can hear enough to use it. First, it helps reduce hearing and emotion system brain hyperactivity. In scientific studies, a significant number of people with hyper ears report their tinnitus is softer or hyperacusis is better after using sleep sound regularly.

Tinnitus Retraining Therapy has used 24 hour sound for tinnitus-hyperacusis since the 1990s, and since then people have also used sleep sound with other treatment approaches. Sleep sound therapy won't change misophonia dislike or fear reactions.

Second, sleep sound helps people with tinnitus-hyperacusis related sleep difficulties or insomnia. The bedroom is the quietest part of any 24-hour period. Tinnitus is most noticeable or loud when a person is trying to fall asleep. This can be a problem at bedtime or if people wake up before they want. It's hard to get to sleep or get back to sleep while listening to tinnitus. Comfortable sleep sound at mixing loudness, or softer, helps make tinnitus less noticeable.

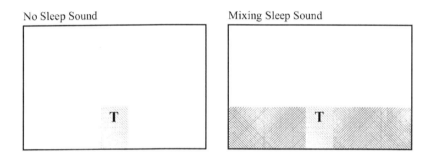

Sleep sound is helpful for shift workers whether they have hyper ears or not. Unwanted outside noise won't sound as loud if using sleep sound. Comfortable sleep sound raises the bedroom noise floor so outside sound isn't as noticeable.

For cochlear implant users, having the CI did not help sleep difficulties, likely because people turn off the CI during sleep.

People with hyper ears fall into two main groups. There is one group of people who "will do anything." These people are open to using sleep sound therapy to help lower brain hyperactivity and help them sleep and cope better.

Then there is the second group. These people say they have difficulties sleeping because of their hyper ears. But when providers recommend sleep sound therapy, their response is, "But I like it quiet."

Jan's View

When I first heard about sleep sound, I was not interested. I thought, I have enough sound from my tinnitus already, thank you very much. The last thing I needed or wanted was more sound. Plus I didn't think I could sleep with sound playing.

More and more science came out on how helpful sleep sound therapy was for hyper ears. I still didn't use it even though I was recommending sleep sound for clients with hyper ears. They told me how much it helped them.

I felt like a hypocrite, so I finally used sleep sound every night. After several months, my tinnitus pitch changed to less annoying, and the volume of my tinnitus dropped. I was so mad at myself. I had wasted many years sleeping in a quiet bedroom that hadn't helped my tinnitus. One of my biggest toolbox regrets is not using sleep sound sooner.

I stopped using sleep sound except for occasional flare-ups. After a long severe flare-up of tinnitus and severe hyperacusis from my 2016 vaping damage, I used sleep sound nightly again. It helped settle things down even though it took many months. I'd rather not wait for another flare-up. So sleep sound is now in my everyday toolbox.

Only certain sound types are used for sleep. Relaxation sound is best for a background soundscape. Sleep sound should be steady, monotonous, and neutral. Not attention grabbing. No silent breaks or a lot of up and down in volume. The sound should be set to run constantly throughout the sleep period. Sleep sound therapy should be used regularly every sleep period for best results.

Coloured noise is most commonly used. White noise is popular, but lower pitched pink or brown noise can be more comfortable to listen to, especially for people with hyperacusis. Different types of music, nature sounds, sound effects, or processed sounds can also be helpful if the sound plays constantly at a fairly constant volume. If there are silent breaks, some people like using a tool combo or custom sound mix, playing soft coloured noise in the background to fill in any gaps.

The sound should be set to a soft comfortable volume, usually partial masking to mixing, or as recommended by your care provider. Set and forget the volume. If you start to use sound therapy for sleep and it makes your hyper ears worse, then turn down the loudness to a softer level. The volume can always be gradually increased over time as your hearing system gets used to the sleep "sound massage." Some sound is better than no sound, especially for people with hyperacusis.

Different sound can be used for falling asleep, including the TV, radio, personal music library, audio books. These distraction sound types can be used on a timer set to turn off after 30 to 60 minutes. After turning off, the relaxation background soundscape should be playing continuously during sleep.

Think about what makes you sleepy since everyone is different. For example, there's an urban legend that the show Bones makes people fall asleep. I didn't believe it until I started watching it on TV. The first episode was fine. I was feeling sleepy by the end of the second episode, and after that I could never stay awake long enough to watch any episodes. I like the characters, plot, and actors so it's strange. But if I'm having trouble falling asleep, at least I can "watch" Bones. I haven't noticed this effect with any other TV show.

There are many device options for sleep, ranging from free if using something you already have, to thousands of dollars for particular sleep therapies. Some devices offer ambient sound, filling the room. Others play sound nearby at the pillow, or directly to the ears. Some people prefer both options, so no matter which ear is flat on the pillow, there is still sound therapy delivered to their ears.

Air Appliances

These have sound in the white to pink noise range like the sound of wind. Some people like using one appliance for multiple purposes, especially if it's something they have. Air purifiers can add sound to a bedroom, and have the added benefit of helping clean the air. Air conditioners, tabletop fans, or ceiling fans cool a bedroom as well as adding sound depending on how loud they are.

Many people with hyper ears like the sound from air appliances. They can be multi-purpose for people sleeping in warm humid environments or people with allergies, asthma, or snoring issues if the sound is comfortable. But there's no way to finely tune the volume of these devices, and filters must be changed or cleaned regularly as directed by the manufacturer. If required, replacement filters add cost.

Jan's View

I had to get an air purifier for my asthma, so I used it for my sleep sound. It has 2 settings for a low and medium volume loudness; both mix with my tinnitus. When I set it to the medium loudness labelled Turbo, I think, Take that, T! I don't know why. It makes me feel better. The air purifier is in a corner of the room facing towards the bed. The sound fills the room evenly since it's a constant loudness.

Over 15 years later, my air purifier is still working fine. It cost about $100 back in the day. It's never cost me for repairs or replacement filters since they're washable. It helps cover up any snoring. Not me, of course, because I don't snore. The air purifier has turned out to be a very helpful low cost tool when I consider how long it's lasted.

For a tool combo, I turn on the air purifier and bedroom ceiling fan for sleeping. The ceiling fan is quieter, and not the same noise frequency range as the air purifier. The fan's noise ripples out from the centre of the bedroom.

The ceiling fan noise mixes with the air purifier noise to create a new sound. Mixing sound is awesome. I was bored after 15 years of sleeping with white noise, so variety is nice plus the added benefit of being a combo.

One of my family members has trouble sleeping because of unwanted noise outside their bedroom window. After another night of no sleep, I suggested they try listening to coloured noise.

"I'M NOT SLEEPING WITH NOISE!" they screamed at me.

I said, "Coloured noise is technically an acoustic definit—"

Slam of bedroom door.

The next day, I tried again. They decided to use an air purifier. It helped them sleep.

I did not tell them, "I told you so."

Water Appliances

If using for sleep, make sure to protect furniture from any water spray or droplets from tabletop fountains. Another option is a fish tank or pet fountain. These are filtered water bowls for pets that are small fountains, so the water is always moving and circulating. The cost depends on features, and what they're made of, e.g. plastic, metal. The plastic ones are lowest cost, but not as long lasting. You can adjust the loudness and water sound with different waterfall setups, depending on the fountain. Replacement filters are extra cost. If you have pets and like the sound of gentle water, this could be a sleep sound option. You could still do sound mixes or combos with other devices.

Bedside Sound Generator (BSG)
These are also called tabletop sound generators, tabletop sound
machines, or white noise machines. Some experts outside the tinnitus-
decreased sound tolerance community bash white noise machines.
These people don't realize how helpful sleep sound therapy is for
people with hyper ears and people doing shift work who have trouble
with insomnia.

Providers often recommend BSG for people with tinnitus-hyperacusis.
More commonly recommended manufacturers include Sound Oasis
and Marsona. These machines offer a variety of relaxing background
sounds including coloured noise and nature sounds.

Sound Oasis has developed different sound and sleep sound therapy
apps, including Tinnitus Sound Therapy Pro app ($6) and free Tinnitus
Therapy Lite app. Apps include white noise and nature sounds.

Lots of other manufacturers make sound machines sold through
different retail and hardware stores. The higher the price, the better the
sound quality, the more sound options, and the longer the track or
audio clip before looping or repeating. If you get a tabletop sound
machine, make sure you can return it if you don't like the sound(s).
Look for these main features:

- Variety of relaxation sounds including white, pink, and/or
  brown noise.
- Volume control for fine-tuning loudness.
- No automatic shut-off; sound therapy should play constantly
  during whole sleep period.
- Battery backup in case electricity goes out, if that's important
  to you.
- Audio input jack or wireless connection so BSG can be used
  with a pillow speaker or sound pillow, if needed.

Audio or Media Devices

These play different relaxation sound types. This includes comfortable sleep sound from a personal music player, smartphone, or Smart TV. Many people like this option instead of buying a separate BSG.

People can set up personal music players or phones with continuous sleep sound, docked, and used on a nightstand beside the bed at a comfortable volume. It's possible to use a computer to take a short track of helpful sound or noise and convert it to loop into a longer playing track on repeat mode.

Jan's View

When I got a new phone in 2020, I permanently docked my old phone on my nightstand. For sleeping, I turn on a brown noise app for sleep sound therapy to mix with my air purifier sound. I think the brown noise helps me fall asleep.

Levo Tinnitus System

As described in the Sound Therapy chapter, the Levo is available through authorized sales distributors, typically audiologists, and was developed by Otoharmonics, founded in 2010 in the US. The Levo tinnitus pitch match sound is used during sleep with an in-ear sound generator. It's for tonal tinnitus, for people with normal hearing or sensorineural hearing loss ≤70 dB thresholds 0.25-8kHz.

A 2017 randomized clinical trial with 60 participants compared benefit of Levo to ambient sound from a bedside sound generator (BSG) with sound type picked by the participant.

Participants using Levo with tinnitus pitch match or white noise showed significantly less tinnitus distress than participants using the BSG. More research was recommended. This research puzzled me. Is Levo a tinnitus therapy approach that should be compared to other tinnitus therapies? Or is it a sleep device that should be compared to other sleep devices? At $5,000, I hope people would get more benefit from the Levo and related counselling than a BSG at about $250 or less.

Smart TV Dark Screen

Smart TV dark screen sleep sound can be used if YouTube is connected on the TV. There are YouTube videos with sleep sounds like white noise, pink noise, fractal music. Look for darkscreen videos. These have 8 to 12 hours of a black screen while the sleep sound is playing so there's no light from the TV to keep the person awake. The Marconi Union no percussion song Weightless is available in 1 hour, 2 hour, or 10 hour versions; it was voted the most relaxing song ever. Check reviews and watch out for poor sound quality in case video sound hasn't been engineered properly.

Sound Pillows

Special pillows can be used with BSG or tabletop sound machines. Manufacturers like Marsona and Sound Oasis make sound pillows compatible with their BSGs. Sound pillows are a pillow with a small speaker inside. When the sound pillow is plugged into the machine, the sound is played through the pillow speaker. Sound pillows bring the sleep sound therapy right by the ear instead of being a backdrop in the room. The person lying on the pillow hears the sound enrichment, and nobody else in the room is bothered by the sound.

Some people find sound pillows very helpful. Typically, only one style of pillow is available, which might not be comfortable for everyone. When breakdowns happen, sound pillows are not usually repairable. People with more severe distress often like to use a sound pillow plus having ambient continuous bedroom sound from a BSG or other device. This way sound therapy reaches the ear lying on the pillow and the ear open to the bedroom soundscape.

Pillow Speaker

Sometimes people make their own sound pillow by getting a flat speaker (e.g. from an audio equipment store) to use inside their regular pillow.

Smart Pillows

These are pillows that stream wireless sleep sound from an audio device to a speaker inside the pillow. Features include built-in relaxation sounds, alarm clock, sleep quality trackers, and snoring monitors that gently vibrate the pillow to get the snorer to change position. Rechargeable batteries last about 2 weeks. Limited pillow styles might not be comfortable for everyone. Cost is about $600 to $700.

SleepPhones®

These are a soft headband with thin removable speakers for sleep sound therapy. It's available in wired or Bluetooth® wireless versions, e.g. at British Tinnitus Association online shop. These can be used with bedside sound generators or other audio sources instead of a sound pillow.

Sleepbuds

These are a pair of soft in-ear sound generating earbuds that fit comfortably in the ears even for restless and side sleepers. The sleepbuds or noise buds are controlled with an app, e.g. volume, sound type, wake up alarm.

There are different soothing and relaxation sound type options. Manufacturers plan to add more sound types in future app updates. These could be a low cost alternative to the Levo Tinnitus System as a sleep sound option, although the pitch match sound type isn't currently available.

Cost is about $50 to $250 depending on the manufacturer. The higher the cost, the better the sound quality. Look for manufacturers with good reputations for making high quality audio products. Look for sleepbuds with rechargeable batteries.

Sleep Sound Apps

There are many apps to help people sleep better, on iOS and Android, for people of all ages. These include some apps mentioned under Sound Therapy Tools. Some free, free with upgrades, by subscription, or at a set price.

As always when choosing apps, consider if the developer is reputable, check user ratings, and best-of lists. Features might include ability to loop tracks, sound mixing, alarm clocks, etc. Some of the descriptions on these apps don't make sense based on hearing or brain science, but that's advertising for you.

When picking sleep sound from an app, keep in mind the usual guidelines: use relaxing or neutral continuous sound without silent breaks or ups and downs in volume. Sound type is based on personal preference. Most apps have coloured noise options, as well as wind and water sound types, nature sounds, no or low percussion music, etc. Some even have city noise at a steady even volume; this could be helpful to train people's brains to get used to sleeping in city noise even when there's other random city noise outside.

With sound mixing, if you pick a sound type on an app with silent breaks like sleep music, you can always mix it with a continuous coloured noise to fill in any gaps, or have a timer to turn the music off after it ends with other ambient relaxation sound continuing to play during the sleep period from the app or a different device.

There are loads of apps for sleep with different sound types and different features. Some popular apps include Calm, Headspace, iAwake, Relax Melodies, Sleep Pillow, Sleep Time, and White Noise. Apps with no percussion music plus binaural beats sleep sound types include iAwake, Relax Melodies, and Sleep Pillow. A popular sleep soundscape at myNoise.net is called Sleeping Dragon.

Being individual, most people won't like every sleep sound option on an app. You have to check them out by listening to them. Start at minimum volume. Be ready to turn off the sound quickly if you hate it or if it makes you cringe or wince. I've tried sleep music on apps that helped me doze off before sudden swells in volume startled me awake. Not going in my toolbox.

Jan's View

I like sound mixing. I used the White Noise app to mix brown noise plus ocean waves and looped it for continuous play. I thought it sounded great until I tried to sleep. The up and down volume of the ocean waves was annoying. The mix was too different from my decades of constant even volume white noise for sleep and only kept me awake. It's still an experiment to figure out what mix or mixes I like most. At least now I have an easy way to mix different sound types when I want.

There's no independent science on sleep sound apps. Tinnitus-hyperacusis scientists are working on developing apps for people with hyper ears. I'm sure these apps will include science-based sleep sound types.

PART VI

HEARING PROTECTION
TOOLS

27

NOISE DAMAGE

The day will come when man will have to fight noise as inexorably as cholera and the plague.

- Nobel Prize winner Robert Koch, 1905 -

Hearing system noise damage can be from repeated exposure over time or from acoustic trauma. As scientists learn more about noise damage to humans, it is clear that noise is unhealthy for cognitive, mental, physical, and hearing health. Even our brain health is at risk.

Researchers have found brain damage in animal models after only 12 hours of damaging noise exposure. Other research shows children's brains don't develop properly if they're exposed at low to moderate noise levels from birth to age 12. This critical quiet maturation period should make parents and care givers think twice about exposing little ones to noise. Authorities and decision makers also need support quiet community policies and regulations to prevent unhealthy noise where children spend time like homes, schools, parks, and hospitals.

Children are more at risk from high level noise damage, because noise-induced hearing loss hurts speech and language development as well as education progress and later job opportunities. Currently the biggest preventable noise risk to children is personal listening starting from as young as 3 years old. Science shows permanent noise-induced hearing loss, tinnitus and hyperacusis appearing by age 9.

Reminder:
Never use personal listening devices at >50% volume, and limit daily listening time.

Ears are ears. Loud is loud. High volume damage hurts hearing systems in all ages whether it's personal listening, sound at work, or outside of work during people's activities or entertainment. Whether the noise exposure is every day, every weekend, or now and then.

Noise is often defined as unwanted sound, e.g. noise from roadwork, construction, leaf blowers. But high volume sound isn't always unwanted. Many people enjoy loud hobbies, e.g. hunting, restoring cars, woodworking, snowmobiling. Others enjoy going to bars, night-clubs, and concerts to socialize or listen to music by their favourite bands. Lots like seeing movies on the big screen at a cinema or personal listening using earbuds or headphones.

There are two ways noise causes hearing system damage: chronic noise damage over time and high level sudden impact noise or acoustic trauma.

CHRONIC NOISE DAMAGE

Misophonia, including phonophobia, isn't caused by loud sound or noise. They're from emotion system hyperactivity—not hearing system damage. The earliest measurable sign of noise damage is speech-in-noise loss (also called hidden hearing loss) despite hearing thresholds within the normal range. Noise damage can also cause temporary and/or permanent tinnitus, hyperacusis, and hearing loss.

By the time people notice hearing difficulties, muffled hearing, pitch distortion, tinnitus, or hyperacusis, the permanent progressive noise damage to the auditory nerves has already happened. Every episode of noise exposure—even if days or months apart—increases risk of early onset permanent sensorineural hearing loss before age 40. Signs of hazardously loud noise include:

- Need to be within arm's length to communicate.
- Must raise voice to be heard.
- Temporary hearing changes after exposure, e.g. muffled hearing, tinnitus, hyperacusis or decreased sound tolerance.

Chronic noise damage happens at much lower loudness levels than the public realizes. Some scientists found brain changes from noise in young people with good hearing. These brain changes are seen in early dementia. The scientists believe the changes happen because young people have hidden hearing loss so they have to concentrate harder at an earlier age to communicate.

Chronic noise can cause invisible, hidden, and/or measurable damage. These are the steps of noise-induced hearing loss caused by occasional or regular exposure to loud sounds or noise:

1. Invisible: connections snap between inner ears and hearing nerves (cochlear synaptopathy).
2. Invisible: permanent progressive hearing nerve rips and tears for about 6 months after the noise exposure.
3. Hidden hearing loss = speech-in-noise loss.
4. Measurable inner ear or cochlea damage.
5. Temporary hearing changes and/or tinnitus-hyperacusis.
6. Permanent hearing changes and/or tinnitus-hyperacusis.
7. Cochlear dead zones: chronic damage to inner ear

structural/sensory parts so specific frequencies no longer processed by hearing system.

8. Musical paracusis where frequencies are heard are off pitch or out of tune; musical diplacusis is where off pitch frequencies are different in each ear.
9. Can you say that again?
10. I left my car blinker on?
11. This music sounds terrible.
12. What was that sweet nothing you whispered in my ear?
13. Pardon?
14. Can you repeat that?
15. Never mind?
16. Stress hormones rise.
17. Heart rate and blood pressure rise .
18. Problems with thinking and memory.
19. Poor work performance.
20. Higher risk of accidents (25% higher in people with tinnitus and high frequency hearing loss)
21. Higher risk of anxiety, depression, psychiatric problems.
22. Higher risk of heart disease: high blood pressure, heart attacks, strokes.
23. Higher risk of diabetes.
24. Higher risk of dementia.

People exposed to noise or music damage often say it's no problem, because they're used to it. Getting used to noise means the hearing system is damaged enough that noise doesn't seem so loud anymore. Getting used to unprotected noise exposure is bad.

ACOUSTIC TRAUMA

Acoustic trauma is noise damage to hearing health from sudden impact loud noise damage. The good news is that experts think noise damage happens differently in the hearing system since damage is instant instead of from chronic noise. This means treatments and possible cure will be different for acoustic trauma than other types of noise damage.

Common acoustic trauma causes include gunfire, accidents and military service especially wartime. People have reported hearing problems, tinnitus, and hyperacusis from acoustic trauma including an air horn blasted beside someone's ear, firecracker practical jokes, high pressure valve release, fireworks, explosions in communities or workplaces, bomb blasts.

It's important to get hearing tested as soon as possible after acoustic trauma. This gives a hearing baseline to compare to for hearing recovery over time. With acoustic trauma, sensorineural hearing thresholds can get better for up to 12 to 16 months after the acoustic trauma. Tinnitus-hyperacusis can get better too, especially if the person gets proper counselling and regularly uses sound therapy and other coping tools as needed.

PUBLIC NOISE EXPOSURE LIMITS

There is a lot of debate over how intense sound levels or noise needs to be before hearing health damage happens. Workplace noise limits of 85 dB or 90 dB daily exposure leave 8% to 25% of workers at risk of permanent noise-induced hearing loss. The 85 dB requirement for hearing conservation programs—recommended for working adults but not updated since 1998—is often wrongly called "safe" and wrongly used for the public.

The goal of public health is to protect the majority of people, including children, elders and people already dealing with illness or disease. More protective public limits are needed, especially since scientists have proven permanent invisible and hidden noise damage to hearing health happening long before any measurable change in hearing thresholds.

The louder the noise, the higher the risk, the faster the damage. For chronic noise, experts like the World Health Organization suggest 70 dB is the maximum daily average exposure limit to prevent permanent noise-induced hearing loss. Noise-induced hearing health damage could still happen below this limit.

Based on noise math, suggested maximum daily listening times to prevent permanent noise damage include:

15 minutes at 90 dB or
30 minutes at 87 dB or
1 hour at 84 dB or
2 hours at 81 dB or
4 hours at 78 dB or
8 hours at 75 dB

Since these exposure-listening time limits likely don't prevent invisible or hidden damage, or prevent tinnitus or hyperacusis, the best policy is no noise exposure. If it can't be avoided, then lower the volume, keep your exposure as short as possible, and/or use hearing protection. In some cases, authorities should require manufacturers or transportation industries to use noise control and make the volume safe for public health.

Chronic Noise Examples

73-95 dB avg—personal listening
75 dB avg—loud restaurant/retail store, vacuum
75-81 dB avg—transit: subways, buses, commuter trains, ferries
80 dB avg—blender, garbage disposal
86 dB avg—transit: subway/train platforms, bus terminals
90 dB avg—lawnmower
81-96 dB avg—stadium college hockey games
85-97 dB avg—stadium semi-pro hockey games
93 dB avg—stadium college football games

91-95 dB avg—stadium National Football League games

96-98 dB avg—pub, bar, nightclub, dance club (amplified music)

100 dB avg—motorcycle, symphony orchestra playing at treble forte, public hand dryers

105 dB avg—stadium pro hockey finals (e.g. Stanley Cup)

105 dB avg—stadium FIFA World Cup soccer training

110 dB avg—jackhammer, rock concert, MRI

120 dB avg—chainsaw

130 dB avg—professional DJ system

140 dB avg—military jet taking off from aircraft carrier

It's hard to identify the level of sudden impact noise that damages the hearing system. It depends on factors including the type of impact, number of impacts, and exposure environment.

Plus experts don't agree on what is safe. Some say 120 dB max should be ok for adults, but it's likely too loud for children. WHO recommends 100 dB max for personal listening and 110 dB max in general. Health Canada recommends 100 dB max for children.

Impact Noise Examples

90 dB max—titanium golf driver hitting ball (in ear canal)

116 dB max—wooden bat hitting slow pitch softball

116 dB max—sports officials/referees whistles

120 dB max—cowbells used by sports fans

123 dB max—aluminum bat hitting slow pitch softball

129 dB max—portable or personal airhorns

130 dB max—vuvuzela (horn used by sports fans)

141 dB max—0.22 rifle (measured 3 cm from shooter's ear)

142 dB max—firecracker at 8 metre distance

155 dB max—balloon popped with pin

155 dB max—consumer fireworks (ground level, 9 feet away)

161 dB max—12 gauge shotgun (3 cm from shooter's ear)

163 dB max—.30-06 rifle (3 cm from shooter's ear)

163 dB max—9 mm handgun (3 cm from shooter's ear)
164 dB max—357 handgun (3 cm from shooter's ear)
165 dB max—balloon blown up until it pops
170 dB max—improvised explosive device, bomb

DAILY SAFE NOISE EXPOSURE

There are different sound level meter apps that let people measure how high the sound levels are around them in their daily life. But noise exposure is based on loudness plus length or duration of exposure.

The problem for the public is that trying to calculate "safe" daily listening to prevent noise-induced hearing loss isn't practical. For example, let's say this is my noise exposure on a particular day:

- 78 dB avg—1 hour on transit.
- 83 dB avg—30 minutes lunch at crowded restaurant with piped in music.
- 78 dB avg—1 hour on transit.
- 76 dB avg—30 minutes shopping at retail store with piped in music.
- 90 dB avg—10 minutes crushing ice cubes making margaritas in blender.

All this noise exposure adds together for noise damage risk. But I can't add the dB or time and divide by 5; dB are logarithmic like the Richter scale for earthquakes. Daily noise exposure is calculated with a complex logarithmic equation.

What was my total exposure that day? I don't know. I don't do logarithmic equations. I leave that for noise experts like acoustical engineers or industrial hygienists. Plus my noise exposure is different every day. Even in the movie Groundhog Day, Bill Murray changed things instead of exactly repeating every day.

Maybe on a different day I have noise exposure at a concert or spend a few hours at a pub. I'd have to do the logarithmic equation again if I wanted to figure out my exposure for that day. It would be hard to figure out my safe listening time before I needed hearing protection. It's a gamble. And nobody should gamble with their hearing.

If it's too loud, protect your hearing. No matter how long you're listening. If you calculate or guesstimate noise plus listening time wrong, worst case scenario is permanent progressive speech-in-noise loss, distorted music, and eventually permanent noise-induced hearing loss.

28

RESTING HEARING & SUPPLEMENTS

I like a quiet life.

- Eric Clapton -

Sometimes people get tinnitus-hyperacusis or hearing loss after chronic noise damage or acoustic trauma. Experts often recommend resting hearing to help recovery. But this does not mean silence.

Science shows if sound therapy starts as soon as possible after symptoms start, it helps lower hearing system hyperactivity. Sound therapy could stop hyper ears from becoming permanent and help hearing return to where it was before the noise happened.

Experts suggest the quiet sound therapy level to rest ears is 45-55 dB. That's the level of a cat loudly purring. The sound of heavy rain on the roof. Chickadees chirping and singing in a garden. A babbling brook. An air purifier or fan. Music turned on low volume, e.g. ≤20% volume for personal listening depending on the device. Conversations without raised voices.

The first 1 to 7 days are key for using 24/7 quiet sound therapy. Sometimes the muffled hearing or hyper ears go away within a day. Sometimes they last longer. A week or more. Keep using quiet sound therapy for as long as you notice worse hearing or any tinnitus-hyperacusis.

If you have a baseline hearing test from before the noise damage or acoustic trauma that's helpful for monitoring hearing thresholds and recovery with time. Hearing system recovery can take up to 12 to 18 months, depending on how severe the acoustic trauma was.

NOISE PROTECTION SUPPLEMENTS

Scientists are researching and supplement companies are selling pills claiming to protect hearing from noise damage or make hearing recover after noise damage. Some of these supplements have the same tinnitus supplement dietary ingredients described in Body Therapy Tools, e.g. antioxidants, magnesium, B12, zinc.

Antioxidants Experts believe antioxidants are the best ingredients to fight noise damage, with different pills having L-Glutathione (called the mother of all antioxidants), D-methionine (an antioxidant in cheese and yogurt), powerful antioxidant ALA (alpha lipoic acid), and antioxidant NAC (N-acetyl cysteine).

NAC is being studied by the US Navy. They're finding hearing system improvement in military personnel who take NAC after acoustic trauma, e.g. improved hearing loss, less tinnitus, and better balance. Scientists are clear that NAC doesn't replace hearing protection. People can use NAC along with hearing protection. Scientists want more specific daily dose information for antioxidants like NAC, based on what's best for an individual person's hearing loss and tinnitus-hyperacusis, as well as their individual noise exposure history and symptoms.

Possibilities for acoustic trauma prevention and treatment look good. Some people recommend taking NAC before and after loud events, e.g. before and after going to a concert, or before and after hunting. People could take it after accidental acoustic trauma to improve any hearing loss, tinnitus-hyperacusis, or balance problems.

It could help people with expected noise exposure loud enough to cause acoustic trauma. You know it's going to happen, but you don't always know when. Like military personnel on active duty in wartime. In that case, a safe daily dose for each individual is the goal. As long as it's safe to take over longer time periods.

Antioxidant formula supplements from your local pharmacy or health store cost less than pills online. Get medical clearance before taking any supplements.

29

HEARING PROTECTION BASICS

Noise: a stench in the ear.

- Ambrose Bierce -

Hearing protection helps protect people's hearing from noise damage. Knowing what we do now about hidden hearing loss and noise risk, it's more important for everyone to protect their hearing from even occasional noise. Hearing healthcare professionals can guide people on selecting suitable hearing protection, and can fit custom hearing protection.

Hearing protection are earplugs or earmuffs that are worn in or over the ears. When wearing properly fit hearing protection, they work by making the noise softer to prevent noise damage. Like sunglasses block out harmful rays of light. You can still see with sunglasses. You should still be able to hear what you need to when wearing hearing protection.

Emergency Finger Plugs

If you stick your index fingertips tight into your ear canals, it can drop sound loudness by 20 to 30 dB. Fingers are a good pair of emergency earplugs. Especially for short annoying sounds like somebody hammering the metal lid on a paint can or in the kitchen when somebody is buzzing up ice cubes in the blender.

If you know a loud sound is coming and you don't want to hear the full volume, finger plugs are handy. Sometimes there isn't time to use finger plugs. Sometimes it isn't socially acceptable to use finger plugs, e.g. elementary school band recital.

We should teach young children how to use their finger plugs when sound is too loud or noisy. Clapping hands over ears or covering ears with hands like earmuffs doesn't lower volume much at all.

Emergency Voice Plugs

Vocal cords also trigger the acoustic reflex that tightens the eardrums. When voice-activated, sound loudness briefly drops by about 15 to 20 dB. Can this protect your hearing from noise trauma? It takes about 0.15 of a second for the acoustic reflex to kick in (pardon the pun). Too late for a sudden loud bang.

But it can help reduce loudness for a bang, bang, bang type sound sequence with 2 to 3 second intervals between each bang. The acoustic reflex isn't meant to protect against long loud sound. Just short bursts of loud sound.

Singing helps give this effect which is why singing along to loud music lowers hearing damage risk. This isn't reliable like using proper hearing protection for music. But helpful in an emergency.

Jan's View

In a concert hall packed with thousands of people, I was looking forward to a charity benefit concert. I hadn't paid too much attention to the musical program itself. Until I heard the skirling as the twelve bagpipers walked in procession up to the stage. Did you know bagpipes are the only instrument with no volume control? They can reach up to 116 dB volume.

All around me, hands reached up to turn down or turn off hearing aids. My emergency finger plugs were up to my shoulders when I realized I couldn't use my finger plugs. It would look too rude. And my arms would get tired. So I used my emergency voice plugs instead.

Every 2 to 3 seconds I would hum. Mmmm pause mmmm pause mmmm pause. Some heads turned and people gave me strange looks. I ignored them. What if I was just a terrible singer, trying to sing along with the bagpipes?

Then 10 snare drummers marched in to join the bagpipers. Did you know snare drums can hit up to 122 dB?

I think my acoustic reflex emergency voice plugs gave me a little hearing protection. At least, that's what I told myself. Before I squirrelled away actual hearing protection everywhere I could think of. Now I have earmuffs and earplugs handy just in case: house, car, pockets, backpack, key chain, purse…

Hearing protection stops noise by sealing or blocking off the ear canals. It can only work if it's worn. The biggest reason people give for not wearing hearing protection is wrong fit. Hearing protection can be the wrong size, wrong style, uncomfortable, didn't meet the person's listening or communication needs, or didn't fit for other reasons.

For example, a 2016 UK study on infantry soldiers working out of a forward operating base in Afghanistan found only about 60% used hearing protection. The solders felt any health benefit was outweighed by the threat of not hearing the enemy in hostile territory. Hearing protection had to meet the soldiers safe listening and communication needs. The scientists recommended properly fit hearing protection and leadership on using hearing protection at the smallest unit level.

How do you get people to use hearing protection when they should? For workers, one-on-one training on individual hearing protection fit and use is best, especially right after their annual hearing test.

For school noise-induced hearing loss prevention programs, a Brazilian systematic review found computer-based hearing protection training worked about the same as videos on how to use hearing protection. About 8% more kids used hearing protection after this type of training.

Kids who took a 4 year program were twice as likely to use hearing protection as kids who didn't take any program. Mixed content worked best to increase hearing protection use: classroom training, giving out hearing protection, noise level testing, hearing testing. Kids who got the mixed content were also more likely to use hearing protection when using firearms than kids who just got hearing testing.

SEALED FIT

Hearing protection must fit like swim goggles.

If real estate is all about location, location, location, then hearing protection is all about fit, fit, fit. If hearing protection doesn't fit a person properly, hearing protection won't protect hearing. It's a bit like fitting shoes; one size and style does not fit all.

Scientists say that hearing protection doesn't protect about 33% of people because they don't fit right even though the user thinks they're wearing them properly. The hearing protection doesn't block noise the way it's supposed to.

That's 33% of workers who think they're protecting their hearing with hearing protection, but are still at risk of noise-induced hearing loss. It's a reason why hearing protection was always supposed to be a last resort for occupational hearing conservation programs. If only there was noise control so workers weren't at risk from noise damage in the first place.

Without professionally fit hearing protection or hearing protection training, poor fit also means 33% of kids and anybody else using hearing protection are still at risk of noise-induced hearing loss. They don't know it doesn't fit and isn't protecting them.

For swim goggles to keep water out there has to be a complete seal. If swim goggles don't seal completely, water will leak or rush in, even through very small openings.

For hearing protection to keep sound waves out, there has to be a complete seal. If the hearing protection doesn't seal sound waves out completely, noise will leak or rush in, even through very small openings. If that happens, the hearing protection doesn't fit you.

Hearing protection has to be sealed the whole time a person is in damaging noise for hearing protection to work. If the seal breaks in noise, it's almost as bad as not wearing any hearing protection at all.

Sometimes people take off their earmuffs or take out their earplugs while they're still being hit with noise. Maybe to talk to somebody or listen to something. Their ears just got drowned with noise. The problem is they're wearing the wrong hearing protection for their individual listening and communication needs. It doesn't fit them.

Fit isn't just about the seal. It's about comfort. If hearing protection isn't comfortable or they can't hear what they need to, people aren't going to use it, or aren't going to wear it the whole time they're in damaging noise.

NOISE REDUCTION

Hearing protection have a Noise Reduction Rating (NRR) on the package or label. The NRR is reported in dB; it's a guide to help you figure out what your noise exposure will be when wearing hearing protection. A way to estimate how much softer the noise will be when you're using that hearing protection, if it fits properly.

The higher the noise hazard, the higher the NRR recommended. Examples of extreme high noise hazard environments include running chainsaws or jackhammers, underground mining, flight deck personnel, e.g. for military jets. In these extremely high noise environments, high noise reduction hearing protection or double hearing protection is usually required.

Double hearing protection (earplugs + earmuffs) is used where verbal communication would be impossible and warning signals would be unheard because of the high intensity of the surrounding noise. This maximum protection should only be used for extreme noise power.

Sometimes people work in noise, and their hearing loss keeps getting worse, even though they're using suitable well fit hearing protection. Often they start trying hearing protection with higher and higher NRR, including double hearing protection. Their hearing loss keeps getting worse. Their hearing keeps getting worse because the cause isn't work noise; it's usually genetic or unknown causes.

HP must fit perfectly to get full NRR.

Lab Noise Reduction Rating

Just like you don't want sunglasses that darken so much it's too hard to see, you don't want hearing protection that blocks so much sound it's too hard to hear what you need to. Studies show hearing protection with moderate NRR is enough for most jobs and most people. Hearing is better protected when people use properly fit hearing protection with moderate NRR than poorly fit hearing protection with high NRR.

NRR is based on lab tests. Fit is easier with earmuffs, so it's easier to get the full NRR. Fit is harder with earplugs. For earplug lab NRR, the tester inserts the earplugs to fit properly on at least 10 subjects. Testers measure the noise reduction with and without earplugs, and average the results to get the NRR.

High noise reduction >24 dB NRR
Moderate noise reduction 17-24 dB NRR
Mild noise reduction <17 dB NRR

Almost all hearing protection has less than 40 dB NRR. Why don't they make hearing protection with higher NRR? If you need that much noise reduction, the noise level is extreme. Hearing protection noise reduction maxes out for sound waves travelling by air conduction. When loud enough, sound waves also travel by bone conduction or vibration of sound through the skull bones to the inner ears. Hearing protection doesn't stop bone conducted noise.

That's why at extreme exposures, hearing protection plus limited exposure times are recommended. Workers using hearing protection can't be in extreme noise for a full shift; there are time limits depending on the noise level. Then workers using hearing protection with "fresh ears" can be rotated in to work in the extreme noise area. Same for extreme noise outside of work, but it's harder to find examples of that.

Real World Noise Reduction Rating

There can be big differences between lab NRR and real world NRR. In the real world, people don't put on hearing protection as well as testers in a lab. So sometimes testers make an untrained subject put on the hearing protection. The untrained person often gets much less protection than the lab NRR. Some hearing protection will have SF (subject fit) NRR or other ratings on the package or labelling.

Some experts recommend doing calculations or derating hearing protection to change the listed lab NRR into expected noise reduction. There are different methods including derating NRR by 25%, 50%, or 70% depending on the hearing protection style.

Studies show about 66% of untrained people using hearing protection will get the lab NRR. When people put in earplugs for NRR testing the way they would in real life, about 33% did such a good job with fit, they got more protection than the lab NRR. About 33% fit well enough to be within plus or minus 5 dB.

The other 33% were more than 5 dB below NRR. That's a big loss of protection. But when they tried a different style of earplug that fit better, the protection was much closer to the listed NRR. Fit, fit, fit.

For workers, keep in mind people aren't as well protected with hearing protection as authorities make it seem. About 33% of workers think their hearing protection fits and protects from noise damage when it doesn't. That's why noise control should be mandatory. Hearing protection should never be the only line of defense.

Don't worry too much over NRR. If hearing protection fits you properly and you wear it all the time in damaging noise, it will soften noise and protect hearing the way it's supposed to.

Fit Testing
Some manufacturers make hearing protection compatible with fit test equipment. These are used for workplace hearing conservation

programs. The fit test measures the amount of noise reduction each worker is actually getting.

LISTENING AND COMMUNICATION NEEDS

Fidelity means how much a sound mimics the sound source. Low fidelity means distortion for sounds or voices. High fidelity sounds clear. It makes a big difference wearing low fidelity hearing protection versus high fidelity hearing protection if you have listening and/or speech communication needs.

When picking hearing protection, fidelity is the first thing to consider. The main difference is high fidelity hearing protection has special filters in the earplug or earmuff cup, and low fidelity earplugs and earmuff cups are solid.

Low Fidelity Hearing Protection

In the past, people thought solid or low fidelity hearing protection with the highest noise reduction was best for everyone. It protected some people from noise-induced hearing loss. But if it blocked out noise and important sounds, people would break the seal, take off or lift up their hearing protection, and noise damage prevention went down the drain. Or they'd refuse to wear it at all.

The problem is solid hearing protection cuts noise the most in the high frequencies. That gives people high frequency hearing loss and sound distortion. It makes it harder to hear speech, music, warning signals, or environmental sounds.

High frequency reduction can make tinnitus-hyperacusis sound louder. Straining to hear while wearing solid hearing protection can make tinnitus-hyperacusis worse, and cause anxiety, stress, and fatigue. If people already have hearing loss, solid hearing protection makes distortion even worse, so it's a big problem, especially if they already have extra distortion from speech-in-noise loss.

If people have listening or communication needs, low fidelity solid hearing protection with high frequency reduction isn't the right fit.

Sunglasses block bright light but the person can still see.

High fidelity hearing protection block loud sound but the person can still hear.

High Fidelity Hearing Protection
People with hearing loss and/or hyper ears usually do best with filtered hearing protection, also called high fidelity, high definition, social, music, or musician's hearing protection. The filters are what make the difference. They lower sound equally at all pitches or frequencies. It's like turning down the volume. This flat pattern of noise reduction prevents distortion, and keeps speech, music, and other sounds clear.

Some manufacturers include more than one filter with their product. Different filters usually have different amounts of noise reduction. So when doing activities, people can decide if they want to use the lower NRR or higher NRR filters. Filters also cut impulse or impact noise automatically.

Some filters are designed for extreme impulse or impact noise, e.g. shooting hearing protection. They let the user hear sound naturally until there's a sudden impact sound like a gunshot. Then the extreme impulse filter kicks in automatically to protect hearing.

STYLES

Ears come in different shapes and sizes so hearing protection comes in different styles and sizes. The hearing protection needs to be comfortable, but also has to seal out noise completely. If one style isn't comfortable or doesn't seal, try a different size or style.

The most common styles are earplugs and earmuffs. Some people like earmuffs better than earplugs or vice versa. Some get a better fit with earmuffs or earplugs, depending on the size of their head, ears, and ear canals. For example, some people have such big outer ears, they can't find earmuffs big enough to fit so they have to use earplugs.

Sometimes people can't use earplugs because their fingers don't have the feeling or movement needed to insert them. Or they have a lot of earwax, chronic ear infections, or middle ear problems so they need to use earmuffs.

It also depends on what other personal protective equipment a person has to use, e.g. hardhat, safety glasses, welding helmet, etc. Temperature also makes a difference. If people are in hot and/or humid noisy areas or working outside in summer, earplugs are more comfortable and help stop skin irritation. If in cold areas or working outside in winter, earmuffs can be more comfortable.

Depending on your activities, you might need more than one style of hearing protection. In the end, pick hearing protection styles that fit, are comfortable, and have the features you need.

EARPLUGS

Earplugs come in different styles with low, moderate, to high noise reduction. This hearing protection blocks the ear canal to lower noise levels. Earplugs can be loose, corded pairs, or on a band (canal caps). They can be pre-made, pre-molded, or custom molded.

Earplug Accessories Include

- Neck cord keeps pairs together.
- Keychain carrying cases.
- Soft or hard carrying cases.
- Replacement ear tips or pods.

Warning:
Never do your own ear impressions for earplugs.

Some online earplug manufacturers get the buyer to make their own earmolds or ear impressions. They use these earmolds to make a pair of "custom" reusable earplugs. Custom is supposed to mean hearing protection is molded from professional in-person ear impressions so earplugs safely fit each individual's ear shape and size. Never make your own ear impressions that might not protect your hearing.

LOW FIDELITY EARPLUGS

Moderate to high noise reduction with distortion. If people have good hearing and no problems with listening or communication needs, these work fine. If they cut too much sound, people feel tired after wearing solid earplugs from straining to hear. They overprotect for everyday sound.

Formable Earplugs $ - $$

Formable earplugs are made of foam, sponge, wax, glass down, or thermoplastic. Cotton, cotton batting, or tissue paper doesn't protect hearing. Foam earplugs were the first type of hearing protection used in the past, designed for male Scandinavian loggers. Most formable earplugs are sized for larger ear canals even if they're sold as one size fits all.

It's possible to find smaller or tapered sizes better for smaller sized ear canals. A mushroom cap or pod style often fits smaller ears well. No-roll foam earplugs are also available that are easier to insert.

Most formable earplugs are sold for a single day's use and then thrown out. If the earplug is still clean after being taken out, some people do re-use them. Don't re-use dirty formable earplugs.

Formable earplugs come in corded pairs and uncorded. It's handy to hang corded pairs around the neck before or after being in the noise hazard. They come in packages of several pairs and large packages, jars, or dispensers. If you go through a lot of formable earplugs, the more in bulk they are, the lower the cost.

For reusable styles like thermoplastic, when the material is heated, the user forms it into the shape of their ear to make a solid plug.

Sealed Fit:

- With earplugs, there needs to be a little suction for there to be a seal. Like a suction cup sticking to a window.
- Follow the manufacturer instructions on how to insert.
- When rolling the formable earplugs thin like a worm between your thumb and fingers, keep rolling when you bring the earplug up to your ear canal.
- Reach other hand over the top of your head, grab the top of your outer ear and pull gently back and up, until your ear canal feels really open and straight. Use a mirror or get somebody to help if you need to. Once you know what your ear canal feels like when open straight, pull the same every time you use earplugs.
- After putting in the earplug, hold your finger against it gently for about 30 seconds to keep most of the expansion inside the ear canal. You want enough sticking out to grab when taking out.
- After the plug is finished expanding, pull very gently on the earplug. Is it sealed snug against your ear canal walls like a suction cup to a window? If it is, you'll feel a bit of resistance. If it shifts or moves, try again.

- If 50% or more of your earplugs are sticking out your ear canals like cigarettes hanging off an ash tray, they're not inserted right.
- When both earplugs are in, say something or hum. If the earplugs are sealed properly, things should sound a bit different, e.g. echo, tone of voice, tinnitus louder. If not, try again.
- If you can't get formable earplugs to fit your ear canals and seal properly, try another size or try a different hearing protection style.

As described in the Sleep Tools section, hearing protection isn't recommended for sleep. People often use formable earplugs or "sleep" earplugs. But too much silence means overactive hearing system from overprotection.

Many retailers are selling formable or sleep earplugs for children and teens. This is a concern for three reasons. Kids under age 12 shouldn't be using earplugs unless fit by an audiologist. Using hearing protection for hours of sleep could cause hyper ears or make hyper ears worse. If environmental community noise is the problem (e.g. airplanes, transit, traffic), the solution is noise control. Not hearing protection.

Canal Caps $ - $$

Canal caps and semi-insert earplugs are pre-molded vinyl or silicone earplugs connected by a plastic or metal band. With less noise reduction than other low fidelity styles, these can work for occasional listening or communication. The band can be worn in different positions:

- Over the head.
- Under the chin.
- Around the neck when not in noise hazard.

Canal caps are quick and easy to get on and off. They're mainly used when people are going in and out of a noisy area without spending much time there, e.g. office staff popping into auto repair shop to ask a question. These would be handy if handed out at cinema theatres for adults going to loud movies.

Sometimes the band makes an unpleasant noise if it's rubbed or knocked. Some manufacturers sell canal caps with quiet bands.

Warning:
Never stretch out the hearing protection band to make it looser.

Canal cap bands are manufactured to give a certain tension or pressure against the earplugs in the ear canals. That's how the seal works.

Canal caps last about 6 to 12 months. They are reusable until the band loses its spring or tension, they lose their pre-formed shape, the material begins to deteriorate, or they can't be cleaned properly.

Sealed Fit:

- Follow manufacturer instructions.
- Without stretching it any wider than you need to, put the band in the position you want and the earplugs in your ears.
- Earplugs are held in place by the band, filling snugly into ear canal entrances.
- If you can't get canal caps to fit your ear canals, try another size or try a different hearing protection style.

Pre-Molded Low Fidelity Earplugs $ - $$
Pre-molded high noise reduction earplugs are usually one piece made of vinyl or silicone. They often have 2 or 3 flanges to fit different sized ear canals from smaller to larger.

Custom Molded Solid Earplugs $$$
Custom molded solid or low fidelity earplugs are prescribed and fit by

an audiologist or hearing healthcare professional. They're made from a professional impression of the wearer's ears. Usually these earplugs are made of medical grade silicone. They come in different colours, similar to hearing aid earmolds. Some custom molded earplugs work two ways: solid low fidelity or filtered high fidelity. These are very useful for people with hyper ears.

3D Printed Custom Molded Solid Earplugs $$$

These earplugs are custom molded for each individual based on a 3D model of the person's ears. Safe lasers and camera tech measure the shape of a person's ear canals for the 3D model. Scans take about 90 seconds. Manufacturers offer in-person scanning events at different locations. 3D earplugs also come in high fidelity, filtered, or social styles.

HIGH FIDELITY EARPLUGS

Soft to moderate sounds still heard. Clear sound quality for listening, communication, or music. Loud noise, including wind or sudden impact noise, filtered or blocked out. High fidelity hearing protection is also called social, filtered, high definition, music, musician's, etc.

These are a good hearing protection option to consider for people who do a lot of work or noisy activities where they want noise reduction plus clear sound quality. For example, people who do a lot of cycling —with loud wind and traffic noise—like filtered earplugs to protect their hearing but can still communicate and hear warning sounds.

Music Inside Earplugs $$ - $$$

Some manufacturers make earplugs that let people listen safely to music while in noisy places. These can be used with different audio sources, e.g. MP3 players. For monaural styles, people usually use the music inside earplug in one ear, and a regular earplug in the other ear.

Pre-Molded High Fidelity Earplugs $ - $$

These can look almost the same as pre-molded solid earplugs. Retail product description should tell you if it's high fidelity or not. These start at around $20. That's a low price to pay to prevent noise-induced hearing loss.

Sometimes these earplugs come with 2 or 3 filters with different amounts of noise reduction, e.g. low, moderate, or high. If they come with a foam tip, it has the most noise reduction. There is no battery to worry about.

This type of earplug doesn't stick out of the ear canals much, and can be used under hats or helmets to lower surrounding noise, including wind noise. With regular use, pre-molded earplugs last about 6 to 12 months. They shouldn't be used if they lose their pre-formed shape, the plastic begins to deteriorate, or they can't be wiped clean.

Sealed Fit:

- Follow manufacturer instructions.
- Gently screw the earplug into your ear canal until one of the flanges fills and seals your ear canal.
- Try the very very very gentle pull for the suction seal test.
- Some pre-molded earplugs will be too small or too large and none of the flanges will seal.
- If you can't get pre-molded earplugs to fit your ear canals and seal properly, try another size or try a different hearing protection style.

Pre-Molded Sound Bounce Earplugs $$ - $$$

Restored Hearing (restoredhearing.com) is an Irish manufacturer who has developed earplugs made with a patented sound absorbing material not used in hearing protection before. Independent testing shows the material is 35 times more effective than other sound absorbing materials. Sound Bounce earplugs cancel noise without electronics. The

Tunable Acoustic Material works by passive noise cancellation, cutting loud noise, but letting soft to moderate sound through clearly.

Pre-Molded Electronic Earplugs $$ - $$$

Pre-molded electronic high fidelity earplugs are similar to pre-molded reusable earplugs except electronic earplugs work off a battery. When turned on, the electronics protect or lower levels when loud sound happens. You should still be able to hear soft to medium loud sounds or speech.

They work for more constant noise and sudden loud impulse sound, whether they're for social, music or other activities.

Some electronic earplugs have an on/off switch. Some won't turn off unless you take the batteries out. Rechargeable batteries are better than throw-away batteries that hurt the environment. Disposable batteries are supposed to become a thing of the past; we don't need more products that use disposable batteries.

Some electronic earplugs may have the same loudness limiting flaws as personal listening headphones and over-the-counter amplifiers. If possible, look for independent test results that they work as advertised.

Unless there's independent evidence, how do you know if electronic earplugs work like the manufacturer claims? How do you know if they meet noise reduction acoustic standards?

One way is independent testing. Some hearing protection is sold for industry, including at safety supply stores. This means the hearing protection meets national and/or international hearing protection standards confirming it does what it's supposed to, e.g. Canadian Standards Association, ANSI, ISO, etc. Look for that on product descriptions or labels.

Does the manufacturer sell to hunting, shooting, and military or law enforcement professionals? Hearing protection should meet strict acoustic standards, although that's not always the case.

User reviews or best-of lists can be helpful, especially if put together by people or organizations who know what they're talking about. But depending on who put together the list, sometimes reviewers look at other features, and don't consider if the electronics really limit sound safely.

Custom Molded Filtered Earplugs $$$
Custom molded filtered or high fidelity earplugs are prescribed and fit by an audiologist or hearing healthcare professional. They're made from professional ear impressions the same as custom molded solid earplugs and two-way solid-filtered.

Because they're prescribed, custom molded earplugs can be fit for children who aren't old enough to safely use other types of earplugs.

Custom earplugs last about 3 to 4 years. They can be wiped clean, so they're reusable until the material starts to shrink, harden, or deteriorate. Usually you can get solid colours, swirls, glitter, metallic, glow in the dark. That would be fun to see at nightclubs, dance clubs, and concerts.

Custom molded earplugs cost more. But they're custom fit for good protection and last longer than other types of earplugs, so the cost is less if averaged over how many months and years they can be used.

Low-High Fidelity Custom Earplugs $$$
For the two-way custom molded earplugs, people can switch the hearing protection from low fidelity solid to high fidelity filtered as needed. This is very helpful for people with hyper ears since it gives the wearer control over how much outside sound is heard in different situations.

The two-way style could be handy for people with misophonia. For example, at meals or places with trigger sounds, people can switch the earplug to solid so they can't hear the soft repeated trigger noise. Nobody needs to know. Switch earplugs back to filtered when the trigger sound isn't happening to get back to hearing sound naturally.

Teachers are at higher risk for hyperacusis than many other jobs. There are different unexpected loud sounds in a school, including kids yelling or screaming, fire alarms, school speaker systems. There's no way to know who's at risk until after hyperacusis has already happened. For prevention, schools could consider providing pre-molded or custom molded filtered earplugs for teachers. They would be useful during regular work days. In emergencies with extended fire alarms, filtered earplugs would still let teachers communicate.

Sealed Fit:

- Earplugs are usually colour coded red for right, blue for left.
- Fit the canal end of the left earplug into your left ear, slightly turning it, until it pops into place. Repeat with right earplug into right ear.
- If they don't fit comfortably, follow-up with the hearing healthcare clinic.

Musician's Earplugs: Pre-molded or Custom Molded $$ - $$$
Some pre-molded and custom molded high fidelity or filtered earplugs are called musician's earplugs. Many musicians and music lovers use them to protect hearing without distortion. These are also good social earplugs, e.g. for watching sports in stands or stadiums.

Professional Musician's Custom Molded Earplugs $$$ - $$$$
Filtered custom molded earplugs were originally designed for professional musicians. Musician's pre-molded or custom molded filtered earplugs are fine for many musicians. But over time, musician's

hearing protection has become more and more high tech, including specialized custom molded earplugs and in-ear monitors.

The goal is preventing noise-induced hearing loss for people and professionals in bands and orchestras. Scientists have studied hearing differences between musicians playing amplified music in rock bands compared to orchestra musicians. They were surprised to find orchestra musicians had worse hearing.

Experts believe this is because orchestra musicians don't get to pick the music they play; there are times they dislike or hate the music. Usually musicians in bands are playing music they wrote and like playing. The emotional reaction to the music changes the noise damage risk.

This is just one more way noise is so complicated. It shows noise risk is lower for recreational music (personal listening or concerts), than for industrial or other unpleasant noise that people don't enjoy listening to. Musicians in bands singing along could also be a factor that lowers risk.

For professional musicians, there are specific musician's hearing protection features for playing different instruments, e.g. guitar versus drums versus violin or flute. For orchestras, other noise control options are also important like noise reducing baffles and placement of orchestra sections. Orchestra musicians are workers like any other workers and have to be protected by occupational noise regulations.

Check out musiciansclinics.com for more detailed musician's hearing protection info and resources. This clinic and website was founded by Canadian audiologist Dr. Marshall Chasin; he's a leading world expert on protecting musician's hearing.

Sports Earplugs: Pre-molded or Custom Molded $$ - $$$
Earplugs are comfortable under hats or helmets for different sports.

This is a good option for high school, college, or professional teams. They protect hearing by cutting crowd noise, but keep clear communication between players. These are also good for people watching from stands or stadiums to protect hearing from crowd, stadium, and field noise while still being able to chat.

There are news reports of coaches playing extremely loud music at practices so athletes "get used" to noise. Causing noise damage to young people's hearing systems is criminal. Don't get them used to noise. Protect their hearing. Filtered pre-molded or custom molded earplugs are a safe option.

Professional teams sometimes pump artificial crowd noise into stadiums to make everything louder and give a so called "home field advantage." The Atlanta Falcons football team were caught doing this; the NFL fined them $350,000 and docked them a 2016 draft pick. You never know what teams are up to; protect your hearing even in the stands or stadiums when watching sports.

Pre-molded filtered earplugs are a lower cost option for people who only play or watch sports occasionally, and for younger teams, since safety supply stores sell them in bulk bags. People who watch or play more often might like the custom molded filtered earplugs option.

Motorsports Aerodynamic Quiet Helmets
Engine noise and wind noise are the biggest risk for people doing motorsports, especially wind noise with motorcycles. Experts recommend people pick an aerodynamic quiet helmet that fits well around the chin and around—not sitting on—outer ears. Fins and ventilation grids on the outside make noise louder. Pick a smooth helmet.

Even with an aerodynamic quiet helmet, there's still risk of hearing damage from engine and wind noise, especially at higher speeds. Don't forget vibration combines with the noise and increases noise-induced hearing loss risk higher than for noise levels alone.

Motorcycle manufacturers including Harley Davidson are developing stealth or quiet electric motorcycles with high power and long ranges before recharging. Hearing protection is likely still needed to cut wind noise.

Motorsports Earplugs: Pre-molded or Custom Molded $$ - $$$
Motorsports include driving motorcycles, All-Terrain Vehicles, dirt bikes, and snowmobiles. For motorsports, riders need to protect hearing, but sometimes need to communicate with each other on the road. Some people riding motorcycles use a solid molded plug in one ear, and a custom molded earplug in the other ear that connects to the helmet communication system.

Some people can hear the helmet speaker, communicate, and listen to music fine using filtered pre-molded or custom molded earplugs under their helmet. Some earplugs are specifically sold for motorsports.

Communication Capability Custom Molded Earplugs $$ - $$$
Custom molded earplugs can be ordered with communication system wireless or plug in capability if needed, e.g. two-way radio, helmet speaker system, radio helmet tech. This is possible for different recreational and work situations.

For example, semi-trailer truck drivers often use a solid earplug in the ear closest to the window to cut wind noise as much as possible, and an earplug with communication capability in the other ear to connect with the truck's communication system, e.g. talk to dispatcher.

Shooting Earplugs: Pre-molded or Custom Molded $$ - $$$
Some people shooting firearms use formable earplugs. These can be fine depending on how good a person's hearing is, and the type of shooting, e.g. target practice, skeet.

Hunters like using extreme impulse filtered shooting earplugs because they can still talk to hunting partners, and can still hear other important sounds while hunting, e.g. prey, predators, other wildlife or people moving around.

Electronic filtered shooting earplugs from reputable manufacturers are an option, but if the battery runs out, there's no protection.

Don't use social or music earplugs for shooting or gunfire. They don't cut enough extreme impulse noise.

3D Printed Custom Molded Social Earplugs $$$
Like 3D printed solid earplugs, these are custom fit to each individual based on a professional in-person scan used to make a 3D model of the person's ears. These earplugs are usually made of medical grade silicone, and come in different colours including solids, fluorescent, and metallic.

Noise reduction depends on the noisy activity. There are specialty models for different consumer target markets, e.g. music, motorsports, shooting, industry, law enforcement.

Combat Arms Earplugs (version 2)
A Minnesota based defense contractor knowingly sold these defective earplugs to the American military. They were used between 2003 and 2015, including by military deployed in Afghanistan and Iraq. The earplugs were too short and could loosen, making the earplugs useless. The defense contractor has to pay $9.1 million dollars to settle claims.

EARMUFFS

Earmuffs come in low to high noise reduction, and low fidelity or high fidelity options. They have cups with a hard shell that reflects sound away from the ear, and a sound absorbent soft cushion to fit snugly around the ears. A plastic or metal headband connects the cups.

Because ears come in so many sizes and shapes, earmuffs come in different sizes and shapes depending on the manufacturer. The cup cushions should fit comfortably against the head with no gaps.

The bigger or bulkier the cup, and the thicker the foam lining, the higher the noise reduction, but the heavier and more uncomfortable the earmuffs will be, especially if wearing for longer periods of time.

Earmuffs styles include:

- Regular profile.
- Thin or low profile.
- Wireless music capability, e.g. Bluetooth.
- AM/FM radio capability.
- Communication capability.
- Over the head.
- Behind the neck.
- Beneath the chin.
- Folding headband.
- Hardhat attached.
- Welding.
- High visibility.
- Camouflage print.
- Intrinsically safe, e.g. electrically insulated.

Earmuff bands are manufactured to have tension or pressure against the head. That's how the cushion seal works. I've seen parents stretch out the headband of their kid's earmuffs; stretching the cups out as wide as possible a few times. Then letting the kid use them instead of throwing them in the garbage.

Destroy the tension, destroy the hearing protection. Hearing protection is destroyed by other changes like drilling holes in the cups for better air circulation. If you change the hearing protection from how the manufacturer made it, it's not going to protect.

Warning:
Never stretch out the earmuff headband to make it looser.

If people break the seal, hearing protection won't work either. This can happen when people slip an earbud cord under the cups so they can listen to music. Even certain hair styles, chunks of hair, or eyeglasses can leave small openings. Broken seal means no protection.

Sealed Fit:

- Without stretching cups any wider than you need to, put on the earmuffs.
- Earmuffs should be held in place by the headband and press lightly and comfortably against the head.
- If you can't get them to fit completely around the outer ears and seal properly, try another size or try a different hearing protection style.

Earmuff Accessories Include

- Eyeglasses: cushioned pads to seal with earmuff cushions and keep noise out.
- Hygiene kit: replacement cushions for earmuff cups.
- Hygiene kit: replacement cushions and foam inserts for earmuff cups.

Earmuffs last about 4 to 5 years; but not the cushions and foam. They should be replaced about every 6 months or as recommended by the manufacturer. They need replacing sooner if the cushion plastic deteriorates or it loses its softness

LOW FIDELITY EARMUFFS

Moderate to high noise reduction with distortion. If people have good hearing and no problems with listening or communication needs, these can work fine. But if they cut too much, people can feel tired after wearing them from straining to listen or hear. This can be a big problem for people with hearing loss, especially at work. They can make tinnitus-hyperacusis sound worse. Solid earmuffs overprotect for everyday sound.

Earmuffs (Standard) $$

Regular earmuffs are low fidelity. The higher the noise reduction, the more sound will be blocked out, the harder it is to hear soft to moderate sounds, and the higher the distortion.

Electronic Earmuffs (Low Fidelity) $$ - $$$

Some electronic earmuffs are low fidelity. The higher the noise reduction, the more sound will be blocked out, the harder it is to hear soft to moderate sounds, and the higher the distortion.

Double Hearing Protection (Formable Earplug + Earmuff)

Double hearing protection is recommended for extreme noise ≥100-105 dB avg. The formable earplug noise reduction rating (NRR) and fit is more important than earmuff NRR. Some people find it a hassle or it's not comfortable to wear earplugs and earmuffs.

If you double up or wear earplugs plus earmuffs at the same time, you can't add NRR dB. Check which hearing protection has the highest NRR. Use that NRR and add 5 for the combined NRR. For example, if the earplug NRR is 33 and earmuff NRR is 24, combined NRR is 38 dB.

Double Cup Earmuff $$ - $$$

These earmuffs can be used instead of double hearing protection for extreme noise reduction. The earmuff has a double cup to give similar noise reduction to a formable earplug plus earmuff. The cups are very heavy, and can slip from head movements. They're not very comfortable.

3D Printed Nanocomposite Earmuffs – Extreme Noise Reduction
Scientists are working on 3D printed nanocomposite earmuffs. These earmuffs have similar extreme noise reduction to double hearing protection or double cup earmuffs. But they are much lighter and more comfortable to wear. It will be interesting to see what direction manufacturers take 3D printed earmuffs, e.g. different NRR, special features, custom printed for individual ears/head.

HIGH FIDELITY EARMUFFS

Filtered, high fidelity or high definition. Soft to moderate sounds still heard. Clear sound quality for listening, communication or music. Loud noise, including wind or sudden impact noise, filtered or blocked out.

These are a good hearing protection option to consider for people who do a lot of work or noisy activities where they want noise reduction plus clear sound quality. Some electronic styles even have safe built-in amplification for people with hearing loss that can also give a bit of sound enrichment under the hearing protection for people with tinnitus-hyperacusis.

Sound Bounce Earmuff Insert $$ - $$$
Restored Hearing (restoredhearing.com) is an Irish manufacturer who developed an earmuff insert made with a patented sound absorbing material. Independent testing at University College Dublin found the earmuff insert is 8 times more effective than regular foam inserts. The Tunable Acoustic Material works without electronics by using passive noise cancellation, cutting loud noise, but letting soft to moderate sound through clearly.

Music Inside Earmuffs $$ - $$$
These earmuffs are compatible with different audio sources, depending on the style, e.g. radio, MP3 players. People like to use

them at work to safely listen to music while wearing hearing protection.

Filtered Earmuffs $$

These have a filter and work similar to filtered earplugs, turning down the volume without distortion. These high fidelity earmuffs are good for people with normal hearing to milder hearing loss. They can be hard to find at retailers.

Electronic Earmuffs (High Fidelity) $$ - $$$

Electronic earmuffs are available in monaural (one external microphone) and stereo or binaural (two external microphones). People who need to locate sound sources while in a noise hazard should use the stereo version. Stereo is also better for people with imbalance. When turned off, electronic earmuff noise reduction is like solid earmuffs.

Make sure you only get electronic earmuffs from reputable manufacturers or retailers. If electronic earmuffs have to meet workplace or other standards, then they should cut noise safely as claimed.

Volume Control Amplification $$ - $$$

Some electronic earmuffs have a knob or button to turn them on. When turned on, a microphone picks up sound outside the earmuff. The electronics measure the sound level and filter automatically as needed.

Electronic earmuffs are great for people with hearing loss since it's hearing protection with safe built-in amplification. For people with moderate to severe hearing loss, especially high frequency, these are a good option. They help people with hearing loss communicate more easily, and hear any other sounds or warning signals they need to hear, while still protecting their hearing.

Push-To-Talk Amplification $$ - $$$

Some manufacturers sell electronic earmuffs with a push-to-talk feature instead of a volume control. When off, the muffs reduce all sound like a solid earmuff. When turned on, they work like any filtered electronic earmuff.

The louder volume only stays on for a few minutes. The person can have a short conversation and then the hearing protection goes back to its usual constant sound reduction.

Some people like push-to-talk more than volume controls.

Communication Capability $$ - $$$
Sometimes in damaging noise, people need to use communication systems like Face-to-Face, two-way radio, Bluetooth, Short Range tech, or other communication devices.

Earmuffs with communication capability allow input directly from communication systems. The connection can be hands-free, hard-wired, or wireless.

Electronic earmuffs with volume wheel and communication capability can boost or amplify soft to moderate sounds. This is helpful for people with hearing loss who need to use communication systems while working in a noise hazard.

Motorsports In-Helmet Earmuffs $$ - $$$
These solid earmuffs are installed inside motorsports helmets, e.g. motorcycle, snowmobile. The muffs are connected with the helmet speaker for safe easy communication or listening to music.

Sports Helmet Communication Systems
Helmet communication or speaker systems are often used by high school, college, and professional sports teams. They're mainly for side-line to athlete communication.

For example, in the National Football League, helmet communication systems let coaches at the sideline communicate with defense, offense, or the quarterback when they're on the field. Teams are only allowed one player on the field at a time with a helmet speaker.

In the NFL, the coach to player speaker system cuts off when the play clock reaches 15 seconds or the ball is snapped, whichever happens first. Other sports can also have rules about when helmet communication systems are used.

These helmets don't always protect hearing. If they don't have built-in hearing protection, filtered pre-molded or custom molded earplugs are good options.

Hearing Protection Communication Headsets $$ - $$$
These headsets let people and teams communicate in loud noise when close by or at a distance. They're commonly used in different industries, e.g. race car driving for communication between in-car units and crew at noisy locations like track side, pits, garages.

Shooting Earmuffs: Filtered or Electronic Filtered $$ - $$$
There are filtered earmuffs and electronic filtered earmuffs designed to protect hearing from extreme impulse or impact noise from gunfire. Some of these use noise cancellation tech. Everyone, including children, doing shooting should always use shooting earplugs or earmuffs.

Like filtered shooting earplugs, people like filtered or high fidelity shooting earmuffs because they can still hear soft to moderate loudness important sounds and speech, but the hearing protection kicks in automatically for gunfire.

When shooting or using firearms, make sure you use hearing protection designed for it. If choosing electronic, look for reputable manufacturers. There are specific options for law enforcement professionals, but they usually have added communication capability for tactical situations.

Tactical Communication and Protective System (TCAPS)

Military professionals need advanced hearing protection with features to protect hearing from extreme noise while keeping situational awareness and clear communication. For example, the US military uses TCAPS high tech electronic hearing protection during training and combat.

TCAPS boosts soft to moderate sounds so military personnel can communicate and safely hear enemy or friendly movement. TCAPS communication compatibility can connect to tactical or two-way radios, smartphones, and other communication gear.

This hearing protection uses noise cancellation tech to cut extreme impulse or impact noise from explosions or blasts. Communication tech works clearly even during extreme noise.

TCAPS looks like an earbud with different sizes of foam inserts and a loop to hold it in place. It's lightweight, comfortable, and can be used with or without other gear.

Noise Cancellation Headsets or Earmuffs $$ - $$$

Noise cancellation hearing protection mainly works for steady, constant, confined noise so it's only used for very specific noise hazards, e.g. military TCAPS headsets, pilot noise cancelling headsets to protect from aircraft noise.

Otherwise, electronic noise cancelling earmuffs or headsets are not for noise damage protection. They make the listening environment more comfortable, e.g. cancel cabin drone from aircraft engine noise, transit noise, background sounds in an open office.

Noise cancellation doesn't work on background speech even though some manufacturers like to make that claim.

Electronic noise cancellation can be helpful in everyday environments for some people with hyper ears when they want to listen more comfortably by lowering ambient background noise. Different headphones and earpieces are available. Noise cancellation systems are sold by different companies and retailers, including stores selling travel or relaxation related products.

Sound quality can vary between manufacturers. Often the higher the price, the better the noise cancellation and fidelity, but lower cost travel ones still work nicely.
Noise cancellation mobile apps are available, but there could be issues, including poor sound quality.

30

CHOOSING HEARING PROTECTION

Hearing protection is a sound investment.

- Author unknown -

When people are using proper hearing protection, it means the hearing protection fits, seals, is comfortable, and still lets the person listen and communicate as needed. No single size or style fits everyone or fits every noisy activity.

For workplaces with damaging noise, employers must provide a hearing protection selection appropriate for individual workers. For some jobs like welders wearing helmets, most will use similar styles and communication features, e.g. earplugs or helmet-mounted earmuffs.

In other workplaces with a variety of noisy jobs, suitable hearing protection typically means more than one brand and noise reduction rating (NRR) of earmuff, and a choice of low fidelity and high fidelity earplugs. Some employers think it's cost-effective to pay or share the cost of custom molded earplugs for every worker.

When workers choose the hearing protection options for earplugs and earmuffs at their workplace, more people use hearing protection than when the employer picks the hearing protection. There will always be some workers who need something different because of their ear or head shape, hearing, or hyper ears.

Jan's View

Once I recommended electronic earmuffs with amplification for a worker with hearing loss.

"Thanks a lot," said the employer in a phone call the next day. "Now I have to get electronic earmuffs for everybody."

No. Workers need suitable hearing protection that fits their needs. Just because one person gets something different doesn't mean everybody else gets it too.

If somebody had a big head and needed extra-large earmuffs, the employer wouldn't have to get extra-large for everybody either.

The best way to see people wearing suitable hearing protection is at loud public events where there are people of all ages. In a world where hearing is valued and protected, everyone should be wearing proper hearing protection just like everyone is supposed to wear seat belts in vehicles.

At a stadium event, children would wear properly sized earmuffs; teens and adults often like earplug styles. But there are always exceptions. Some people with hearing loss could be wearing filtered or electronic earplugs to help make communication easier. People with middle ear or other hearing conditions could be wearing earmuffs, as well as the people who just like earmuffs better.

There's still some stigma until hearing protection becomes the norm. If somebody at a concert wore earmuffs, would it make the band mad? Would people make stupid comments? Would people make stupid comments if they saw someone using earplugs? Possibly. But people shouldn't judge other people's hearing protection style. People need to use whatever gives them a comfortable sealed fit that meets their age, medical, listening, and communication needs.

HEARING AIDS IN NOISE

Some people wear hearing aids in noisy areas or wear earmuffs over their hearing aids. But hearing aids and loud noise don't go together. If turned on, hearing aids aren't designed to block out sound enough to work as hearing protection. If turned off, hearing aids are not hearing protection. It can also be hot and humid under an earmuff. Not good for hearing aid electronics.

There is one possible exception. If you have more severe hearing loss and wear Behind-The Ear style hearing aids with solid earmolds, the earmolds could act like hearing protection when the hearing aids are turned off.

If the earmolds have vents or holes, turning off the hearing aids won't likely protect hearing. That's where electronic earmuffs with built-in volume control or push-to-talk amplification can help by blocking noise, but safely boosting loudness of incoming soft to medium volume sounds, music, or voices.

GENERAL AGE GUIDELINES

Science shows impaired brain development in children exposed to environmental noise from birth to age 12. Hearing seems normal, but sounds and speech aren't processed normally as the child grows older. Entertainment noise may also be high risk. Parents and care givers should seriously consider not exposing newborns or young children to any noise when not absolutely necessary.

Earplugs are not recommended for children under age 12 unless prescribed and fit by an audiologist. It's best if kids don't stick things in their ears. Ears are also not at adult size yet so store bought protection likely won't fit properly. Hearing healthcare clinics fit and/or sell prescription, custom, or over-the-counter hearing protection for all ages.

For wearing hearing protection, age birth to 3 years old is a grey area. In the past, parents didn't usually have to worry about noise damage to their baby's hearing. Now it's more common to see babies and toddlers with over-the-head style earmuffs on at loud public places, e.g. movies, stadium events, concerts.

The headbands have a slight spring tension to keep the muffs sealed in place against the head. Is the slight weight or pressure safe for the baby's head?

Babies are born with 2 soft spots (fontanelles) on their head where skull bones haven't fused together and hardened yet. This gives room for the baby's brain to grow inside the skull. The back soft spot is usually finished fusing closed when babies are about 3 months old. The top soft spot is usually finished fusing closed when babies are about 2 to 3 years old.

0 – 3 months

- Avoid damaging noise, if possible.
- Get medical clearance from family doctor or ear specialist.
- Be very careful with baby's fragile head.
- Prescription hearing protection fit by hearing healthcare professional.

3 months – 3 years

- Avoid damaging noise, if possible.
- Get medical clearance from family doctor or ear specialist.
- Be very careful with baby or toddler's fragile head.
- Prescription hearing protection fit by hearing healthcare professional.

Age 3-12

- Prescription earmuffs that seal comfortably around ears, fit by hearing healthcare professional.
- Prescription canal caps or earplugs that seal comfortably in ears, fit by hearing healthcare professional.

Age 12 +

- Prescription or over-the-counter earmuffs that seal comfortably around ears.
- Prescription or over-the-counter canal caps or earplugs that seal comfortably in ears.

HEARING PROTECTION KIT

We have first aid kits at home. Emergency kits in the car. Why not hearing protection kits? The biggest reason people don't use hearing protection is that they don't have any to use.

Whether it's for one person or a family, a Hearing Protection Kit means you have hearing protection to grab when you need it. A Hearing Protection Kit makes sure you have the proper hearing protection for different activities. The Hearing Protection Kit could be in a plastic container, drawer, or cupboard set aside for hearing protection and gear like safety goggles.

At home, hearing protection could be hung or placed where it's needed if that makes you more likely to use it, e.g. with the chainsaw or near power tools. Hearing protection could be stored in a vehicle or carried along in a key chain case so it's always handy.

Jan's View

My Hearing Protection Kit has several pairs of tapered formable earplugs on a cord that fit my ears well. Some pairs are for home when using noisy equipment like my "50% quieter" leaf blower.

I have pre-molded music earplugs, about $20 online, for everyday noise, transit, loud sports events, or music shows, e.g. Symphony of Zelda orchestra concert. I also take pairs of foam earplugs with me to concerts in case I'm not comfortable listening with high fidelity earplugs.

If you have hyper ears, sometimes you have to play around with hearing protection for everyday noise. At concerts or loud events, I don't notice if my filtered earplugs make my tinnitus louder. At home in a quiet TV room, my tinnitus gets loud if I use my filtered earplugs for watching movies with gunfire.

One trick that helps me is to only use a filtered earplug in one ear. I sit where the no earplug ear is towards the wall, and my earplug ear is facing into the room for the TV or people talking. My tinnitus doesn't get as loud as with two earplugs. There no noise hazard or risk of noise damage, so the earplug is only for listening comfort.

A home Hearing Protection Kit should include enough styles and sizes of hearing protection needed to fit each person for different activities, as well as portable hearing protection for unexpected loud noise, if possible.
A family Hearing Protection Kit might include:

- Prescription earmuffs or earplugs to fit each child up to age 12.
- High fidelity earplugs for everyone over 12, if safe to use.
- Key chain cases so people can carry earplugs with them.
- Formable earplugs or pair of regular earmuffs for loud household chores, e.g. using power tools.
- A few pairs of formable earplugs and pre-molded filtered earplugs in the vehicle first aid kit.
- Other hearing protection as needed.

It's usually best to have extra pairs of earplugs, canal caps, and/or earmuffs, just in case. It's also a good idea to have replacement soft cup cushions, cup foam inserts, and eyeglass cushions if needed for earmuffs.

RETAIL SALES

Hearing protection range in cost from lowest with formable and pre-molded earplugs to highest for custom molded and electronic ear protection. You can get hearing protection from different stores or retail outlets, but some will have better selections than others.

Pharmacies usually only have low fidelity hearing protection like formable earplugs. Big box retail, hardware, and online stores have hearing protection styles from different manufacturers who may or may not be reputable.

Safety supply stores usually have the best range of styles including canal caps. There is bulk pricing for formable and pre-molded earplugs as well as other products. Safety stores have earmuff hygiene kits and other hearing protection accessories that work with brands they sell.

If hearing protection manufacturers sell to safety supply stores, it means their hearing protection meets specific standards. Look for these manufacturers at other retailers too. Common brands include 3M, Aearo, Bilsom, Condor, E.A.R., Elvex, Etymotic Research, Honeywell, Howard Leight, Moldex, MSA, Peltor, Tasco.

If you're checking out hearing protection, best-of lists can be helpful. The product descriptions should have the info you need to figure if the hearing protection is low or high fidelity, and what special features or options it has.

The higher the NRR, the less likely the hearing protection is high fidelity. Sometimes pre-molded solid and filtered flanged earplugs look similar. If the NRR is high, and the description doesn't say anything about high definition, high fidelity, music, or filters, then it's not filtered.

For custom molded earplugs if it's filtered you'll be able to see the tiny round filter on the outside of the hearing protection. If the earplug is completely solid, it's not filtered.

Filtered earmuffs that work without electronics are hard to find, but they'll also have some type of filter system you can see on the outside of the cups, and the description will say something about cutting loud noise while keeping soft to moderate sounds clear.

Don't believe all the product descriptions, especially for online

retailers that aren't safety supply stores. I've seen foam earplugs advertised as great for work and music. Not factual. Foam distorts music
because of its high frequency noise reduction. I've seen lots of foam or
pre-molded earplugs advertised as noise cancelling just because they
reduce noise. Not factual. Noise cancelling is very specific tech
whether it's something that works with electronics or not.

Custom could be by an industrial hearing protection salesperson who
does individually molded ear impressions for everyone at a workplace
at risk of noise-induced hearing loss. It could be trained hearing protection professionals going to different venues or trade shows to do 3D
ear impressions for earplugs. Audiologists and hearing healthcare
professionals do impressions for custom earmolds at their clinics.

HEARING PROTECTION SUMMARY

The best hearing protection is what you'll wear the whole time you're
exposed to hazardous noise, without lifting it up or taking it off. Fit, fit,
fit. Comfortable seal like for swim goggles. Noise reduction, filters,
and features that are right for your listening and communication needs,
like well fit sunglasses. Consider the cost and recharging time of
batteries for electronic products that don't work if the battery is dead.
Don't do your own ear impressions. Consider more than one style for
your Hearing Protection Kit.

Low Fidelity Hearing Protection

- Finger plugs.
- Canal caps.
- Formable earplugs.
- Solid pre-molded or custom molded earplugs.
- Two way low-high fidelity custom molded ear plugs popular
  for people with tinnitus or decreased sound tolerance.
- 3D printed solid earplugs.

- Earmuffs, including some electronic earmuffs.
- Double hearing protection.
- Double cup earmuffs.
- 3D printed nanocomposite earmuffs .

High Fidelity Hearing Protection

- Also called high definition, social, music, sports, musician's.
- Pre-molded filtered earplugs.
- Custom molded filtered earplugs.
- Two way low-high fidelity custom molded ear plugs popular for people with tinnitus or decreased sound tolerance.
- Electronic pre-molded or custom molded earplugs.
- 3D printed filtered earplugs.
- Filtered earmuffs.
- Electronic earmuffs, volume control or push-to-talk.
- Electronic noise cancellation.

Specialty Hearing Protection

- Music inside earplugs or earmuffs, e.g. radio, MP3.
- Musician's custom molded filtered earplugs, in-ear monitors.
- Motorsports pre-molded or custom molded filtered earplugs, in-helmet earmuffs.
- Shooting earplugs or earmuffs, including electronic.
- Communication capability.
- Helmet communication systems.
- Hearing protection communication headsets.
- Military, e.g. Tactical Communication and Protective System (TCAPS).
- Law enforcement, filtered with communication capability.

31

OVERPROTECTION

Silence is the sharper sword.

- Samuel Johnson -

People with tinnitus-hyperacusis often notice loud sounds or noisy environments make their hyper ears worse. It's not always possible to lower the volume or walk away from noise. Some people wear hearing protection to limit the sound getting to their ears.

When sound can cause noise damage, then using hearing protection is good. The most common problem is overprotection, especially for a person with hyperacusis. Overprotection is when a person wears hearing protection that cuts too much sound for their exposure. Blocking out as much sound as possible no matter how loud the sound is, or wearing hearing protection all the time just in case a loud sound happens.

Overprotection makes tinnitus-hyperacusis worse. More silence means higher hearing system hyperactivity. The solution is not to wear hearing protection unless needed. When you do need to wear hearing protection, don't overprotect your ears by blocking out too much sound.

Just like modern sunglasses can automatically adjust for the surrounding brightness, modern hearing protection can automatically adjust for the surrounding loudness. Hearing protection can protect from constant sound or occasional sound. Modern hearing protection can lower the volume safely without overprotecting. If there's a sudden loud sound, modern hearing protection kicks in automatically to cut the loudness. Wearing suitable hearing protection with the right fit and features, there won't be overprotection.

One of the biggest challenges for people with hyperacusis is overprotection. With hyperacusis, everyday sounds hurt. What do you do if something hurts? The logical thing to do is avoid it.

"It hurts when I do this, Doc."

A classic answer is, "Then don't do it."

People with hyperacusis start avoiding sound that hurts. They often use low fidelity hearing protection to block out unwanted everyday sound that isn't loud enough to damage hearing. Solid earplugs or heavy earmuffs. This is overprotection for everyday sounds.

In more severe cases, sometimes people use double hearing protection. They want the highest noise reduction to make everything as soft as possible. Thinking it will help their hyperacusis when it only makes hyperacusis worse. Unless you're in extreme noise, where everybody is required to wear high noise reduction hearing protection, then it's likely overprotection is happening.

Are you underground hard rock mining? Are you at a sawmill or on a flight deck with military jets in operation? Are you fracking? If not, you likely don't need double hearing protection.

If you're going about your daily activities at home or in your community with no hazardous loud noise exposure, it's overprotection to use low fidelity hearing protection. The more hearing is protected with low fidelity Two way low-high fidelity custom molded ear plugs popular for people with tinnitus or decreased sound tolerance., the more hyperacusis gets worse. It's a vicious cycle.

Imagine being locked in a cell with no light for a week. Only darkness to see. When the person gets out, light is painfully bright. Too much darkness made their eyes oversensitive to light. With normal light exposure, vision sensitivity returns to normal.

Too much silence causes the same problem for hyperacusis. Part of hyperacusis therapy is to wean off low fidelity hearing protection and bring sound back into their lives, using soft comfortable relaxation sound therapy. This helps lower hearing system hyperactivity so hyperacusis gets better.

If a person has been overprotecting their ears, they can't just stop using hearing protection instantly. That's very painful and difficult. You have to wean off silence. Slowly add sound. Regular everyday sound.

Weaning To Filtered Earplugs
If you've been overprotecting your ears, the goal is switching to filtered earplugs for everyday noise so you have clear communication and hear soft to moderate safe sound. Loud noise, even sudden impulse noise, is automatically filtered out. Options include:

- Social earplugs aka music, musician's, high fidelity, high definition.
- Pre-molded filtered or electronic filtered.
- Custom molded filtered or electronic filtered.

- Two-way solid-filtered earplugs have high noise reduction option for all sound when needed.

People can only use earplugs if it's medically safe, so get clearance first from your family doctor or ear specialist. See what your audiologist prescribes for your individual needs. For more complicated cases, care providers often consult with each other or team up, e.g. Meniere's, vestibular conditions, middle ear conditions, severe tinnitus-hyperacusis. Your care providers might recommend certain styles, depending on your hearing condition and hyper ears.

When weaning off hearing protection, a slow change combined with regular counselling and guidance to discuss any concerns is usually most comfortable. If you work in hazardous noise, then your audiologist can help guide you on any adjustments you need to make for work while you are going through treatment.

These are a few examples of weaning; they're not meant to replace the advice of your audiologist or professional care provider. Most people will need more than one style of hearing protection handy to go through the weaning process. Keep a selection so you have different styles or noise reductions to prevent noise damage when needed for different loud activities.

Example A – No Hazardous Noise

- Double hearing protection: foam earplugs under earmuffs
- Custom molded two-way earplugs (set to solid) under earmuffs
- Custom molded two-way earplugs (set to solid).
- Custom molded two-way earplugs (set to filtered).

This person is wearing double hearing protection for their regular daily personal and work activities. First they could wean off the foam earplugs by gradually switching over to wearing custom molded two-way earplugs underneath the earmuffs. The two-way earplugs could be set to solid or high noise reduction.

They could wean off the earmuffs by wearing them for less and less time each day as they worked towards only using the custom molded two-way earplugs. Once they're used to the custom earplugs on solid, they could slowly wean earplugs over to filtered noise reduction.

A different person might want to phase out using the earmuffs first. They could gradually wear the earmuffs less and less time each day working towards wearing only the foam earplugs. Then they could switch over to using the custom molded filtered earplugs instead of the foam plugs. They could phase out the foam earplugs by wearing them for less and less time each day and work up to just wearing the custom molded earplugs on solid and then filtered.

Example B –Hazardous Work Noise

- Double hearing protection: foam earplugs under earmuffs.
- Foam earplugs under electronic earmuffs (turned off).
- Electronic earmuffs (turned off).
- Electronic earmuffs (turned on).

This person doesn't need double hearing protection for their work noise exposure. Their audiologist recommended electronic earmuffs. First they could wean off foam earplugs by spending more and more time only using electronic earmuffs (turned off). When electronic earmuffs are turned off, they lower noise like regular low fidelity earmuffs.

Once they're only using the earmuffs, they could start wearing electronic earmuffs turned on when they need to hear voices or equipment sounds, or for at least 5 to 15 minutes per shift. The goal would be to eventually wear the earmuffs turned on to a comfortable volume for as much of the shift as possible to keep the ears "exercised" with safe soft to moderate sound, e.g. very gradually increase amount of time turned on each shift even if only by 15 minutes over a work week.

A different person might switch to just earmuffs and then wean over to electronic earmuffs turned off, and then turned on gradually over time.

Sound Therapy

To help lower hearing and emotion system hyperactivity causing hyperacusis, it's important to start using sound therapy along with weaning off low fidelity hearing protection. It can be a challenge to add in more sound daily. More discomfort or pain can happen when the cars process more sound, just like muscles can hurt when we exercise after a period of low activity.

When first adding hyperacusis sound therapy, the volume is at the softest level where it's just loud enough to hear. If you can only listen for 5 minutes at a time, it's still better than overprotection silence. Very slowly increase the volume and amount of daily time you spend listening to sound naturally—and with gentle relaxation sound therapy —over a period of days, weeks, and months, depending on how severe the hyperacusis is to start with.

How much sound and how fast depends on each individual person, and what your hearing healthcare provider recommends.

Social Earplugs

Many people with hyperacusis also have misophonia or phonophobia. They're upset, scared, or afraid about random trigger sounds or painful loud sounds that might happen when they're out and about with no hearing protection. That's where high fidelity or two way low-high fidelity earplugs are a good option.

Imagine a person with hyperacusis going to the mall. If a retail store or restaurant has piped in music that's too loud or there is a sudden unexpected loud noise, filtered earplugs automatically lower the loudness to safe levels.

For example, at a recent trip to Walmart, there were baby screams, an adorable child rolling by in a cart chanting, "me want CAKE CAKE me want CAKE CAKE..." There were crashes and beeps from metal carts and forklifts used for stocking shelves. Beeps from scanners and loud store announcements. These are all normal sounds to hear there. But if these sounds aren't comfortable, social hearing protection is a safe option to filter them out.

Image a teen with hyperacusis. By wearing high fidelity earplugs, they can hear fine at school. They'll still be able to communicate. But if the halls are noisy between classes, somebody yells, a fire alarm bell goes off, or a noisy message comes through the school speaker system, the loudness will be cut automatically.

There's even more control over volume with two-way filtered earplugs. A touch to the earplugs quickly changes hearing protection from clear high fidelity sound to high noise reduction any time.

High fidelity or filtered earplugs keep sound safe, comfortable—and most importantly—won't overprotect or make hyperacusis worse even if used regularly. High fidelity pre-molded or custom molded earplugs —including the two way low-high fidelity style—are a realistic, inconspicuous, practical option.

They're also handy at home for blow drying hair or running a blender if those sounds are uncomfortable. If there's no listening or talking, low fidelity like regular earplugs or earmuffs is also fine. Work with your hearing healthcare professionals to choose what's best for you.

10

COPING TOOLBOX SUMMARY

Great works are performed, not by strength, but by perseverance.

- Samuel Johnson -

- Communication.
- Hyperactive hearing system.
- Hyperactive emotion system.
- Neuroplasticity.
- Ethical science.
- Definitions.
- Outcome measures.
- Hearing healthcare providers.
- Shared decision making.
- Coping tools.
- Tool combos.
- Cost-benefit analysis.
- Distraction.
- Relaxation.

- Sound.
- Mind.
- Body.
- Sleep.
- Habituation.
- Cognitive.
- Behavioural.
- Mindfulness.
- Noise damage.
- Noise control.
- Hearing protection.
- Universal hearing healthcare.
- Target market.
- Electronics fails.
- Cure ale.
- False advertising.
- Buyer beware.
- Don't believe everything you read.

I hope you enjoyed Tinnitus Toolbox-Hyperacusis Handbook. It was an emotional roller coaster to research and write. When I started the first draft in 2016, I never realized all the good and bad I'd end up discovering in Hyper Ears World. Please visit my website for a full reference list.

Thank you so much for reading Tinnitus Toolbox-Hyperacusis Handbook and spending time with me. I hope you found at least 1 new coping tool or learned at least 1 new thing about tinnitus, hyperacusis, decreased sound tolerance, or hearing health.

Quiet cheers,

Jan L. Mayes

11

ASSOCIATIONS & ORGANIZATIONS

Seize fate by the throat.

- Ludwig van Beethoven -

Association websites have tinnitus and decreased sound tolerance facts, how to manage or cope better, the latest research or cure news, local care providers, and other resources. International associations and organizations include:

British Tinnitus Association
tinnitus.org.uk

Action on Hearing Loss
actiononhearingloss.org.uk

American Tinnitus Association
ata.org
Help Network Listing: People can talk to or email volunteers with

tinnitus and decreased sound tolerance for support, guidance and resources.

Tinnitus Advisors: in 2018, ATA is launching a Tinnitus Advisors program. Distressed callers will be able to speak to an audiologist who can answer tinnitus and decreased sound tolerance questions and help them find local care providers.

Australian Tinnitus Association
tinnitus.asn.au

Canadian Hearing Society
chs.ca

Acouphènes Québec
acouphenesquebec.org

Asociación de Personas Afectadas por Tinnitus
acufenos.org

France Acouphènes
france-acouphenes.org

Deutsche Tinnitus-Liga e.V.
tinnitus-liga.de

LIFELINES & HELPLINES

If you're not in crisis, don't use helplines. If you're feeling emotional distress or despair and need crisis support, there are websites, live chat, and helplines or lifelines to call or text in different countries including:

Action on Hearing Loss

- Helpline Telephone: 0808 808 6666

- Helpline Textphone: 0808 808 9000
- Email: tinnitushelpline@hearingloss.org.uk

Australia

- lifeline.org.au or contact 13 11 14

British Tinnitus Association

- Helpline Telephone: 0800 018 0527

Canada

- Canada National Suicide Prevention Lifeline: 1-800-273-TALK (8255)
- Or Text Telephone: 1-800-799-4889
- Association Québécoise de Prévention du Suicide (French): 1-866-APPELLE
- Kids Help Phone: 1-800-668-6868
- Or Live Chat counselling at kidshelpphone.ca

United Kingdom

- Contact 116 123

United States

- US National Suicide Prevention Lifeline: 1-800-273-TALK (8255)
- Crisis Text Line 741741

Wikipedia (wikipedia.org) has a complete List of Suicide Crisis Lines by country. Depending on the country, this list includes specific lines for kids, youth, and the military community.

To people feeling really down or thinking of killing themselves, don't do it. It's not your time. If you've tried to hurt or kill yourself in the past like I have, we're far more likely to have suicidal thoughts again than someone who isn't a suicide survivor. It's like riding a bike. It's easy to jump back on and ride downhill to barking dogs, the dungeon, living hell, or whatever it's like for you.

Contact emergency services. Call a suicide or tinnitus helpline or lifeline. Talk to somebody about how you're feeling, e.g. doctor, therapist, friends, family. There is help.

You are not alone.

In the past 20 years, people have used new coping tools, therapies, aids, and devices to cope better, including me. Something can be done. And the cure is getting closer every year.

My3 App
The website lifelineforattemptsurvivors.org for the My3 mobile app has support and resources for people living with suicidal thoughts and suicide attempts. The app helps people plan to stay safe by picking 3 others they'll reach out to if they're thinking about suicide. At first I thought I didn't have 3 so that was depressing. But I have 3 if I include my doctor plus a helpline and a lifeline in my network. Some people might have a counselling therapist, close friend or family member in their 3. It's good to include a helpline and/or lifeline since they're there 24/7.

ABOUT THE AUTHOR

Jan L. Mayes has been writing and blogging horror fiction and tinnitus-hyperacusis non-fiction for over 10 years. Her background in linguistics, audiology and adult education—combined with over 30 years of experience coping with ghosts, hyper ears and plotting murders—have given her a broad base from which to approach many topics.

She is an international award winner for her self-help tinnitus-hyperacusis non-fiction books including a 2013 Eric Hoffer Award and 2019 International Book Award.

Jan is a member of The Writer's Path writing club. She lives in the Pacific Northwest of Canada. She enjoys reading, cookies, quiet activism, and deadheading, as should all right thinking people.

author@janlmayes.com
www.janlmayes.com
Jan L. Mayes Blog
Goodreads Jan L. Mayes Author Page
Twitter @janlmayes
Jan's Facebook Author Page
Jan's Pinterest
Jan's Instagram
Books2Read by Jan L. Mayes

ALSO BY JAN L. MAYES

My paperback and ebooks are available at bookstores, subscription services, and some libraries. For more info check out my website janlmayes.com or visit:

Goodreads

Books2Read

Fiction

Doctor Bell Anthology: Tinnitus Terror Tales

Regretfully Invited: 13 Short Horror Stories

Poetry

Gossamer: A Poetry Collection

Non-Fiction

Tinnitus Toolbox-Hyperacusis Handbook

Tinnitus Treatment Toolbox

Manufactured by Amazon.ca
Bolton, ON